AF801368

New Anti-cancer Drug Development and Evaluation

Yongchang Zhang • Nong Yang
Editors

New Anti-cancer Drug Development and Evaluation

Springer

Editors
Yongchang Zhang
Hunan Cancer Hospital/The Affiliated Cancer Hospital of Xiangya School of Medicine
Central South University
Changsha, China

Nong Yang
Department of Medical Oncology, Lung Cancer and Gastrointestinal Unit, Hunan Cancer Hospital/The Affiliated Cancer Hospital of Xiangya School of Medicine
Central South University
Changsha, China

ISBN 978-981-97-7273-5 ISBN 978-981-97-7274-2 (eBook)
https://doi.org/10.1007/978-981-97-7274-2

© The Editor(s) (if applicable) and The Author(s), under exclusive license to Springer Nature Singapore Pte Ltd. 2024
This work is subject to copyright. All rights are solely and exclusively licensed by the Publisher, whether the whole or part of the material is concerned, specifically the rights of translation, reprinting, reuse of illustrations, recitation, broadcasting, reproduction on microfilms or in any other physical way, and transmission or information storage and retrieval, electronic adaptation, computer software, or by similar or dissimilar methodology now known or hereafter developed.
The use of general descriptive names, registered names, trademarks, service marks, etc. in this publication does not imply, even in the absence of a specific statement, that such names are exempt from the relevant protective laws and regulations and therefore free for general use.
The publisher, the authors and the editors are safe to assume that the advice and information in this book are believed to be true and accurate at the date of publication. Neither the publisher nor the authors or the editors give a warranty, expressed or implied, with respect to the material contained herein or for any errors or omissions that may have been made. The publisher remains neutral with regard to jurisdictional claims in published maps and institutional affiliations.

This Springer imprint is published by the registered company Springer Nature Singapore Pte Ltd.
The registered company address is: 152 Beach Road, #21-01/04 Gateway East, Singapore 189721, Singapore

If disposing of this product, please recycle the paper.

Preface

Oncology has emerged as a pivotal research field in medicine, with malignant tumors becoming a central focus due to their significant impact on human health and life. Recognizing their role as a major threat to humanity, numerous countries have invested heavily in tumor research, encompassing both basic and clinical studies. Recent years have witnessed rapid progress in various aspects of oncology, including tumor genesis, genetics, molecular epidemiology, and advancements in traditional treatments like surgery, radiotherapy, and chemotherapy. Notably, the introduction of multidisciplinary comprehensive treatment approaches, along with innovative therapies and clinical practices, has marked significant strides in this field. Despite these advancement, the journey toward groundbreaking discoveries in prevention, diagnosis, and treatment of malignant tumors remains arduous, presenting vast areas yet to be explored and challenges to be overcome.

Clinical trials are pivotal in the discovery and development of new therapies, acting as the foundation for objective, evidence-based medical advancements. These trials have evolved significantly, translating biological understanding of cancer into therapeutic opportunities. Defined as scientific research methods to evaluate the safety and efficacy of new drugs, treatments, medical devices, or interventions, clinical trials undergo various stages, from basic research to human patient testing, before approval and clinical application. Their primary objectives are to assess the clinical efficacy of treatments or drugs, including their impact on symptoms, disease progression, pain attenuation, survival prolongation, and quality of life improvement, and to evaluate the safety compared to standard treatments.

As the bedrock of modern medical practice, clinical trials provide essential scientific evidence for medical decision-making, ensuring the scientific integrity and efficacy of healthcare. The future of clinical trials promises a more dynamic, adaptive, and patient-centered approach. Emphasizing patient input and global learning, these trials aim to address relevant issues, improve cancer control, and advance personalized treatments.

This book delves into the development and trajectory of clinical trials for new cancer drugs. It aims to provide readers with a historical perspective on cancer drug research and development, fostering a deeper understanding of this critical field.

Changsha, China Yongchang Zhang

Acknowledgment

We would like to express our gratitude to Dr. Dongjun Qin for his valuable assistance in editing and language proofreading. This work was financially supported by the National Natural Science Foundation of China (82222048).

Contents

1 **Transformations and Challenges in Cancer Treatment** 1
Jinye Mi, Fang Wu, and Nong Yang
1.1 The First Revolution: Chemotherapy 2
1.2 The Second Revolution: Targeted Therapy 3
1.2.1 Advantages of Targeted Therapy 5
1.2.2 Challenges for Targeted Therapy 6
1.2.3 EGFR-Targeted Therapy in Lung Cancer 7
1.3 The Third Revolution: Immunotherapy 13
1.3.1 Key Milestones in the History of Tumor Immunotherapy Since the 1960s 16
1.3.2 Challenges for Tumor Immunotherapy 17
1.3.3 Top Ten Challenges 20
1.3.4 Precision Oncology Medicine: Challenges and Changes in the Evaluation of New Anticancer Drugs 21
References 24

2 **Drug(gable) Targets Discovery** 27
Yizhi Li and Siqi Xiang
2.1 Approved Targeted Therapy in Lung Cancer 28
2.1.1 EGFR 28
2.1.2 ALK 31
2.1.3 ROS1 32
2.1.4 KRAS 33
2.1.5 BRAF 34
2.1.6 MET 36
2.1.7 RET 38
2.1.8 PD-1/PD-L1 39
2.2 Target Identification to Targeted Therapies 41
2.2.1 Screening and Identification of Molecular Targets 42
2.2.2 Drug Development Based on the Targets 43
2.2.3 Therapeutic Targets Test in Preclinical Settings 44

2.3 Challenges in Clinical Trials 47
2.4 Antitumor Mechanism and Discovery of Biomarkers 48
References 49

3 Preclinical and Translational Study Design 53
Liang Zeng, Xing Zhang, and Hongzhi Ma
3.1 Preclinical Evaluation 54
3.1.1 Safety Pharmacology 56
3.1.2 Pharmacokinetics 57
3.1.3 General Toxicology 58
3.1.4 Reproductive Toxicity 58
3.1.5 Genetic Toxicity 59
3.1.6 Carcinogenicity 59
3.1.7 Immunotoxicity 59
3.1.8 Light Safety 59
3.2 Nonclinical Data Supporting Clinical Trial Design and Marketing 60
3.2.1 Determining the Initial Dose of Medication for Humans 60
3.2.2 Dose Escalation and Maximum Dose in Clinical Trials 60
3.2.3 Toxicological Study Duration and Protocol to Support Early Clinical Trials 60
3.2.4 Duration of Toxicological Studies to Support Subsequent Clinical Trials and Marketing 61
3.2.5 Combined Use of Drugs 61
3.2.6 Support Nonclinical Studies in Pediatric Populations 62
3.2.7 Binding Drugs 62
3.3 Preclinical Study Results of Vedolizumab Monoclonal Antibody 64
3.3.1 Immune Checkpoint Inhibitors 64
References 74

4 Clinical Trials 77
Huan Yan, Ting Li, and Lianxi Song
4.1 Definition of Clinical Trials 78
4.1.1 Clinical Trial Monitor 78
4.1.2 Ethics Committee 79
4.1.3 The Start a Clinical Trial 79
4.1.4 Data Management 79
4.1.5 Power Analysis and Sample Size Calculation 80
4.1.6 Statistical Analysis Plan 80
4.1.7 Ethical Consideration 81
4.1.8 Overview of Conducting a Clinical Trial 81
4.1.9 Basic Concepts of Clinical Trials 81

4.1.10 Phases of Clinical Trials ... 84
4.1.11 Clinical Trial Design ... 87
4.2 Innovation in Oncology Clinical Trial Design ... 88
4.2.1 Basket Trials ... 89
4.2.2 Umbrella Trials ... 89
4.2.3 Platform Trials ... 89
4.3 Highlight of Clinical Trial Results ... 92
4.3.1 When the Results Are Positive ... 93
4.3.2 When the Result Is Negative ... 94
References ... 95

5 Small-Molecule Compounds ... 99
Lingli Liu, Yuanze Sun, and Dan Yang
5.1 Targeted Protein Kinase ... 99
5.1.1 First-Generation EGFR TKIs ... 100
5.1.2 Second-Generation EGFR TKIs ... 102
5.1.3 Third-Generation EGFR-TKIs ... 103
5.1.4 Fourth-Generation EGFR TKIs ... 105
5.2 Targeted PD-1/PD-L1 Signaling Pathway ... 105
5.2.1 Direct Interaction Blocking Between PD-1 and PD-L1 ... 107
5.2.2 Inhibiting the Transcription and Translation of PD-L1 ... 108
5.2.3 Promoting Degradation of PD-L1 Protein ... 108
5.2.4 Conclusion and Outlook ... 109
References ... 109

6 Antibodies ... 115
Zhe Huang, Jingyi Li, and Miaomiao Zhang
6.1 Immune System and Its Role in Cancer ... 115
6.2 Antibody and Its Biological Function ... 117
6.3 Antibodies in Cancer Treatment ... 118
6.3.1 mAbs in Cancer Treatment ... 119
6.3.2 Bispecific Antibodies for Cancer Treatment ... 122
6.3.3 Antibody-Drug Conjugates (ADCs) for Cancer Treatment ... 125
6.3.4 ICIs for Cancer Treatment ... 128
6.4 Examples of Combination Therapies for Cancer Treatment ... 132
6.5 Challenges and Outlook ... 134
6.6 Conclusion ... 136
References ... 137

7 Cell-Guided Drugs ... 141
Haoyue Qin and Guowei Zhou
7.1 Adoptive Cell Therapy (ACT) ... 142
7.2 LAK Therapy ... 142
7.3 CIK Therapy ... 144

7.4 Tumor-Infiltrating Lymphocyte Therapy 145
7.4.1 Introduction 145
7.4.2 Implementation Procedure of TIL Therapy 146
7.4.3 Development Progression of TIL Therapy. 146
7.4.4 Optimization of TIL Therapy. 147
7.4.5 TIL-Related Clinical Trials and Drugs 148
7.4.6 Future Prospects of TIL Therapy 149
7.5 TCR-Gene Engineered T Cells Therapy 149
7.5.1 Introduction 149
7.5.2 Implementation of TCR-T Therapy 150
7.5.3 Evolution of TCR-T Therapy. 151
7.5.4 Optimization of TCR-T Therapy 152
7.5.5 TCR-T-Related Clinical Trials and Drugs 152
7.5.6 Future Prospects of TIL Therapy 153
7.6 CARs-Mediated Cell Immunotherapy 154
7.6.1 Introduction 154
7.6.2 Implementation of CARs Therapy. 155
7.6.3 Development Progression of CARs Therapy. 156
7.6.4 CARs-Related Clinical Trials and Drugs. 158
7.6.5 Prospects of CARs Therapy. 160
7.7 NK Cell Therapy 161
7.7.1 Introduction 161
7.7.2 Implementation of NK Cell Therapy 162
7.7.3 Development Progression of NK Cell Therapy 163
7.7.4 NK Cell Therapy-Related Clinical Trials and Drugs. 164
7.7.5 Prospects of NK Cell Therapy 164
7.8 Summary 166
References. 166

8 Gene-Guided Drugs 173
Yuda Zhang and Tian Xu
8.1 Definition of Gene Therapy 173
8.2 Techniques of Gene Therapy 174
8.2.1 AAV Vector Delivery Technology 174
8.2.2 CRISPR Gene Editing Technology 174
8.2.3 Single/Double-Base Editing Technique. 176
8.2.4 Oncolytic Virus Genetic Modification Technology 176
8.3 Process for Gene Therapy Drug Development 177
8.3.1 Virus Vector Design and Optimization 177
8.3.2 Proof of Concept for Viral Vectors Through In Vitro and In Vivo Experiments 179
8.3.3 Drug Clinical Evaluation 179
8.3.4 Current Status of Gene Therapy Drugs in China. 180
8.4 Representative Gene Therapy Drugs Developed in China. 181
8.4.1 Gendicine. 181
8.4.2 Oncorine. 182

8.5 Gene Therapy Drugs Under Clinical Trials 182
8.6 Gene Therapy Adverse Events 184
References 184

9 Biosimilar 187
Ya Wang, Qinqin Xu, and Xiangyu Zhang
9.1 Trastuzumab Biosimilar 189
9.2 Bevacizumab Biosimilar 190
9.3 Denosumab Biosimilar 192
9.4 Rituximab Biosimilar 193
9.5 Cetuximab Biosimilar 195
9.6 Pertuzumab Biosimilar 195
References 195

10 New Insights on Success and Failed Drugs 199
Ziyi Sun and Yuling Zhou
10.1 Successful Drugs 199
10.1.1 Targeted Therapy 199
10.1.2 Immunotherapy 205
10.2 Failed Drugs 209
10.2.1 Targeted Therapy 210
10.2.2 Inadequate Number of Patients 210
10.2.3 Immunotherapy 211
10.3 Conclusion 212
References 212

11 The Road from Laboratory to Patient 217
Yongchang Zhang and Yangqian Chen
11.1 Overview 218
11.2 Drug Discovery 219
11.2.1 Target Discovery and Validation 219
11.2.2 Lead Compound Identification and Optimization 220
11.3 Preclinical Development 223
11.3.1 Clinical Trials 223
11.4 Approval to Launch 225
11.5 Conclusion 227
11.5.1 The Importance of New Antitumor Drugs 227
11.5.2 Eliminate the Lag in Drug Approval: Concerns and Efforts 227
11.5.3 Trends in Oncology Drug Innovation in China 229
References 231

Editors and Contributors

About the Editors

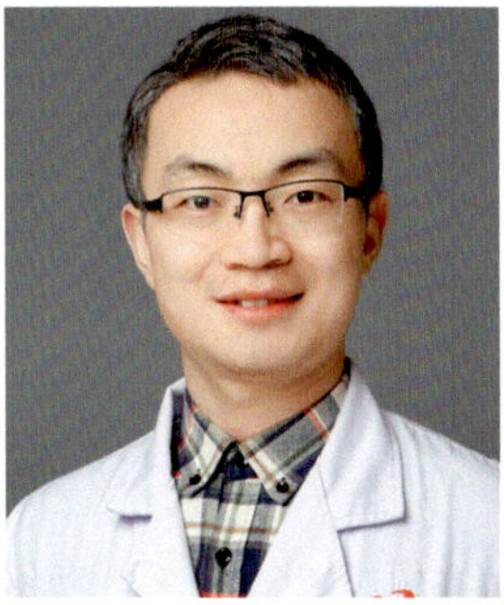

Yongchang Zhang is an Associate Chief Physician, Professor, and Honorary Professor at Central South University and Hunan Normal University. He currently serves as the Director of the Early Clinical Research Center and the Anticancer New Drug Research Ward at Hunan Provincial Cancer Hospital. Additionally, he is the Deputy Chief of the Lung-Gastrointestinal Internal Medicine Department and the Director of the Hunan Provincial Key Laboratory of Precision Diagnosis and Treatment for Lung Cancer.

Dr. Zhang specializes in the precision diagnosis and treatment of malignant tumors and the development of new drugs, with significant contributions to the clinical treatment and translational research of lung cancer. Over the past 5 years, Dr. Zhang has published over 100 peer-reviewed papers in leading oncology journals. Dr. Zhang has received funding from the National Natural Science Foundation of China for Outstanding Young Scientists and has been recognized as a Leading Talent in Science and Technology Innovation by Hunan Province. Dr. Zhang's primary research focus is on conducting clinical studies of new anticancer drugs, with a particular emphasis on targeted therapy and immune resistance in lung cancer and gastrointestinal malignancies. He has led more than 10 IND studies, including Phase I–IV clinical trials of new drugs, as well as studies on novel cell immunotherapy, BE/PK, and healthy subjects. He excels in clinical trials of novel anticancer drugs, including new immune checkpoint inhibitors, novel ADC drugs, cell immunotherapy (CART, TILs), and tumor vaccines. His dedication to finding a cure for advanced malignant tumors brings hope to patients.

Dr. Zhang serves as a Standing Committee member of the Integrated Rehabilitation Committee for Bone and Soft Tissue Tumors of the Chinese Anti-Cancer Association, a member of the Oncology Respiratory Disease/Oncology Precision Treatment Committee of the Chinese Anti-Cancer Association, and a member of the Palliative Care/Malignant Mesothelioma Committee of the Chinese Anti-Cancer Association. He is also a Council Member of the Young Scientists Association in Hunan Province, Chairman of the Young Committee of the Precision Medicine Professional Committee of the Hunan Province Anti-Cancer Association, and Vice Chairman of the Young Committee of the Oncology Internal Medicine Professional Committee of the Hunan Medical Association.

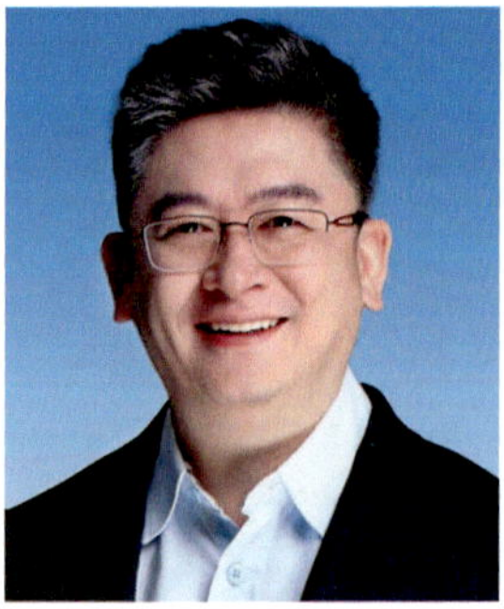

Nong Yang is the Vice President of the Second People's Hospital of Hunan Province, China. He is a Chief Physician and a Doctoral Supervisor. Additionally, he holds positions as a Long-Term Expert at Hainan Cancer Hospital, Hainan Chengmei Hospital, and Hainan Tropical Cancer Research Institute. He also serves as the Director of the Hunan Province Clinical Medical Research Center for Respiratory Cancer, the Director of the Key Laboratory for Precision Diagnosis and Treatment of Lung Cancer, and a Chief Expert of the National Science and Technology Major Project. Furthermore, he acts as an Evaluation Expert for the Center for Drug Evaluation (CDE) under the National Medical Products Administration of China. In 2022, Dr. Yang was included in the Top 100 Scholars List for Academic Influence in Chinese Lung Cancer Research (ranked 54th), and in 2020, he was ranked 12th in terms of academic influence in Chinese lung cancer research.

Dr. Yang specializes in precise immunotherapy, targeted therapy, and chemotherapy for lung and gastrointestinal cancers. He has accumulated a wealth of successful cases in these areas, particularly in dealing with complex and drug-resistant cases. His research focuses on precise immunotherapy, targeted therapy, and chemotherapy for lung and gastrointestinal cancers. Dr. Yang has contributed to the development of several clinical guidelines and consensus reports, including those of the Chinese Society of Clinical Oncology and the Chinese Medical Association. He has been involved in the development of guidelines for clinical trials conducted by the CDE for multiple anticancer drugs. As the principal investigator or leading PI, he has designed, organized, and participated in nearly 400 phase I–III clinical trials, with over 40 ongoing clinical studies.

Over the past 5 years, Dr. Yang has published more than 43 academic papers, with a cumulative impact factor exceeding 375.23. Notably, his research has revealed the molecular mechanisms underlying primary resistance to ALK fusion lung cancer targeted therapy, specifically the fusion of reciprocal and non-reciprocal ALK partners. This achievement has been incorporated into the Chinese Society of Clinical Oncology's consensus interpretation of testing reports, and he was invited to contribute to the ASCO ALK Fusion Lung Cancer Testing Guidelines.

Contributors

Yangqian Chen, M.D. Department of Medical Oncology, Lung Cancer and Gastrointestinal Unit, Hunan Cancer Hospital/The Affiliated Cancer Hospital of Xiangya School of Medicine, Central South University, Changsha, China

Department of Medical Oncology, Graduate Collaborative Training Base of Hunan Cancer Hospital, Hengyang Medical School, University of South China, Hengyang, China

Yan Huan, M.D. Department of Medical Oncology, Lung Cancer and Gastrointestinal Unit, Qinghai University, Changsha, China

Zhe Huang, M.D. Department of Medical Oncology, Lung Cancer and Gastrointestinal Unit, Hunan Cancer Hospital/The Affiliated Cancer Hospital of Xiangya School of Medicine, Central South University, Changsha, China

Jingyi Li, M.D. Department of Medical Oncology, Lung Cancer and Gastrointestinal Unit, Hunan Cancer Hospital/The Affiliated Cancer Hospital of Xiangya School of Medicine, Central South University, Changsha, China

Ting Li, M.D. Department of Medical Oncology, Lung Cancer and Gastrointestinal Unit, Hunan Cancer Hospital/The Affiliated Cancer Hospital of Xiangya School of Medicine, Central South University, Changsha, China

Yizhi Li, M.D. Department of Pharmacy, The Second Xiangya Hospital, Changsha, China

Lingli Liu, M.D. Medical College, Hunan University of Medicine, Huaihua, China

Hongzhi Ma, M.D. Department of Medical Oncology, Lung Cancer and Gastrointestinal Unit, Hunan Cancer Hospital/The Affiliated Cancer Hospital of Xiangya School of Medicine, Central South University, Changsha, China

Jinye Mi, M.D. Department of Infectious Diseases, Zhuzhou Central Hospital, Zhuzhou, China

Haoyue Qin, M.D. Department of Medical Oncology, Lung Cancer and Gastrointestinal Unit, Hunan Cancer Hospital/The Affiliated Cancer Hospital of Xiangya School of Medicine, Central South University, Changsha, China

Lianxi Song, M.D. Department of Medical Oncology, Yiyang Central Hospital, Yiyang, China

Yuanze Sun, M.D. Department of Medical Oncology, Lung Cancer and Gastrointestinal Unit, Hunan Cancer Hospital/The Affiliated Cancer Hospital of Xiangya School of Medicine, Central South University, Changsha, China

Ziyi Sun, M.D. Department of Oncology, Beijing Electric Power Hospital, Beijing, China

Fang Wu, M.D. Department of Hematology and Oncology, Hunan Provincial Children's Hospital, Changsha, China

Siqi Xiang, M.D. Department of Biochemistry and Immunology, Medical Research Center, Institute of Medicine, Jishou University, Jishou, China

Qinqin Xu, M.D. Qinghai Provincial People's Hospital, Xining, China

Tian Xu, M.D. Department of Medical Oncology, Lung Cancer and Gastrointestinal Unit, The Second Xiangya Hospital, Changsha, China

Wang Ya, M.D. Department of Medical Oncology, Lung Cancer and Gastrointestinal Unit, Hunan Cancer Hospital/The Affiliated Cancer Hospital of Xiangya School of Medicine, Central South University, Changsha, China

Dan Yang, M.D. Department of Medical Oncology, Lung Cancer and Gastrointestinal Unit, Hunan Cancer Hospital/The Affiliated Cancer Hospital of Xiangya School of Medicine, Central South University, Changsha, China

Nong Yang Department of Medical Oncology, Lung Cancer and Gastrointestinal Unit, Hunan Cancer Hospital/The Affiliated Cancer Hospital of Xiangya School of Medicine, Central South University, Changsha, China

Department of Medical Oncology, Lung Cancer and Gastrointestinal Unit, Hunan Second People's Hospital, Changsha, China

Liang Zeng, M.D. Department of Medical Oncology, Lung Cancer and Gastrointestinal Unit, Hunan Cancer Hospital, The Affiliated Cancer Hospital of Xiangya School of Medicine, Central South University, Changsha, China

Miaomiao Zhang, M.S. Department of Medical Oncology, Lung Cancer and Gastrointestinal Unit, Hunan Cancer Hospital/The Affiliated Cancer Hospital of Xiangya School of Medicine, Central South University, Changsha, China

Xiangyu Zhang, M.D. Department of Respiratory and Critical Care Medicine, The Third Xiangya Hospital, Changsha, China

Xing Zhang, M.D. Department of Medical Oncology, Lung Cancer and Gastrointestinal Unit, University of South China, Changsha, China

Yongchang Zhang Department of Medical Oncology, Lung Cancer and Gastrointestinal Unit, Hunan Cancer Hospital/The Affiliated Cancer Hospital of Xiangya School of Medicine, Central South University, Changsha, China

Yuda Zhang, M.D. Department of Medical Oncology, Lung Cancer and Gastrointestinal Unit, Hunan Cancer Hospital/The Affiliated Cancer Hospital of Xiangya School of Medicine, Central South University, Changsha, China

Guowei Zhou, M.D. Xiangya Hospital, Central South University, Changsha, China

Yuling Zhou, M.D. Department of Medical Oncology, Lung Cancer and Gastrointestinal Unit, Hunan Cancer Hospital/The Affiliated Cancer Hospital of Xiangya School of Medicine, Central South University, Changsha, China

Abbreviations

5-FU	5-Fluorouracil
6MP	6-Mercaptopurine
AACR	American Association for Cancer Research
AAV	Adeno-associated virus
ACT	Adoptive cell therapy
Act D	Actinomycin D
ADCC	Antibody-dependent cellular cytotoxicity
ADCP	Antibody-dependent cellular phagocytosis
ADCs	Antibody–drug conjugates
ADM	Adriamycin
ADME	Absorption, distribution, metabolism, and excretion
AEs	Adverse events
AK104	Cadonilimab
ALK	Anaplastic lymphoma kinase
ALL	Acute lymphoblastic leukemia
ALT	Alanine aminotransferase
AM	Aminomethylene
AMD	Age-related macular degeneration
AML	Acute myeloid leukemia
APCs	Antigen-presenting cells
API	Active pharmaceutical ingredient
Ara-C	Cytosine arabinoside
ARMS-PCR	Amplification refractory mutation system-polymerase chain reaction
ASCO	American Society of Contemporary Ophthalmology
ASOs	Antisense oligonucleotides
AST	Aspartate transaminase
ATP	Adenosine triphosphate
AUC	Area under the curve
$AUC_{0\text{–}t}$	Area under the curve from time zero to the last measurable concentration

AUC_{inf}	Area under the concentration–time curve from zero to infinity
AUC_{last}	Area under the concentration–time curve to the last observable concentration
B16F10	Mouse melanoma cell
BAC	Bacterial artificial chromosome
BCL	B-cell lymphoma
BCMA	B-cell maturation antigen
BET	Bromodomain and extraterminal domain JQ1
BiTEs	Bispecific T cell engagers
BLM	Bleomycin
BM	Brain metastasis
BMS	Borane dimethyl sulfide complex
BRAF	V-raf murine sarcoma viral oncogene homolog B
BRD4	Bromodomain-containing protein 4
CAFs	Cancer-associated fibroblasts
CAR	Chimeric antigen receptor
CAR-NK	Chimeric antigen receptor NK cell
CAR-T	Chimeric antigen receptor T
CDC	Complement-dependent cytotoxicity
CDE	Center for Drug Evaluation
CFDA	China Food and Drug Administration
ChIP	Channel intrinsic protein/chromatin immunoprecipitation
CHO	Chinese hamster ovary
CHOP	Cyclophosphamide, adriamycin, oncovin, and prednisolone
CI	Confidence interval
CIK	Cytokine-induced killer
CIT	Cancer immunotherapy
CL	Clearance
CLL	Chronic lymphocytic leukemia
Clog P	Octanol–water partition coefficient
CLS	Capillary leak syndrome
C_{max}	Peak serum concentration
Cmax	Maximum plasma concentration
C-MET	Cellular-mesenchymal epithelial transition factor
CML	Chronic myeloid leukemia
CNS	Central nervous system
CR	Complete response
CRS	Cytokine release syndrome
CSCO	Chinese Society of Clinical Oncology
CSF	Cerebrospinal fluid
CTL	Cytotoxic T lymphocytes
CTLA-4	Cytotoxic T lymphocyte-associated antigen-4
CTX	Cyclophosphamide
CyR	Cytogenetic response
DALYs	Disease-specific disability-adjusted life years

DAMPs	Damage-associated molecular patterns
DAR	Drug-to-antibody ratio
DARTs	Dual-affinity re-targeting molecules
DC	Dendritic cell
DCR	Disease control rate
DCs	Dendritic cells
DDP	Cisplatin
DLBCL	Diffuse large B-cell non-Hodgkin's lymphoma
DLT	Dose-limiting toxicity
DMC	Data Monitoring Committee
dMMR	Mismatch repair-deficient
DRR	Drug Registration Management Regulations
DSMB	Data Safety Monitoring Board
DVD-Ig	Dual-variable domain Ig
ECG	Electrocardiogram
ECM	Extracellular matrix
EDC	Electronic data capture
EGF	Epidermal growth factor
EGFR	Epidermal growth factor receptor
EMA	European Medicines Agency
EML4	Echinoderm microtubule-associated protein-like 4
EMT	Epithelial–mesenchymal transition
ERBB2	Epidermal growth factor receptor 2
ERK	Extracellular regulated protein kinase
ESCC	Esophageal squamous cell carcinoma
ESMO	European Society for Medical Oncology
ES-SCLC	Extensive-stage small cell lung cancer
FasL	Fas ligand
FDA	Food and Drug Administration
Gal-9	Galectin-9
GM-CSF	Granulocyte-macrophage colony-stimulating factor
GPC3	Glypican-3
GPC3-CART	Glypican 3 (GPC3)-directed CAR T cells
GPRC5D	G Protein-coupled receptor, Class C Group 5 Member D
GTPase	Guanosine triphosphatase
GVHD	Graft-versus-host disease
GWAS	Genome-wide association studies
HCC	Hepatocellular carcinoma
HDR	Homologous recombination repair
HER	Human epidermal growth factor receptor
HER2	Human epidermal growth factor receptor 2
HGF	Hepatocyte growth factor
HIP1R	Huntingtin-interacting protein 1-related
HL	Hodgkin's lymphoma
HLA	Human leukocyte antigen

HMGB1	High mobility group box 1
HNSCC	Head and neck squamous cell carcinoma
HPV	Human papilloma virus
HR	Hazard ratio
HTS	High-throughput screening
IC_{50}	Half-maximal inhibitory concentration
ICB	Immune checkpoint blockade
ICH	International Council for Harmonisation
ICI	Immune checkpoint inhibitor
IDMC	Independent Data Monitoring Committee
IFN-γ	Interferon-γ
Ig	Immunoglobulin
IgA	Immunoglobulin A
IgB	Immunoglobulin B
IgV	Immunoglobulin variable
IL	Interleukin
IND	Investigational New Drug
IO	Immuno-oncology
IQR	Interquartile range
IrAEs	Immune-related adverse events
IRC	Independent Review Committee
IRCC	International registry on CIK cells
IRRC	Independent Review Radiology Committee
iRT	Immune checkpoint radiotherapy
ITAMs	Immunoreceptor tyrosine-based activation motifs
ITIM	Immunoreceptor tyrosine-based inhibitory motif
ITSMs	Immunoreceptor tyrosine-based switch motifs
ITT	Immunoglobulin tail tyrosine
IV	Intravenous
JAK3	Janus kinase 3
JAMA	The Journal of the American Medical Association
Kd	Dissociation constant
KRAS	Kirsten rat sarcoma viral oncogene
LAG-3	Lymphocyte activation gene-3
LAK	Lymphokine-activated killer
LHON	Leber's hereditary optic neuropathy
LMP1	Latent membrane protein 1
LN-144	Lifileucel
mAb	Monoclonal antibody
MAGE	Melanoma antigen genes
MAPK	Mitogen-activated protein kinase
MART-1	Melanoma antigen recognized by T cells
mCRC	Metastatic colorectal cancer
mDFS	Median disease-free survival
mDoR	Median duration of response

MDSCs	Myeloid-derived suppressor cells
MHC	Major histocompatibility complex
MIBC	Muscle-invasive bladder cancer
MLV	Moloney leukemia virus
MMAE	Microtubule inhibitor monomethyl auristatin E
mOS	Median overall survival
mPFS	Median progression-free survival
MSI	Microsatellite instability
MSI-H	Microsatellite instability high
MSLN	Mesothelin
MTC	Medullary thyroid carcinoma
MTD	Maximum tolerated dose
mTOR	Mammalian target of rapamycin
MTX	Methotrexate
NAMPT	Nicotinamide phosphoribosyltransferase
NCCN	National Comprehensive Cancer Network
NCT	National Clinical Trial
NDA	New Drug Application
NEJM	New England Journal of Medicine
NHEJ	Non-homologous end joining
NIH	National Institutes of Health
NK	Natural killer
NKT	Natural killer T cells
NMPA	National Medical Products Administration
NOAEL	No-observed-adverse-effect level
NOEL	No-observed-effect level
NR	Not reached
NRCTs	Non-randomized trials
NSCLC	Non-small cell lung cancer
NST	Non-severe toxic dose
ODD	Orphan drug designation
ORR	Objective response rate
ORRs	Overall response rates
OS	Overall survival
PBMCs	Peripheral blood mononuclear cells
PD	Pharmacodynamic
PD-1	Programmed death protein 1
PD-L1	Programmed cell death 1 ligand 1
PD-L2	Programmed cell death 1 ligand 2
PDCD1	Programmed cell death 1
PDX	Patient-derived xenograft
PFS	Progression-free survival
PI3K	Phosphoinositide 3-kinase
PICO	Population, intervention, comparator, and outcomes
PK	Pharmacokinetic

PKB/AKT	Protein kinase B
pM	Picomolar
pMHC	Peptide–MHC complex
PPP	Platinum-based chemotherapy pre-treated patient
PR	Partial response
PTC	Papillary thyroid carcinoma
QD	Once-daily
R&D	Research and development
R/M NPC	Recurrent/metastatic nasopharyngeal carcinoma
r/r FL	Refractory or relapsed follicular lymphoma
r/r iNHL	Relapsed or refractory indolent non-Hodgkin's lymphoma
r/r LBCL	Relapsed/refractory large B-cell lymphoma
rAAV	Recombinant adeno-associated virus
RANKL	Receptor activator of nuclear factor kappa-B ligand
RAS	Rat sarcoma
RAS-GTP	RAS activation bodies
RC48	Disitamab vedotin
RCC	Metastatic renal cell carcinoma
RCTs	Randomized controlled trials
RNA	Ribonucleic acid
RO5	Lipinski's rule of five
RPTK	Receptor protein tyrosine kinase
RTKs	Receptor tyrosine kinases
SAP	Statistical analysis plan
SAR	Structure–activity relationship
SB3	Samsung Bioepis Ltd
scFv	Single-chain Fv
SEC-HPLC	Size exclusion high-performance liquid chromatography
SHP-1	Src homology phosphatase 1
SHP-2	Src homology phosphatase 2
siRNA	Small interfering RNA
STAT3	Signal transducer and activator of transcription 3
$T_{1/2}$	Half-life
TAA	Tumor-associated antigen
TAK-788	Mobocertinib
TAMs	Tumor-associated macrophages
TCGA	The Cancer Genome Atlas
TCR	T cell receptor
TCR-T	T cell receptor-gene engineered T cells
T-DXd	Trastuzumab deruxtecan
TEAE	Treatment-emergent adverse event
TIGIT	T cell immunoglobulin and ITIM domain
TILs	Tumor-infiltrating lymphocytes
TIM-3	Mucin-domain containing-3
TK	Tyrosine kinase

TKIs	Tyrosine kinase inhibitors
Tmax	The median time to reach maximum concentration
TMB	Tumor mutational burden
TME	Tumor microenvironment
TNF-α	Tumor necrosis factor-alpha
TPP-1	Triphenylphosphine compound
TPS	Tumor proportion score
TRAEs	Treatment-related adverse events
Treg	Regulatory T cell
TRK	Tropomyosin receptor kinase
UR2	The Manchester University Tumor Virus type 2
V_d	Volume of distribution
VEGF	Vascular endothelial growth factor
VH	Variable regions of the heavy
VL	Variable regions of the light
VLB	Vinorelbine
VSIG9	V-set and immunoglobulin domain-containing protein 9
VSTM3	V-set and transmembrane domain-containing protein 3
WUCAM	Washington University Cell Adhesion Molecule

Chapter 1
Transformations and Challenges in Cancer Treatment

Jinye Mi, Fang Wu, and Nong Yang

Abstract The chapter on cancer treatment evolution traces the journey from chemotherapy, the earliest form of treatment with nonspecific action and significant side effects, to the more refined targeted therapy, which heralds precision medicine by focusing on specific molecular targets for enhanced efficacy and fewer side effects. It culminates with the latest advancement, immunotherapy, which revolutionizes cancer treatment by employing the body's immune system, offering potential cures and long-lasting responses. This chapter underscores the shift towards increasing specificity and personalization in cancer therapy, highlighting the transformative impact these developments have had on patient outcomes and the ongoing quest for more effective, patient-centered treatments.

Keywords Cancer treatment · Chemotherapy · Targeted therapy · Immunotherapy · Challenge

In the United States, there has been a notable decrease in cancer mortality over the past three decades [1] (Fig. 1.1). The approval and widespread adoption of targeted therapies and immunotherapies have played an undeniable role in this positive trend. Nonetheless, it's vital to acknowledge that research and development (R&D)

J. Mi
Department of Infectious Diseases, Zhuzhou Central Hospital, Zhuzhou, China

F. Wu (✉)
Department of Hematology and Oncology, Hunan Provincial Children's Hospital, Changsha, China
e-mail: wufang@hnca.org.cn

N. Yang
Department of Medical Oncology, Lung Cancer and Gastrointestinal Unit, Hunan Cancer Hospital/The Affiliated Cancer Hospital of Xiangya School of Medicine, Central South University, Changsha, China

Department of Medical Oncology, Lung Cancer and Gastrointestinal Unit, Hunan Second People's Hospital, Changsha, China

© The Author(s), under exclusive license to Springer Nature Singapore Pte Ltd. 2024
Y. Zhang, N. Yang (eds.), *New Anti-cancer Drug Development and Evaluation*,
https://doi.org/10.1007/978-981-97-7274-2_1

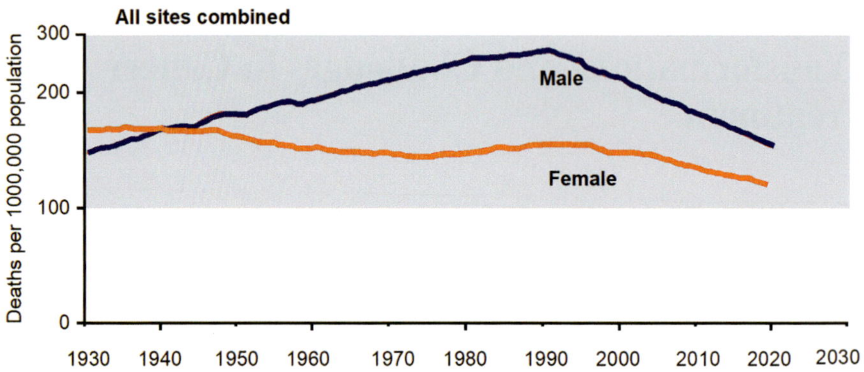

Fig. 1.1 Trends in cancer mortality in the United States from 1930 to 2020

for new drugs is both costly and time-consuming. Reports indicate that despite substantial investments in drug discovery and repurposing, approximately 97% of candidate anticancer drugs fail to gain approval after undergoing comprehensive clinical trials [2].

As an increasing number of molecular targets pivotal to cancer biology are being identified, a wide variety of new anticancer agents have emerged, some of which are currently undergoing clinical trials. These agents can be categorized primarily into two groups: small molecules and humanized monoclonal antibodies. Both types have shown promising inhibitory capabilities [3].

In the evolution of contemporary medicine, three fundamental therapies have been cornerstones in cancer treatment: surgery, radiation therapy, and pharmacological therapy [4]. Notably, pharmacological therapy has undergone three revolutionary phases in recent decades.

1.1 The First Revolution: Chemotherapy

Cytotoxic chemotherapeutic agents were initially developed in the 1940s, with nitrogen mustard being employed in the treatment of lymphoma and demonstrating considerable efficacy as early as 1943. In 1948, Sydney Farber demonstrated that the utilization of folic acid antagonists, such as aminopterin, led to temporary remissions in children with acute lymphoblastic leukemia (ALL). This breakthrough served as a cornerstone for the development of contemporary chemotherapy in cancer treatment.

Subsequent to these initial breakthroughs, the development of novel anticancer drugs has yielded significant advancements in chemotherapeutic agents. In the 1950s, the discovery of several agents, including 5-fluorouracil (5-FU), 6-mercaptopurine (6MP), methotrexate (MTX), cyclophosphamide (CTX), actinomycin D (Act D), among others, marked a pivotal step forward [5]. Notably, MTX was the first chemotherapeutic agent to demonstrate the capability in the treatment of choriocarcinoma. In the 1960s, the discovery of several chemotherapeutic agents that are widely used today marked a significant milestone in cancer treatment. These agents included vinorelbine (VLB), adriamycin (ADM), cytosine arabinoside (Ara-C), bleomycin (BLM), and cis-platinum (DDP). The introduction of combination chemotherapy regimens during this period played a crucial role in advancing the treatment of ALL and Hodgkin lymphoma, resulting in favorable outcomes. By the 1970s, the use of combined chemotherapies for specific tumors had become more established, with the clinical application of cisplatin and ADM. This marked advancement facilitated a shift in the goals of palliative chemotherapy toward radical treatment. Moreover, the 1980s witnessed the introduction of taxoids and camptothecin, derived from plants, which found extensive application in clinical practice [6].

Chemotherapy drugs, while diverse in their types, share a common goal in their mechanisms of action. Despite the specifics of each drug, they universally work to disrupt DNA integrity and impede DNA replication. They also target microtubules within the mitotic spindle and inhibit mitosis. This action collectively hinders cancer cell proliferation, invasion, and metastasis, ultimately leading to the destruction of cancerous tissues and cells.

Chemotherapy has become an essential component in cancer treatment, demonstrating its potential to achieve curative outcomes in certain chemotherapy-sensitive tumors, such as ALL, chorionic epithelial cell carcinoma, and testicular carcinoma. Moreover, in cases of advanced breast cancer, chemotherapy has effectively extended the survival of patients with chemotherapy-sensitive tumors [3]. Nonetheless, it's crucial to note that certain kinds of tumors display resistance to current chemotherapy drugs, and regrettably, chemotherapy has not proven successful in prolonging the lifespan of patients affected by these tumors.

A primary drawback of chemotherapy drugs is their non-selectivity, affecting many normal dividing cells, including vital stem cells, in addition to cancer cells. This phenomenon explains the pronounced side effects of chemotherapy on rapidly dividing cells, such as those in bone marrow, liver, and gastrointestinal epithelium. It's crucial to maintain precise control over chemotherapeutic drug dosages. Insufficient doses might not effectively eliminate cancer cells, while excessive doses can cause severe side effects, inflicting irreversible harm on patients, and sometimes leading to death [3].

1.2 The Second Revolution: Targeted Therapy

The discovery of DNA's double helix structure has profoundly deepened our understanding of life. Genetic mutations have been identified as foundational contributors to numerous diseases, including cancer. This realization prompted researchers to contemplate the feasibility of targeting these mutations for treatment, given that cancer cells originate from genetic alterations. Surgical procedures, radiotherapy, and chemotherapy lacked selectivity, resulting in significant damage to healthy cells during the course of treatment. Over the years, there has been a notable transition from traditional cytotoxic drugs to tumor-targeting drugs that specifically target abnormal signaling pathways within tumor cells [7, 8]. This transition has ushered in a new era of tumor therapy, emphasizing the development of drugs that precisely target distinct molecular markers implicated in the aberrant signaling pathways of cancer cells [9]. Dubbed "biological missiles," targeted drugs are engineered to selectively affect cancer cells, inducing their destruction, while sparing adjacent healthy tissues and cells. Transformative approach offers substantial promise in improving the effectiveness and precision of tumor treatments, heralding a hopeful future in the fight against malignancies.

In 1987, scientists first acknowledged the biological role of epidermal growth factor receptors (EGFRs) in the proliferation and metastasis of non-small cell lung cancer (NSCLC) [10]. In 1997, a landmark breakthrough occurred when the US Food and Drug Administration (FDA) approved rituximab for treating refractory B-cell non-Hodgkin lymphoma cases that were resistant to traditional therapies [11]. Subsequently, the focus in cancer treatment research pivoted to targeted drugs, ushering in a new era of innovative targeted medications. In 2013, the National Cancer Institute unveiled a landmark database, the most expansive to date, of cancer-related genetic variants. This invaluable resource significantly propelled research into targeted drug therapies and serves as a robust repository, catalyzing deeper insights into malignancies [1].

Targeted drugs, often composed of small molecules, are engineered to efficiently penetrate cells, enabling them to primarily target intracellular components. Many cancer patients have distinct molecular targets that specific drugs can address, making them ideal candidates for targeted therapies. Yet, pinpointing these targets usually requires genetic testing to determine their presence and gauge the patient's potential response to the drug. Genetic testing of tumors typically involves a biopsy, in which doctors remove a portion of the tumor for analysis, which carries inherent risks contingent upon the tumor's size and location. Despite their considerable benefits, molecular-targeted drugs have unveiled certain limitations. These drugs meticulously target specific genes, rendering their efficacy vulnerable to any mutations within the targeted gene. Consequently, many cancer patients develop resistance to these drugs within a few years of starting targeted therapy. Additionally, the development of such drugs is not only time-intensive but also financially burdensome, often putting them out of reach for many cancer patients [12].

Targeted therapy seeks to develop agents that specifically interfere with the key molecules pivotal to cancer biology. These agents function by impeding tumor cell proliferation, disrupting the cell cycle, facilitating tumor cell differentiation, suppressing tumor cell metastasis, inducing tumor cell apoptosis, and restraining tumor angiogenesis. The overarching objective is to achieve successful tumor treatment through these intricate mechanisms. The concept of a "magic bullet" was proposed by Paul Ehrlich over a century ago. Over a century ago, Paul Ehrlich introduced the concept of a "magic bullet," which entailed using antibodies to selectively deliver cytotoxic drugs to tumor cells, sparing healthy ones. In 1975, Georges Kohler and Cesar Milstein pioneered hybridoma technology, laying the foundation for the development of monoclonal antibody drugs. Their revolutionary work has earned them the Nobel Prize in 1984. Since the 1980s, molecular targeted therapy in cancer treatment has experienced remarkable progress, alongside rapid advancements in biology, genetics, epigenetics, and other fundamental research areas. A pivotal moment came in 1997 when the US FDA approved rituximab, the world's first molecular-targeted drug, specifically for CD20-positive indolent lymphoma. This landmark achievement propelled the field forward, fostering the development of an extensive array of targeted therapies aimed at combatting various types of malignancies [11].

Since then, numerous tumor molecular targeting drugs have gained global approval and market presence. These drugs predominantly encompass monoclonal antibodies and small-molecule inhibitors. Notably, the EGFR family stands out a prominent target, with widely utilized monoclonal antibodies including cetuximab, trastuzumab [13, 14], and pertuzumab [3] specifically designed to target EGFR. Additionally, EGFR-targeting tyrosine kinase inhibitors (TKIs) such as gefitinib [15, 16], afatinib [17], and osimertinib [18] have gained substantial recognition and are frequently employed in clinical settings. Over time, targeted therapy has undergone significant advancement and has been applied in the treatment of diverse forms of malignancies.

1.2.1 Advantages of Targeted Therapy

A standout benefit of targeted therapy is its exceptional selectivity, drastically reducing harm to healthy tissues and cells. It demonstrates outstanding efficacy with fewer adverse reactions in comparison to chemotherapy and radiotherapy, thus earning its recognition as a "highly efficiency, low-toxicity" treatment modality.

Rituximab is a high-purity monoclonal antibody specifically developed to target the CD20 antigen of B cells. In the context of indolent lymphoma, the initial use of rituximab in combination with the CHOP chemotherapy regimens [CTX + vincristine (VCR) + doxorubicin (ADM) + prednisone (PDN)] yielded a remarkable 90% response rate and demonstrated the overall survival (OS) benefit in elderly patients. To date, the efficacy of the combination treatment strategies, comprising targeted therapy and chemotherapy, has demonstrated remarkable outcomes compared to chemotherapy alone in treating both indolent and advanced lymphomas, regardless of the age of the patient [11].

Imatinib, the first TKI, is known for its selective inhibitory impact on Bcr-Abl tyrosine kinase and has depicted remarkable effectiveness in the treatment of chronic myeloid leukemia (CML). Imatinib alone has demonstrated the capacity to induce a clinical hematological complete response (CR) in 98% of CML patients, along with a cytogenetic response (CyR) in 53% of cases. It is noteworthy that imatinib stands as the first signal transduction inhibitor approved by the US FDA, highlighting its revolutionary impact on cancer treatment.

Subsequently, gefitinib earned US FDA approval, establishing itself as the inaugural potent EGFR-TKI to achieve this distinction. Its advent brought about a transformative shift in the treatment landscape for NSCLC. In its phase III clinical trial, gefitinib demonstrated an impressive single-agent objective response rate (ORR) of 71.2% and a 12-month progression-free survival (PFS) rate of 24.9%. The groundbreaking efficacy data highlighted a remarkable 26% reduction in disease progression risk. Conclusively, these results cement gefitinib as the first-line therapy in lung cancer patients with EGFR mutations [18].

Trastuzumab stands out as the earliest approved targeted therapy among anti-HER2 drugs, serving as a pivotal cornerstone in the management of HER2-positive breast cancer. Notably, both single-target therapy and the combination of trastuzumab with pertuzumab in combination with chemotherapy have produced substantial survival benefits for patients with HER2-positive breast cancer. The CLEOPATRA study, focusing on first-line treatment, highlighted exceptional results with combined dual-target chemotherapy. The study reported a median overall survival (mOS) rate of 57.1 months and an impressive 8-year survival rate of 37% [3]. These findings highlight the transformative impact of targeted therapeutic drugs in significantly enhancing patient outcomes. Moreover, their favorable safety profiles mark the dawning of a new era in cancer treatment.

1.2.2 Challenges for Targeted Therapy

Targeted therapy in tumors has become increasingly common in clinical practice, offering significant benefits to numerous patients. Despite its notable advancements, several challenges persist, particularly concerning molecularly targeted drugs. These noncytotoxic agents display considerable disparities in individual tolerance and blood concentration levels. As a result, discerning the optimal effective dosage and balancing it between the minimum effective dose and the highest tolerable amount through traditional clinical trials presents a substantial hurdle. To navigate this challenge, it's vital to adopt an "individualized titration" approach for treatment dosages, which focused on the content of target-related biomarkers. This tailored approach helps pinpoint patient subgroups poised to benefit significantly from targeted drugs, thereby optimizing therapeutic outcomes.

While single-targeted therapies often have limited impact on many tumors, there's a growing inclination toward combination regimens to amplify efficacy. Still, determining the optimal dosage, sequencing of combined drugs, and understanding the effectiveness and potential side effects of multidrug treatments necessitate large-scale, multicenter randomized clinical studies. In recent years, large-scale sequencing studies of whole tumor genomes, unveiling the intricate and highly heterogeneous nature of tumor genotypes in most malignancies [19]. The driver mutations in tumors prove to be challenging for targeted therapy. The presence of such diverse and complex tumor gene mutations presents significant challenges in the selection of appropriate therapeutic targets. Consequently, targeted therapies for most malignant tumors still face substantial obstacles, necessitating the exploration of novel targets.

Drug resistance poses another significant challenge in tumor-targeted therapy, as highlighted by anti-HER2 therapy. Alterations in the HER2 gene itself can lead to acquired resistance. These changes encompass variations in HER2 expression at mRNA or protein levels, shifts in HER2 gene copy number, and mutations within HER2 that hinder the binding of targeted agents [20]. While trastuzumab, a groundbreaking targeted drug in anti-HER2 breast cancer treatment [21], has demonstrated remarkable efficacy, nearly 70% of patients with HER2-positive metastatic breast cancer exhibit inherent resistance, and virtually all patients develop secondary resistance following an initial positive response [22]. Therefore, finding solutions to overcome drug resistance has emerged as a critical issue in anti-HER2 targeted therapy.

Further studies are warranted to holistically assess the efficacy, safety, and cost-effectiveness of combining targeted drugs with chemotherapy agents or other targeted therapies. There is a pressing need for continuous development of novel drugs that possess high efficacy, low toxicity, and reversible drug resistance. Notably, antibody-drug conjugates (ADCs) exemplify such drugs, holding significant clinical therapeutic promise with the aim to benefit a broad spectrum of tumor patients [23].

1.2.3 EGFR-Targeted Therapy in Lung Cancer

Among the predominant driver genes in lung cancer, KRAS accounts for 32% of cases, closely followed by EGFR at 11%. The EGFR, an integral component of the tyrosine kinase receptor family expressed in various tumor types, including lung cancer, orchestrates crucial roles in tumor proliferation, invasion, metastasis, and angiogenesis by activating pivotal oncogenic signaling pathways, notably the RAS-RAF-MEK and PI3K-Akt-mTOR pathways. EGFR inhibitors have notably improved the OS of patients with advanced lung cancer.

1.2.3.1 First-Generation EGFR-TKIs

1.2.3.1.1 Gefitinib

In first-line treatment, three studies (IPASS, WJTOG3405, and NEJ002) demonstrated that gefitinib significantly improved PFS and ORR compared to chemotherapy in patients with advanced EGFR-mutated NSCLC [24], although no significant difference in OS was observed. Additionally, a phase IV study reported a median progression-free survival (mPFS) of 9.7 months and an ORR of 50.0% for patients with advanced EGFR-mutated NSCLC undergoing gefitinib first-line therapy, while the CTONG1304 study demonstrated that gefitinib maintained its effectiveness when readministered to NSCLC patients who had previously shown progression on chemotherapy [15, 24, 25].

1.2.3.1.2 Erlotinib

The primary evidence supporting for the use of erlotinib in the first-line treatment of NSCLC is derived from the ENSURE, OPTIMAL, CTONG0802, and EURTAC studies. These studies collectively indicate erlotinib demonstrates improved mPFS and ORR when compared with platinum-containing dual-agent chemotherapy. However, there is no observed OS benefit associated with its use [18].

1.2.3.1.3 Icotinib

Icotinib has been primarily studied in the Chinese population. The CONVINCE study offers compelling evidence that icotinib improved mPFS in comparison to chemotherapy as a first-line treatment for patients with advanced NSCLC with an EGFR mutation. Additionally, findings from the ICOGEN study suggest that icotinib demonstrates non-inferiority in terms of PFS when compared to gefitinib in second-line treatment [26].

1.2.3.2 Second-Generation EGFR-TKIs

1.2.3.2.1 Afatinib

The research on afatinib in NSCLC primarily stems from the LUX series studies, notably Lux-Lung 3, Lux-Lung 6, Lux-Lung 7, and Lux-Lung 8, among others. In the context of first-line therapy, afatinib has demonstrated superior PFS benefits compared to chemotherapy, along with improved ORR and an enhanced quality of life for patients. It has also exhibited significant efficacy against rare EGFR mutations, such as G719X, S768I, and L861Q. Moreover, afatinib has shown prolonged PFS, and OS in comparison to gefitinib or erlotinib. The LUX-Lung 8 study further solidified the role of afatinib in the second-line treatment of lung squamous cell carcinoma. Additionally, afatinib has proven effective in providing clinical benefits to patients without T790M mutations, who display resistance to first- and second-generation EGFR-TKIs [27].

1.2.3.2.2 Dacomitinib

The efficacy of dacomitinib in the first-line treatment of advanced NSCLC proved notably superior to gefitinib, demonstrating a mPFS of 14.7 months, a mOS of 34.1 months, and an OS rate of 56.2% at 30 months. Similarly, studies such as

ARCHER 1009 and BR.26 have highlighted comparable efficacy of dacomitinib and erlotinib in second-line and subsequent treatments.

1.2.3.3 Third-Generation EGFR-TKIs

1.2.3.3.1 Osimertinib

Osimertinib, an irreversible inhibitor that targets the EGFR receptor via binding to the Cys797 residue at the ATP site, has shown significant promise in various lines of therapy for NSCLC. In first-line therapy, the FLAURA study demonstrated that osimertinib substantially improved survival outcomes, with a mPFS of 18.9 months in the osimertinib group compared to first-generation EGFR-TKIs. Although the ORRs were comparable, osimertinib demonstrated a median duration of response (mDoR) of 17.2 months and a mOS of 38.6 months. Patients with rare EGFR mutations experienced varying survival outcomes, with a mOS of 8.9 months, including 19.3 months for L861Q. A notable case involved a patient with a 19-exon insertion who achieved a partial response (PR) lasting 16.8 months post-treatment. However, the clinical benefit observed in patients with rare EGFR mutations was lower compared to those with sensitive mutations, emphasizing the necessity for further prospective studies to confirm these findings. In second-line therapy, the AURA study demonstrated that osimertinib was significantly superior to chemotherapy in patients harboring T790M mutations who had progressed after EGFR-TKIs treatment, with an impressive ORR of 62%, a disease control rate (DCR) of 90%, and a mPFS of 12.3 months in the osimertinib group. Furthermore, in third-line treatment, osimertinib has demonstrated notable advantages over docetaxel plus bevacizumab, as indicated by significantly improved mPFS and ORR in NSCLC patients.

1.2.3.3.2 Almonertinib

Almonertinib stands as the sole domestically developed third-generation EGFR-TKI available in China. In a phase II study, almonertinib demonstrated promising clinical benefits in patients with locally advanced or metastatic NSCLC bearing EGFR T790M mutation. The study results revealed an ORR of 52%, a DCR of 92%, and a mPFS of 11 months. These findings highlight the potential efficacy of almonertinib in advanced or metastatic NSCLC bearing EGFR mutation [28].

1.2.3.3.3 Other Third-Generation EGFR-TKIs

Furmonertinib and abivertinib represent two domestically developed third-generation EGFR TKIs in China. These EGFR-TKIs have demonstrated promising efficacy in patients with the T790M mutation. Abivertinib, in particular, has exhibited promising results in the treatment of asymptomatic brain metastasis (BM) in patients with NSCLC. Moreover, several other third-generation EGFR inhibitors, including but not limited to AZD3759, TAS-121, and ASP8273, are currently under development [29].

1.2.3.4 Fourth-Generation EGFR TKIs

EAI045, the first fourth-generation EGFR inhibitor, binds to the ATP site independently of Cys 797, thereby surmounting resistance in patients with T790M/C797S mutation. Preclinical studies have demonstrated the substantial synergistic effect of EAI045 when combined with cetuximab for the treatment of EGFR triple mutant (L858R/T790M/C797S) NSCLC.

JBJ-04-125-02 is a small-molecule allosteric inhibitor evolved from EAI045, boasting heightened inhibitory efficacy. Preclinical studies have demonstrated the superior tumor inhibition effects of JBJ-04-125-02 as a standalone agent. In comparison to EAI045 + cetuximab, the combination of ocitinib + JBJ-04-125-02 shows diminished toxicity and amplified antitumor activity.

Brigatinib, a selective dual-target inhibitor (ALK/EGFR), has exhibited an ORR of 25% in patients carrying acquired resistance mutations, including EGFR T790M. Encouraging results outcomes have been observed from the combination of brigatinib with cetuximab in patients with EGFR/C797S/T790M triple mutant NSCLC. These findings underscore the potential of brigatinib to surmount C797S resistance and establish itself as a fourth-generation EGFR-TKI.

1.2.3.5 Changes for EGFR-Targeted Therapy

1.2.3.5.1 Combination Therapy

(a) Antivascular drugs

Compared to first-line erlotinib monotherapy, the combination of erlotinib and bevacizumab has demonstrated improved survival outcomes in patients with NSCLC, as evidenced by a 1-year PFS rate of 55%. However, the benefits in terms of PFS did not lead to OS improvement. The RELAY study further revealed that the addition of ramucirumab to erlotinib led to significant improvements in PFS and DCR among NSCLC patients, compared to EGFR-TKI monotherapy. Notably, the combination of afatinib and bevacizumab exhibited promising clinical efficacy in NSCLC patients with EGFR mutation-acquired resistance, demonstrating a DCR of 90.7%.

(b) Chemotherapy

In first-line treatment, compared with chemotherapy or gefitinib monotherapy, the combination of chemotherapy and gefitinib significantly improved PFS and OS in NSCLC patients. In a study focusing on EGFR-sensitive mutated lung cancer conducted, PFS, ORR, and DCR in the pemetrexed + carboplatin + icotinib group were notably superior to icotinib monotherapy. In second-line therapy, the addition of gefitinib to chemotherapy did not yield a notable improvement in mPFS compared to chemotherapy alone, and it even led to worse OS in patients with NSCLC. These findings suggest that the use of first-generation EGFR-TKIs alongside chemotherapy following tumor progression may result in compromised clinical outcomes. However, another study found that the use of preceding EGFR-TKIs in combination with S1 chemotherapy was safe and effective for patients exhibiting resistance to first-generation EGFR-TKIs [30]. Moreover, regardless of the sequence of treatment, erlotinib in combination with chemotherapy has demonstrated significant improvement in survival benefits.

(c) Immunotherapy

In patients with advanced EGFR-mutated NSCLC, the combination of nivolumab and erlotinib yielded an ORR of 15%. The PFS rate at 24 weeks reached to 48%, and the DoR extended up to 38.2 months. Notwithstanding the favorable efficacy demonstrated by the combination of immunotherapy and EGFR-TKIs, it is worth noting that the incidence of adverse events (AEs) was also high. Therefore, the exploration of additional biomarkers beyond PD-L1 may prove beneficial in identifying suitable patients for combination immunotherapy.

(d) Different EGFR inhibitors

In a phase Ib study, the combination of afatinib and cetuximab demonstrated effectiveness in patients with acquired resistance to first-generation EGFR-TKIs and experiencing progression following afatinib treatment, with an ORR of 11% and mPFS of 2.9 months.

(e) Other

The combination of erlotinib with the antihormonal drug improved PFS and OS. Moreover, erlotinib combined with tivantinib (MET inhibitor) has shown improved patient survival and was better tolerated than erlotinib alone. Findings from the ECOG-ACRIN 1512 study revealed that PFS was significantly prolonged in both cabotinib monotherapy and erlotinib + cabotinib combination treatment when compared with erlotinib monotherapy.

1.2.3.5.2 Adjuvant/Neoadjuvant Therapy.

(a) Neoadjuvant therapy

The CTONG1104 study compared the effectiveness of gefitinib and chemotherapy in postoperative patients. The gefitinib group exhibited a significantly prolonged median disease-free survival (mDFS) compared to the chemotherapy, although no significant difference was observed in OS. In addition, erlotinib demonstrated notable improvements in various aspects, including an increase in the radical resection rate to 68.4%, the pathological response rate to 21.1%, ORR to 42.1%, mDFS to 10.3 months, and OS to 51.6 months. The INN06 study indicated that 51.3% of patients underwent cetuximab + cisplatin + docetaxel achieved PR before surgery, 8% confirmed pathological CR after surgery, mPFS was 22.5 months, and mOS was not achieved, with the 5-year OS rate reaching 58%.

(b) Postoperative adjuvant therapy

According to the EVAN's study, erlotinib demonstrated an improvement in the 2-year DFS rate when compared to chemotherapy. In the SELECT study, although the mDFS and mOS were not achieved in the erlotinib group, there was an improvement in the 2-year DFS rate, along with a reduction in the recurrence rate when compared with historical data. Notably, patients who received erlotinib upon relapse experienced enduring benefits. Moreover, the latest findings from the ADAURA study showed that the DFS rates with ocitinib at 1, 2, and 3 years were 97%, 89%, and 79%, respectively, significantly higher than those in the placebo group. The risk of tumor recurrence or death was reduced by 79%, with promising prospects for the OS results.

1.2.3.5.3 Challenges for EGFR-TKIs Resistance

A vast majority of patients encounter disease progression within 24 months following treatment with EGFR-TKIs. Resistance mechanisms can be classified into two categories: EGFR-dependent and EGFR-independent resistance. Approximately one-third of patients who develop resistance to third-generation EGFR-TKIs manifest secondary EGFR mutations, with the most prevalent mutations found at residues C797, L718, and L792 [31, 32].

(a) EGFR-Dependent Resistance

More than 50% of EGFR-dependent resistance is attributed to the T790M mutation, against which oechtinib acts as an inhibitor, while the C797S point mutation is the common oechtinib resistance mutations. In patients with EGFR del19/C797S/T790M triple mutation-mediated resistance, the combination of brigatinib and cetuximab has shown significant synergy. Currently, EAI045 and JBJ-04-125-02 are classified as fourth-generation EGFR-TKIs which specifically designed to target the C797S mutation. In recent years, exon20 insertion mutations have garnered attention as a focal point in EGFR resistance. The ORR, DCR, and mPFS of amivantamab in patients with exon20 insertion mutations patients were 36%, 67%, and 8.3 months respectively. Other effective drugs in this context include poziotinib, TAK-788, and luminespib.

(b) EGFR-Independent Resistance

The primary mechanisms entail the activation of MET and HER2 signaling pathways, while other resistance mechanisms include disruptions in the PI3K/Akt/mTOR, RAS-MAPK signaling pathways, epithelial-mesenchymal transition (EMT), and small-cell phenotypic transformation. In a phase Ib clinical study, we demonstrated robust antitumor activity of osimertinib + savolitinib (MET-TKI) in patients with MET amplification, boasting an ORR of 64% (including PR) and a mPFS up to 9.1 months. Capmatinib + gefitinib showed promising efficacy in NSCLC patients harboring EGFR mutations and MET amplification, yielding an overall ORR of 27% and an ORR of 47% in patients with MET copy number ≥6.

EGFR-TKIs resistance presents a significant clinical challenge for patients with EGFR mutations, emphasizing the critical need to overcome this resistance. Central nervous system (CNS) involvement stands out as the most frequent site of disease progression, with ocitinib demonstrated superior blood-brain barrier penetration and anti-brain metastases activity compared to other EGFR-TKIs. Approximately 50% of patients undergoing treatment with first- and second-generation EGFR-TKIs inevitably develop resistance, primarily attributed to the T790M mutation. Ocitinib has shown PFS benefits in subsequent second-line therapy for patients with the T790M mutation. Beyond the prevalent T790M resistance mutation, it's vital to delve deeper into other resistance mechanisms. It is necessary to investigate additional resistance mechanisms and develop novel inhibitors, with the aim of enhancing the prognosis of NSCLC patients with EGFR mutation. Additionally, exploring the potential of combination therapy holds significant promise in this context [32].

1.3 The Third Revolution: Immunotherapy

Due to the constraints of targeted therapies and their current inability to effectively combat all forms of cancer, efforts have pivoted toward exploring the human body's innate cancer-fighting mechanism-the immune system. This recognition has prompted a surge in investigations into the drawbacks associated with targeted drugs, fostering an intensified exploration of the potential of the immune system as a promising avenue to surmount these limitations and achieve holistic cancer treatment strategies.

Tumor immunotherapy is widely recognized as the third revolution in cancer therapy, distinguished by its unparalleled application and remarkable efficacy, which sets it apart from conventional treatment modalities. Tumor immunotherapy has its origins since the late nineteenth century, but significant progress has been made over the past 30 years. The pivotal moment in its history can be traced back to 1893 when a New York surgeon named William Coley encountered a patient with a recurring sarcoma behind his left ear. Despite surgical removal, the tumor exhibited poor wound healing. Interestingly, the patient developed a streptococcus pyogenic infection in the wound, accompanied by a high fever. Remarkably, the tumor began to shrink and eventually receded. This extraordinary case intrigued Coley, leading him to hypothesize that the infection had stimulated the patient's immune defenses, resulting in tumor regression. Motivated by this observation, Coley cultured a streptococcal abscess from another patient and injected the live bacteria to the patient. While some patients exhibited improvement, others tragically succumbed to the infection. Consequently, he experimented with inactivated bacteria, formulating a blend of inactivated *Streptococcus pyogenes* and *Serratia marcescens*, known as Coley toxin. Despite the discontinuation of further development due to adverse reactions and other factors, Coley toxin undoubtedly marked the beginning of a new era in tumor immunotherapy.

Australian immunologist Macfarlane Burnet, along with others in the late 1950s, proposed the "immune surveillance theory." This theory posited that the immune system serves as a vigilant sentinel, capable of discerning between "self" and "non-self," including the recognition of tumor antigens as "non-self," prompting their clearance by lymphocytes. This laid a crucial theoretical foundation for tumor immunotherapy. A simple yet vivid analogy describes the body as a country, with the immune system acting as the protective army and police force. In this analogy, external bacteria and viruses symbolize foreign adversaries that may sporadically invade. Similarly, internal cells can mutate into tumors, akin to the emergence of saboteurs within the population. However, the existence of a robust defense system allows the body to fend off external threats while maintaining internal stability. Internally, the immune system can accurately discern "self" and "non-self," facilitating precise elimination, a process fundamentally distinct from external interventions like chemoradiotherapy. This process, known as "immunoediting," not only eliminates certain tumor cells but also reshapes the tumor's antigenicity. A recent study demonstrating the potent influence of immunoediting on tumor immune escape analyzed 258 regions from 88 early-stage untreated NSCLC using RNA sequencing and histopathological analysis to evaluate tumor-infiltrating lymphocytes. The intricate relationship between tumors and the immune system poses a challenging dilemma in the exploration of tumor immunotherapy strategies. With the widespread adoption of high-throughput and high-bandwidth detection and analysis methods, various "omics" studies have substantially enriched the biological data pertinent to tumor immunology. Large biological databases are experiencing explosive growth with an exponential increase in data. In addition, advancements in machine learning and artificial intelligence algorithms have provided tools for processing biological big data. These advancements have made it feasible to integrate multiple "omics" data and construct complex and comprehensive "tumor-immunity" interaction models. Constructing a more comprehensive interaction model between tumors and the immune system using systemic theory is an inevitable trajectory for future development.

A significant distinction between immunotherapy and conventional tumor treatment modalities, such as surgery, radiotherapy, and chemotherapy, is the pronounced impact of individual variations on therapeutic outcomes. Several studies have underscored the close association between the efficacy of immune checkpoint inhibitors and various aspects, including tumor mutation burden, tumor lymphocyte infiltration, and tumor neoantigens. These factors are highly personalized, exhibiting significant diversity among patients and the potential for dynamic changes during the course of immunotherapy. The individual variation likely contributes significantly to the relatively low clinical response rates observed in immunotherapy. Among the factors contributing to individualized differences in tumors, the generation of tumor antigens through random mutations in tumor cells plays a pivotal role. Clinical analyses have demonstrated a strong correlation between the quality of neoantigens and patients' response to immunotherapy, as well as their OS.

In recent years, the rapid advancements of high-throughput sequencing technology have provided an effective tool to unveil the personalized differences in tumors, enabling the swift discovery of highly individualized neoantigens. Extensive high-throughput sequencing data have indicated that, despite their personalized characteristics, neoantigens are pervasive across all types of tumors. Human immune cells can recognize these neoantigens and elicit antitumor immune responses, thereby contributing to complete or partial tumor regression. Consequently, the exploration of therapeutic strategies targeting tumor neoantigens has emerged as a significant developmental focus in tumor immunotherapy. However, the clinical application of personalized therapy remains constrained due to the limitations of conventional pathological analyses and other techniques, which often fail to effectively identify tumor antigens.

In 1984, tumor biotherapy, also referred to as immunotherapy, was officially recognized as the fourth therapeutic approach, standing alongside surgery, radiotherapy, and chemotherapy. Over the past three decades, immunotherapy has great attention due to its therapeutic potential. Diverse immunotherapeutic techniques primarily strive to "boost positive immune regulation and curb negative immune regulation," echoing the fundamental principles of traditional Chinese medicine, which emphasize the concept of "strengthening Yang and subduing Yin,"

More than four decades later, in 2002, American tumor biologist Robert Schreiber proposed the "tumor immunoediting theory," underscoring the immune system's dual capability of eliminating tumor cells and fostering tumor growth. According to this theory, the dynamic interplay between the immune system and tumors can be divided into three distinct stages: "elimination, equilibrium, and escape." This conceptual framework not only deepens the comprehension of tumor immunotherapy but, more importantly, provides a novel strategy for its implementation.

Tumor immunotherapy possesses three pivotal advantages. Firstly, it offers a broader treatment window, making it possible in the treatment of advanced cancers with extensive metastasis. This attribute is particularly advantageous for patients who have undergone standard therapies, as immunotherapy has shown remarkable efficacy even in advanced cases. Secondly, immunotherapy exhibits promising prognoses and significant "survival trailing effects." Patients who respond positively to immunotherapy have a substantial likelihood of achieving long-term, high-quality survival, setting it apart from chemotherapy and targeted therapies. Thirdly, immunotherapy demonstrates a broad-spectrum effectiveness that can be applied across various types of cancer, offering the potential for concurrent treatment of multiple diseases. However, it is essential to acknowledge that immunotherapy is not without side effects, as T-cell infiltration, cytokines, and autoantibodies are among the contributing factors to these potential adverse effects [33].

1.3.1 Key Milestones in the History of Tumor Immunotherapy Since the 1960s

In the 1960s, researchers established critical role of cellular immunity, emphasizing its significance in combating tumors, distinguishing it from humoral immunity. In the 1980s, Dr. Rosenberg played a pivotal role in the field of cytokine and cellular adoptive immunotherapy, making significant breakthroughs that revolutionized the understanding and treatment of various cancers. His success in treating advanced tumors using lymphokine-activated killer cells and interleukin-2 (LAK/IL-2) therapy not only marked a significant breakthrough but also paved the way for a transformative approach in the field.

In 1992, IL-2, a pivotal cytokine for T-cell function, received approval for the treatment of metastatic kidney cancer, followed by its approval for the treatment of metastatic melanoma.

The year 1997 marked a significant milestone as rituximab, the world's first monoclonal antibody for tumor treatment, received approval from the US FDA for the treatment of non-Hodgkin's lymphoma [34].

In 2008, Russia approved the first tumor vaccine, oncophage, for the treatment of kidney cancer.

In 2010, the US FDA granted approval for sipuleucel-T, a dendritic cell vaccine designed to stimulate tumor-specific immunity, for the treatment of prostate cancer.

In 2011, the US FDA approved ipilimumab, an immunomodulator that inhibits the negative immune regulation of T cells, for the treatment of melanoma.

Immunomodulatory checkpoint inhibitors, including anti-CTLA-4 monoclonal antibodies and PD-1/PD-L1 monoclonal antibodies, have demonstrated remarkable efficacy across various tumor types, leading to their clinical approval for widespread application [35, 36].

The application of adoptive cell immunotherapy, especially tumor-infiltrating lymphocytes (TILs) and genetically modified T cells, such as chimeric antigen receptor T (CAR-T) cells, has yielded remarkable outcomes in patients with melanoma and leukemia.

The joint awarding of the Nobel Prize in Physiology or Medicine in 2011 to Bruce Beutler, Jules Hoffmann, and Ralph Steinman, for their groundbreaking contributions to innate immunity activation and the discovery of dendritic cells.

In 2012, Carl H. June gained global attention for his successful application of CAR-T therapy to cure leukemia in 6-year-old Emily.

In late 2013, *Science* magazine ranked cancer immunotherapy as the number one breakthrough among all scientific disciplines.

In 2014, the US FDA approved the PD-1 antibodies Keytruda (pembrolizumab) and Opdivo (nivolumab) [37].

In 2015, former US President Jimmy Carter announced that his tumor had been effectively treated with Keytruda, a PD-1 antibody, which stands as a notable example of the successful application of immunotherapy in cancer treatment.

In 2016, the US FDA granted approval to Tecentriq (atezolizumab), a PD-L1 monoclonal antibody, for the treatment of locally advanced or metastatic urothelial carcinoma in patients who experienced disease progression following platinum-based chemotherapy or within 12 months of receiving platinum-based chemotherapy before or after surgery.

In 2017, the US FDA approved two CAR-T-cell therapies, Kymriah and Yescarta. Kymriah received approval for the treatment of recurrent or refractory B-cell precursor ALL in children and young adults up to 25 years of age. Yescarta was approved for the treatment of certain types of large B-cell lymphoma in adults who have not responded to or have relapsed after at least two other treatment regimens.

1.3.2 Challenges for Tumor Immunotherapy

Tumor immunology still faces challenges despite the remarkable progress in detection and analysis techniques. The high heterogeneity of tumors, the intricate nature of the immune system, and the complex interaction between tumors and the immune system hindered a comprehensive analysis of the primary driving factors that affect tumor immunity.

While tumor neoantigens capable of inducing T-cell responses are present in the majority of tumor patients, the stochastic nature of T-cell activation, coupled with tumor heterogeneity and immunosuppression within the tumor microenvironment, presents a persistent challenge in identifying which tumor neoantigens can elicit an effective antitumor immune response [38] (Fig. 1.2).

Additionally, tumors can circumvent immune surveillance during their growth by undergoing immunoediting, often characterized by HLA heterozygosity loss or the downregulation of tumor neoantigen expression. Such evasion mechanisms frequently result in the failure of anticipated antitumor immune therapies and can contribute to tumor recurrence following tumor immunotherapy.

Despite considerable advancements, tumor immunology still faces significant challenges in thoroughly understanding and effectively utilizing tumor immunity for therapeutic strategies. Persistent research is imperative to overcome these challenges and improve the outcomes of tumor immunotherapy.

The concept of the tumor immunophenotype, which categorizes tumors into immune-inflamed, immune-excluded, and immune-desert types based on their interaction with immune cells, has significant implications for the efficacy of tumor immunotherapy. While the influence of genetic and environmental factors on the immunophenotype is widely acknowledged, precise determinants shaping these phenotypes remain a critical area of investigation. Tailoring immunotherapy strategies to specific immunophenotypes represents a promising avenue for future precision immunotherapy, urging further studies in exploration of the underlying factors driving diverse immunophenotypic responses.

Antitumor drug discovery heavily depends on preclinical models for elucidating mechanisms of action, optimizing delivery methods and therapeutic dosages, and

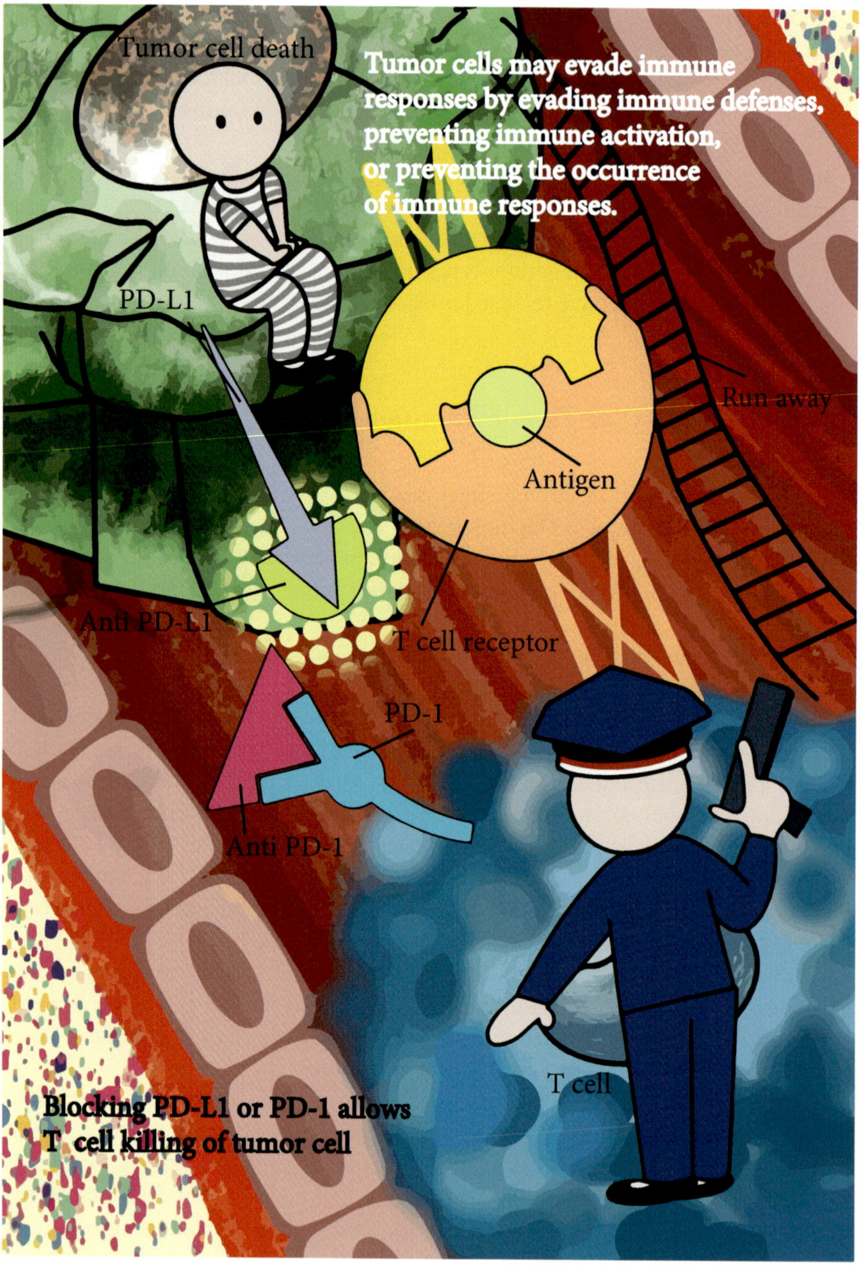

Fig. 1.2 Immunotherapy for antitumor

ensuring safety. These preclinical models have significantly advanced tumor therapy research. However, when studying precise tumor immunotherapy, the dearth of effective animal models often poses a significant obstacle in preclinical studies. The prevailing issue with conventional preclinical models lies in their inability to recapitulate the tumor immune-related characteristics that significantly influence the human cancer immune response. While genetically engineered mice with tumor suppressor gene knockout models partially emulate human tumor pathogenesis, they fail to mirror the continuous accumulation of mutations seen during human tumor evolution. Additionally, these models generally represent genetically stable tumors, which often exhibit limited responses to immunotherapy. Consequently, the lack of robust preclinical models has constrained the translation of preclinical research, leading to the need to address critical scientific queries through model experiments during clinical trials. Nonetheless, due to the intricate interactions of the immune system, optimizing the dose, administration interval, and timing of immunotherapy poses a significant challenge in clinical trials due to the extensive range of optimization regimens. Consequently, the field of tumor immunotherapy necessitates the development of more refined preclinical models that faithfully reflect the complex immunobiological traits of human tumors.

The advancement of precision tumor immunotherapy critically relies on interdisciplinary collaboration. Tumor immunotherapy research represents a multifaceted endeavor encompassing both fundamental scientific inquiry and technical complexities. The integration of tumor immunotherapy, particularly precision tumor immunotherapy, poses significant challenges for clinical and regulatory research. With the expanding scope of immunotherapy, an increasing number of therapeutic modalities are being combined with immunotherapy. This has led to the emergence of over 1000 novel combined therapy regimens in clinical practice, including radiation therapy, chemotherapy, and surgery. Existing clinical study endpoints in tumor research, such as ORR, PFS, and OS, may not be ideally suited for assessing tumor immunotherapy; therefore, suitable clinical endpoints for tumor immunotherapy research necessitates further exploration and optimization. In pursuit of novel clinical protocols for immunotherapy research, Bristol-Myers Squibb, Inc., has designed a pioneering phase II trial, known as the Fast Real-time Assessment of Immuno-oncology Integrated Therapies Program (FRACTION). FRACTION serves as an overarching study framework, incorporating adaptive trial designs and facilitating the evaluation of multiple tumor immunotherapy combinations [39]. The program employs a comprehensive approach, enrolling specific tumor types in successive studies through subprotocols introduced over time, thereby facilitating the assessment of promising combinations tailored to patients with distinct malignancies.

Tumor immunotherapy, as an evolving technology intricately linked to the advances in tumor immunology, presents unique regulatory challenges distinct from conventional therapeutic drugs. Currently, different countries employ diverse regulatory approaches for governing immunotherapy products and technologies, broadly classified into two distinct paradigms. The first regulatory approach involves seeking regulatory approval from drug regulatory departments, treating immunotherapy as a product subject to clinical access regulation. The second approach considers immunotherapy as a medical technology, with health authorities regulating it, and medical institutions being able to make clinical decisions within the legal framework.

Regardless of the regulatory approach, the distinctive characteristics of immunotherapy necessitate the development of detailed strategies to meet its complex clinical research requirements. As the field evolves and expands, establishing comprehensive and tailored regulatory frameworks specifically designed for immunotherapy becomes increasingly critical. These frameworks should account for the unique attributes of immunotherapy, ensuring its safe and effective application in clinical settings.

With the rapid progress in tumor immunology, novel tumor immunotherapy strategies continue to emerge, and personalized therapy has gained significant prominence in tumor treatment. However, the development of tumor immunotherapy still confronted with challenges. To expedite the healthy advancement of tumor immunotherapy, it is imperative to foster close collaboration among institutions, medical facilities, and governments. A comprehensive framework for the progression of tumor immunotherapy need be designed through top-level coordination, ensuring a synchronized and effective approach to drive progress in this area.

1.3.3 Top Ten Challenges

In 2020, Daniel S. Chen published an article titled "Top Ten Challenges in Cancer Immunotherapy" in *Immunity* [40]. The article delineates ten critical challenges faced by tumor immunotherapy, such as concerns regarding the reliability of preclinical study results and the identification of optimal combinations of immunotherapy-based treatments for individual patients. Tackling these challenges requires a collaborative effort between basic researchers and clinicians, along with the pooling of resources to enhance the comprehension of the intricate interactions between tumors and the immune system. The list serves to highlight crucial obstacles in the field, urging collaborative initiatives and fostering further research advancements. It is worth noting that the list presents the challenges in a sequence from basic research to clinical development, without prioritizing any particular issue. Given the intricate nature of cancer immunotherapy (CIT), coordinated efforts and collaboration undoubtedly play a pivotal role in propelling advancements in this field:

(1) Development of preclinical models that can effectively translate to human immunity.
(2) Determining the primary drivers of cancer immunity.
(3) Understanding organ-specific tumor immune contexture specific to various organs and tumors.
(4) Understanding the molecular and cellular factors influencing primary and secondary immune escape.
(5) Elucidating the benefit of endogenous versus synthetic immunity.

(6) Efficient assessment of cancer immunotherapy combinations in early-phase clinical studies.
(7) Comprehensive characterization of the effects of steroids and immune suppression on cancer immunotherapy and autoimmune toxicities.
(8) Maximizing personalized approaches through composite biomarkers.
(9) Developing improved regulatory endpoints tailored for cancer immunotherapy.
(10) Optimizing long-term survival with multi-agent cancer immunotherapy combination regimens [40].

The ten challenges of antitumor immunity listed here need to be overcome to propel the field of tumor immunotherapy forward, with further technological advancements poised to play a crucial role. As the field has evolved over recent years, the pursuit of integrating various components of cancer research has persisted. Ongoing collaboration is needed to foster diverse ideas and perspectives in the field.

1.3.4 Precision Oncology Medicine: Challenges and Changes in the Evaluation of New Anticancer Drugs

The introduction and implementation of precision medicine programs have propelled contemporary medicine into an era of extensive integration of medical data. Diverse sources of information including genomics, proteomics, metabolomics, epigenetics, microbiology, environment, behavior, clinical examinations, and traditional Chinese medicine have contributed to the exponential growth of medical data. The knowledge system of precision medicine has surpassed the capacity of individual physicians, and the rapid pace of knowledge updates has outgrown the capabilities of the traditional medical education system. Consequently, the clinical application of precision medicine in cancer treatment increasingly relies on information technology.

E.g. 1. Anticancer Drug Evaluation: Gefitinib
Gefitinib (Iressa) stands as a pioneering targeted drug for lung cancer, heralding the era of precision medicine and emphasizing the importance of biomarkers in diagnostic testing and patient selection. Launched by AstraZeneca in Japan in 2002, the drug received conditional US FDA approval in 2003. This decision was based on two phase III clinical trials, DEAL1 and IDEAL2, emphasizing response rates over survival outcomes. The US FDA greenlit gefitinib as a third-line treatment for NSCLC patients who either didn't respond to chemotherapy or developed metastasis.

After its initial US FDA approval, the efficacy of gefitinib in treating advanced or metastatic NSCLC was further explored. The phase III SEL trial, which encompassed 169 patients, failed to showcase any marked improvement in overall survival with gefitinib in comparison to a placebo. This led the US FDA in 2005 to restrict gefitinib's use for new patients, essentially sidelining it from the US market. That same year, AstraZeneca also decided to pull the European listing for gefitinib. In a subsequent move, AstraZeneca voluntarily retracted gefitinib from the US market in 2011.

Since 2004, researchers have observed a notable effectiveness of gefitinib among Asians and nonsmokers, linking its efficacy to a higher prevalence of EGFR mutations in these groups. This discovery shed light on gefitinib's mechanism of action and helped identify patient subgroups that might benefit most from this targeted therapy.

The NTEREST compared gefitinib with docetaxel in the second-line treatment of NSCLC. The study found that among patients with EGFR mutations, the objective response rate of gefitinib compared with docetaxel was significantly higher in patients with the presence of EGFR mutations, compared to docetaxel, gefitinib demonstrated a significantly higher ORR (42% for gefitinib vs. 21% for docetaxel; $P = 0.04$) and a longer PFS (7.0 months for gefitinib vs. 4.1 months for docetaxel; $P = 0.0001$). The results suggested that gefitinib was not inferior to docetaxel and could be considered for the second-line treatment of NSCLC.

The IPASS study, a randomized, open, parallel phase III study of first-line treatment compared oral gefitinib (250 mg) once daily monotherapy with paclitaxel/carboplatin chemotherapy. The findings of the IPASS study suggested longer PFS of gefitinib in Asian, nonsmoking, and adenocarcinoma populations (HR 0.74, 95%CI 0.65–0.85; $P < 0.0001$) [24]. In a subgroup analysis of biomarkers conducted within the NTEREST study, it was found that gefitinib treatment led to longer PFS in EGFR-positive subjects (HR 0.48, 95% CI 0.36–0.64, $P < 0.0001$). Conversely, among subjects negative for EGFR mutations, the PFS was significantly shorter with gefitinib compared to chemotherapy (HR 2.85, 95% CI 2.05–3.98; $P < 0.0001$). These findings suggest that gefitinib notably benefits EGFR-positive subjects, while mutation-negative subjects may not experience of benefit and could potentially achieve better outcomes with chemotherapy.

In the WJTOG3405, NEJ002, and IPASS studies, gefitinib consistently showed significant improvements in PFS and ORR for advanced EGFR-mutated NSCLC patients compared to chemotherapy. These findings established gefitinib as a first-line therapy for advanced or metastatic NSCLC with EGFR-sensitive mutations. Consequently, the European Union approved gefitinib in 2009 for all NSCLC treatment lines with EGFR mutations. By 2015, gefitinib made its return to the US market.

E.g. 2. Evaluation of New Anticancer Drugs: Pseudoprogression in Immunotherapy

During immunotherapy, some patients show an immune-related response, such as an increase in tumor size or new lesions. However, a biopsy often reveals necrosis or inflammatory cell infiltration, eventually leading to a decrease in tumor load. This unusual clinical response is known as pseudoprogression. It's thought to arise from the activation of immune cells by immune checkpoint inhibitors, causing these cells to gather on or within the primary tumor and micrometastases. Differentiating pseudoprogression from genuine tumor progression is a considerable challenge.

When pseudoprogression arises, its resemblance to tumor recurrence can significantly hinder treatment, potentially reducing patient survival if misjudged.

The likelihood of spurious progression varies among different types of cancer, as evidenced by clinical trial data demonstrating varying incidences of pseudoprogression across different tumor types. For instance, melanoma patients receiving immunotherapy exhibit an incidence of pseudoprogression ranging from 2.78% to 9.69%, while NSCLC patients show an incidence of 1.81–5.77%, and renal cell carcinoma patients demonstrate an incidence of 2.86–8.82%. Consequently, in the majority of cases, the increase in tumor size is generally attributed to treatment failure and genuine progression rather than spurious progress.

Pseudoprogression typically manifests within the initial weeks of immunotherapy, with occasional cases observed up to 12 weeks. However, occurrences beyond the treatment duration are less common. Pseudoprogression can be classified into early pseudoprogression and delayed pseudoprogression based on the timing of tumor shrinkage. Early pseudoprogression is characterized by an increase of ≥25% on imaging assessment within 12 weeks following the initiation of immunotherapy, while delayed pseudoprogression refers to an increase of ≥25% in imaging assessment after the initial 12-week period.

While cytotoxic chemotherapeutic drugs and molecular targeting drugs directly attack tumor cells and reduce the lesion, immunotherapy functions by stimulating and mobilizing the body's immune system through active or passive methods. By activating immune cells, immunotherapy aims to restore the normal antitumor immune response, disrupt immune suppression, and enhance tumor immunity. This process is designed to reinitiate the tumor-immune cycle, bolster the infiltration of immune cells surrounding the tumor tissue, sustain an effective local immune response in the lesion, and eradicate tumor cells. The approach offers strong specificity and long-lasting effects. As a consequence, some patients may not immediately observe tumor shrinkage. Instead, in the initial stages of treatment, the lesion may briefly enlarge or even give the appearance of new lesions, followed by subsequent shrinkage or disappearance. Alternatively, some patients may experience persistent tumor lesions after receiving immunotherapy, yet exhibit alleviated clinical symptoms and prolonged survival periods. In such cases, patients may undergo pseudoprogression, where the tumor lesions initially enlarge and then subsequently shrink in response to immunotherapy.

Histopathological analysis indicates a significant influx of T cells following tumor cell death at the initial stages of immunotherapy. However, the presence of PD-L1 and CTLA-4, expressed by tumor cells or antigen-presenting cells (APCs), leads to the deactivation of these T cells. Administration of anti-PD-1/PD-L1/CTLA-4 immune checkpoint inhibitors effectively reactivates these T cells, prompting their infiltration into the tumor lesions for the elimination of tumor cells. This process leads to the release of numerous antigens that attract immune cell infiltration from the surrounding tissue, leading to local tissue edema and necrosis. Consequently, as more tumor cells perish, additional antigens are released, further attracting infiltrating inflammatory cells. However, the contraction of the tumor tissue may cause the rupture of local diseased blood vessels, resulting in bleeding.

Consequently, this event triggers a recurrence of inflammation, leading to lesion exudation and edema. The accumulation of necrotic products from deceased tumor cells within the local lesions can potentially metastasize to other organs through the blood and lymphatic systems, consequently causing a partial enlargement of tumor lesions or the development of new infiltrating lesions.

References

1. Siegel RL, Miller KD, Wagle NS, Jemal A. Cancer statistics, 2023. CA Cancer J Clin. 2023;73:17–48.
2. Wong CH, Siah KW, Lo AW. Estimation of clinical trial success rates and related parameters. Biostatistics. 2019;20:273–86.
3. Swain SM, Miles D, Kim SB, et al. Pertuzumab, trastuzumab, and docetaxel for HER2-positive metastatic breast cancer (CLEOPATRA): end-of-study results from a double-blind, randomised, placebo-controlled, phase 3 study. Lancet Oncol. 2020;21:519–30.
4. Muthusamy B, Patil PD, Pennell NA. Perioperative systemic therapy for resectable non-small cell lung cancer. J Natl Compr Cancer Netw. 2022;20:953–61.
5. Smyth EC, Gambardella V, Cervantes A, Fleitas T. Checkpoint inhibitors for gastroesophageal cancers: dissecting heterogeneity to better understand their role in first-line and adjuvant therapy. Ann Oncol. 2021;32:590–9.
6. Goodman J, Walsh V. The story of taxol: nature and politics in the pursuit of an anti-cancer drug. Cambridge University Press, New York; 2001.
7. Devarakonda S, Morgensztern D, Govindan R. Genomic alterations in lung adenocarcinoma. Lancet Oncol. 2015;16:e342–51.
8. Saijo N, Takeuchi M, Kunitoh H. Reasons for response differences seen in the V15-32, INTEREST and IPASS trials. Nat Rev Clin Oncol. 2009;6:287–94.
9. Hanahan D, Weinberg RA. Hallmarks of cancer: the next generation. Cell. 2011;144:646–74.
10. Weinberg RA, Weinberg RA. The biology of cancer. W.W. Norton & Company, New York; 2006.
11. Coiffier B. Rituximab therapy in malignant lymphoma. Oncogene. 2007;26:3603–13.
12. Mingge X, Jingyu W, Qi L, et al. Promoting access to innovative anticancer medicines: a review of drug price and national reimbursement negotiation in China. Inquiry. 2023;60:469580231170729.
13. Balduzzi S, Mantarro S, Guarneri V, et al. Trastuzumab-containing regimens for metastatic breast cancer. Cochrane Database Syst Rev. 2014;2014:Cd006242.
14. Maximiano S, Magalhães P, Guerreiro MP, Morgado M. Trastuzumab in the treatment of breast cancer. BioDrugs. 2016;30:75–86.
15. Song Y, Wu YL, Cao LJ, et al. Efficacy and safety of gefitinib as third-line treatment in NSCLC patients with activating EGFR mutations treated with first-line gefitinib followed by second-line chemotherapy: a single-arm, prospective, multicenter phase II study (RE-CHALLENGE, CTONG1304). Am J Clin Oncol. 2019;42:432–9.
16. Li XN, Qiu D, Pan X, Hou XX. Mutation of the epidermal growth factor receptor gene and its impact on the efficacy of gefitinib in advanced non-small cell lung cancer. Int J Clin Exp Med. 2015;8:5397–405.
17. Jiang Y, Fang X, Xiang Y, et al. Afatinib for the treatment of NSCLC with uncommon EGFR mutations: a narrative review. Curr Oncol. 2023;30:5337–49.
18. Shah R, Lester JF. Tyrosine kinase inhibitors for the treatment of EGFR mutation-positive non-small-cell lung cancer: a clash of the generations. Clin Lung Cancer. 2020;21:e216–28.
19. Gelatti ACZ, Drilon A, Santini FC. Optimizing the sequencing of tyrosine kinase inhibitors (TKIs) in epidermal growth factor receptor (EGFR) mutation-positive non-small cell lung cancer (NSCLC). Lung Cancer. 2019;137:113–22.

20. Giordano SH, Temin S, Kirshner JJ, et al. Systemic therapy for patients with advanced human epidermal growth factor receptor 2-positive breast cancer: American Society of Clinical Oncology clinical practice guideline. J Clin Oncol. 2014;32:2078–99.
21. Maadi H, Soheilifar MH, Choi WS, et al. Trastuzumab mechanism of action; 20 years of research to unravel a dilemma. Cancers (Basel). 2021;13:3540.
22. Barok M, Joensuu H, Isola J. Trastuzumab emtansine: mechanisms of action and drug resistance. Breast Cancer Res. 2014;16:209.
23. Zolot RS, Basu S, Million RP. Antibody–drug conjugates. Nat Rev Drug Discov. 2013;12(4):259–60.
24. Hida T, Ogawa S, Park JC, et al. Gefitinib for the treatment of non-small-cell lung cancer. Expert Rev Anticancer Ther. 2009;9:17–35.
25. Fukuoka M, Yano S, Giaccone G, et al. Multi-institutional randomized phase II trial of gefitinib for previously treated patients with advanced non-small-cell lung cancer. J Clin Oncol. 2023;41:1162–71.
26. Zhao Q, Cheng J, Chen P, et al. Icotinib: efficacy in different solid tumors and gene mutations. Anti-Cancer Drugs. 2020;31:205–10.
27. Westover D, Zugazagoitia J, Cho BC, et al. Mechanisms of acquired resistance to first- and second-generation EGFR tyrosine kinase inhibitors. Ann Oncol. 2018;29:i10–9.
28. Chen W, Zhang L, Shen H, et al. Successful administration of low-dose almonertinib in a patient with lung adenocarcinoma after osimertinib-induced interstitial lung disease: a case report and literature review. Anti-Cancer Drugs. 2023;34:460–6.
29. Tan CS, Kumarakulasinghe NB, Huang YQ, et al. Third generation EGFR TKIs: current data and future directions. Mol Cancer. 2018;17:29.
30. Lin Y, Wang X, Jin H. EGFR-TKI resistance in NSCLC patients: mechanisms and strategies. Am J Cancer Res. 2014;4:411–35.
31. Du X, Yang B, An Q, et al. Acquired resistance to third-generation EGFR-TKIs and emerging next-generation EGFR inhibitors. Innovation (Camb). 2021;2:100103.
32. Wu SG, Shih JY. Management of acquired resistance to EGFR TKI-targeted therapy in advanced non-small cell lung cancer. Mol Cancer. 2018;17:38.
33. Postow MA, Sidlow R, Hellmann MD. Immune-related adverse events associated with immune checkpoint blockade. N Engl J Med. 2018;378:158–68.
34. Weiner GJ. Rituximab: mechanism of action. Semin Hematol. 2010;47:115–23.
35. Chen DS, Mellman I. Elements of cancer immunity and the cancer-immune set point. Nature. 2017;541:321–30.
36. Boussiotis VA. Molecular and biochemical aspects of the PD-1 checkpoint pathway. N Engl J Med. 2016;375:1767–78.
37. Malmberg R, Zietse M, Dumoulin DW, et al. Alternative dosing strategies for immune checkpoint inhibitors to improve cost-effectiveness: a special focus on nivolumab and pembrolizumab. Lancet Oncol. 2022;23:e552–61.
38. Sanmamed MF, Chen L. A paradigm shift in cancer immunotherapy: from enhancement to normalization. Cell. 2018;175:313–26.
39. Sharma P, Goswami S, Raychaudhuri D, et al. Immune checkpoint therapy-current perspectives and future directions. Cell. 2023;186:1652–69.
40. Hegde PS, Chen DS. Top 10 challenges in cancer immunotherapy. Immunity. 2020;52:17–35.

Chapter 2
Drug(gable) Targets Discovery

Yizhi Li and Siqi Xiang

Abstract The dramatic rise in global cancer incidence and mortality rates underscores the urgent need for effective cancer treatment strategies. This situation highlights the critical importance of discovering druggable targets for various cancer types, including lung cancer. The concept of druggable targets has revolutionized cancer treatment, pivoting toward a more personalized approach. By understanding specific molecular mechanisms underlying different cancers, researchers have been able to identify key targets for treatment. This strategy has been particularly successful in the treatment of non-small cell lung cancer (NSCLC), where kinase inhibitors targeting specific pathways, like EGFR, ALK, and PD-1/PD-L1, have shown significant efficacy. The success in NSCLC serves as a model for other cancer types, demonstrating the potential of targeted therapy in improving patient outcomes. The chapter underscores the necessity of continuous research in molecular testing and drug discovery to expand the arsenal of targeted treatments.

Keywords Druggable targets · NSCLC · EGFR · ALK · PD-1/PD-L1

The incidence and mortality rates of lung cancer are rapidly escalating worldwide, underscoring its position as a particularly aggressive malignancy that jeopardizes global health and longevity. The disease's stealthy progression results in about 85% of patients being diagnosed at advanced stages. In 2022, the United States recorded 1,918,030 new cancer diagnoses and 609,360 fatalities. Alarmingly, lung cancer was responsible for roughly 350 daily deaths, making it the foremost cancer-related cause of death [1]. Non-small cell lung cancer (NSCLC) is the most common subtype of lung cancer, accounting for 85% of all newly diagnosed cases [2]. Lung

Y. Li
Department of Pharmacy, The Second Xiangya Hospital, Changsha, China

S. Xiang (✉)
Department of Biochemistry and Immunology, Medical Research Center, Institute of Medicine, Jishou University, Jishou, China
e-mail: xiangsiqi@hnca.org.cn

© The Author(s), under exclusive license to Springer Nature Singapore Pte Ltd. 2024

Y. Zhang, N. Yang (eds.), *New Anti-cancer Drug Development and Evaluation*,
https://doi.org/10.1007/978-981-97-7274-2_2

adenocarcinoma, the most subtype of lung cancer, frequently exhibits oncogenic driver mutations. This characteristic makes molecular testing an invaluable tool in devising treatment strategies for NSCLC patients. The US Food and Drug Administration (FDA) has approved several therapeutic agents for the treatment of NSCLC. Notably, kinase inhibitors have been pivotal in targeting and modulating EGFR, ALK, ROS1, KRAS, BRAF, MET, RET, and PD-1/PD-L1 pathways [3].

2.1 Approved Targeted Therapy in Lung Cancer

2.1.1 EGFR

EGFR is a glycoprotein that belong to the tyrosine kinase receptor family. EGFR regulates multiple pathways associated with cell growth, proliferation, division, and death. Mutated EGFR proteins remain constantly activated, thereby becoming a cancerous trigger that promotes abnormal cell proliferation. Common mutation sites of the EGFR gene are found on exons 18, 19, 20, and 21. Specifically, mutations in exon 19 account for about 45%, and the L858R point mutation on exon 21 represents approximately. These two mutations are referred to as sensitive mutations. In contrast, mutations like G719X, S768I, and L861Q are deemed rare (Fig. 2.1). Notably, in the Asian population, 40–60% of lung cancer patients have EGFR mutations.

In 1984, F.J. Hendler discovered that epidermal growth factor (EGF) could promote the growth of benign and malignant cells in culture, suggesting that the EGF receptor might be a good marker for epidermoid malignancies [4]. Later, in 1988, S. Ozawa found that the EGF receptor binding capacity was higher in tissues from esophageal and lung cancers compared to other cancer types, including pancreatic cancer, colorectal cancer, breast cancer, and gastric cancer. These findings support the notion that the increase in EGF receptor levels may play a role in the development of human esophageal and lung cancers.

It has been indicated that EGFR exon 20 insertion mutations constitute 4.8% of EGFR-mutant NSCLC and 2.3% of all NSCLC patients [5]. In 2021, the US FDA approved mobocertinib (TAK-788) for the treatment of adult NSCLC patients with EGFR exon 20 insertion mutations. This approval was based on positive outcomes observed in a phase I/II trial, which primarily focused on two cohorts: a platinum-based chemotherapy pre-treated patient (PPP) cohort and an EXCLAIM cohort. The PPP cohort comprised 114 NSCLC patients with EGFR exon 20 insertion mutations who previously undergone platinum-based chemotherapy. The EXCLAIM cohort consisted of 96 NSCLC patients with EGFR exon 20 insertion mutations who had received prior treatment. The data showed that in the PPP cohort, the independently assessed objective response rate (ORR) was 28%, the disease control rate (DCR) was 78%, and the median progression-free survival (PFS) was 7.3 months. Similarly, the EXCLAIM cohort exhibited an ORR of 25%, a DCR of 76%, and a median PFS of 7.3 months [6].

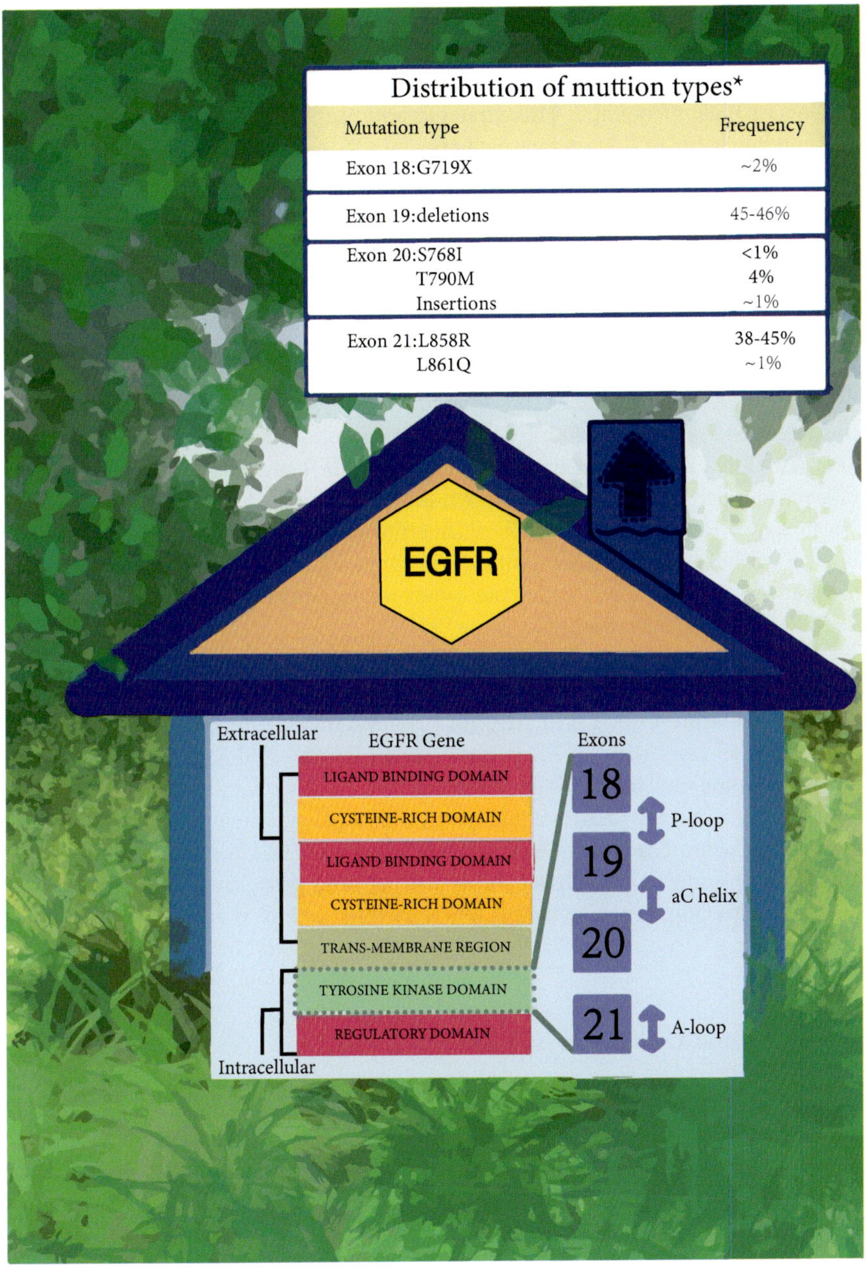

Fig. 2.1 Mutation types for EGFR

EGFR-targeted therapy for EGFR has profoundly reshaped the treatment landscape for EGFR-mutant NSCLC. EGFR-specific medications are now integrated into adjuvant therapy post-surgery and span multiple treatment stages, from first to subsequent lines of therapy. This strategic approach has markedly enhanced survival outcomes for EGFR-mutant patients, with those at advanced stages often had survival times beyond 3 years. To date, four generations of EGFR-specific drugs have been introduced, with the first three generations seeing widespread clinical use.

2.1.1.1 First-Generation EGFR-TKIs

Gefitinib (Iressa) stands as the trailblazing EGFR-targeted drug approved for clinical application in lung cancer. It's especially favored as a primary treatment for advanced NSCLC patients with EGFR exon 19 deletions and EGFR exon 21 mutations (L858R). In the first-line treatment of EGFR-mutated NSCLC, gefitinib achieves an ORR of 67%, indicating two-thirds of patients treated observe a reduction in tumor size by at least 30%. Furthermore, with a median progression-free survival (mPFS) rate of 10.9 months during initial gefitinib treatment, it's evident that half of the patients can anticipate tumor management without any further progression for nearly 11 months.

Erlotinib, known commercially as Tarceva, emerged as the second EGFR-targeted drug for lung cancer treatment, developed and manufactured by Roche-Genentech. It's prescribed primarily for first-line treatment of advanced NSCLC, specifically in cases with EGFR exon 19 deletions and EGFR exon 21 mutations (L858R). Compared to gefitinib, erlotinib has a higher incidence of grade 3–4 adverse events, notably diarrhea and rash. Additionally, a great number of patients undergoing erlotinib treatment require dose adjustment and treatment cessation.

First-generation EGFR-TKIs exhibit distinct drug properties, including reversible binding to their targets, which is less tenacious, and the possibility of off-target effects.

2.1.1.2 Second-Generation EGFR-TKIs

Afatinib, commercially known as Giotrif (or Gilotrif in some areas), is a second-generation irreversible EGFR/HER2 inhibitor manufactured by Boehringer Ingelheim in Germany. It has demonstrated favorable therapeutic outcomes against rare EGFR mutations, such as EGFR G719X, S768I, and L861Q, and offers promising control over brain metastases. While it also demonstrates therapeutic potential for squamous cell lung cancer, its ability to inhibit the T790M resistance mutation remains limited.

Dacomitinib, commercially known as Vizimpro, is a pan-EGFR inhibitor that also targets HER2 and HER4. Based on findings from the ARCHER 1050 study, it is the only first-line monotherapy to have demonstrated superior overall survival (OS) benefits compared to first-generation targeted drugs. This efficacy is particularly notable in Asian populations and patients with the L858R mutation. Importantly, many patients tolerate dacomitinib well, even when doses are reduced, allowing them to complete their treatment without compromising survival benefits.

Second-generation EGFR-TKIs possess distinct characteristics. They act as irreversible inhibitors, forming permanent bonds with their targets. Compared with first-generation EGFR-TKIs, these drugs exhibit promising efficacy against certain specific mutations, like G719X, L861Q, and S768I. Moreover, their target spectrum is broad, inhibiting not just EGFR but also engaging HER2.

2.1.1.3 Third-Generation EGFR-TKIs

Osimertinib has demonstrated efficacy in treating T790M-mediated resistance observed in first- and second-generation EGFR-targeted therapies; it's also used in first-line treatments and postoperative adjuvant therapy. Additionally, third-generation targeted drugs, such as amivantamab and mobocertinib, both of which were domestically developed in China, owe their origins to structural adjustments made to the osimertinib framework. Given the similarity in their molecular structures, cross-drug resistance is anticipated. Hence, if a patient develops resistance to one of these drugs, there's a substantial chance of resistance when transitioning to either of the other two. The primary resistant mutation noted is C797S, presenting an obstacle that future, fourth-generation EGFR-targeted therapies need to surmount.

Third-generation EGFR-TKIs offer a unique set of features. Beyond targeting a range of both common and rare sensitive mutations, they also target certain resistant gene mutations. With prolonged treatment using first- and second-generation EGFR-TKIs, acquired resistance often manifests, largely attributed to the T790M mutation in the EGFR gene. Yet, third-generation medications, notably osimertinib, can counteract this T790M-mediated resistance. Furthermore, osimertinib exhibits effectiveness against the sensitive sites targeted by first- and second-generation counterparts.

2.1.2 ALK

ALK, or anaplastic lymphoma kinase, is a gene that interacts with various receptor tyrosine kinases (RTKs). When the ALK gene undergoes rearrangement, it produces a fusion gene leading to the formation of a fusion protein. This protein merges the amino-terminal of echinoderm microtubule-associated protein-like 4 (EML4) with the carboxy-terminal of ALK, retaining the full intracellular tyrosine kinase (TK) domain of ALK. Aberrant expression of this domain triggers self-phosphorylation, subsequently activating downstream signaling pathways, such as RAS/MAPK, PI3K/AKT, and JAK/STAT3. This activation prompts malignant transformation and unrestrained cell proliferation. As such, ALK positivity serves as a diagnostic marker to identify the presence of NSCLC.

In 2007, Dr. Hiroyuki Mano identified a fusion between the ALK gene and the EML4 gene in lung cancer patients in Japan, shedding light on a new therapeutic avenue for advanced NSCLC [7]. In that same year, Manabu Soda developed transgenic mice to specifically express EML4-ALK in their alveoli. The findings showed that ALK inhibitors significantly decreased their tumor burden in comparison with those left untreated. While most of the untreated mice succumbed within a month, the mice treated with the ALK inhibitor showed no EML4-ALK/3T3 cell infiltration in their lungs and had prolonged survival. These results underscored the critical role of EML4-ALK as the solitary driver mutation in NSCLC and that its in vivo inhibition can considerably reduce the severity of lung cancer [8].

The prevalence of ALK positivity, predominantly resulting from ALK rearrangement, in advanced NSCLC is between 3% and 5%. While it's a relatively infrequent target, its high activity has garnered considerable research interest. The therapeutic horizon for ALK-positive advanced NSCLC has been broadened with the progression of ALK inhibitors. The advent of first-generation ALK inhibitors like crizotinib, complemented by second-generation inhibitors, like ceritinib and alectinib, and the third-generation inhibitor, brigatinib, has considerably extended the life expectancy for patients with ALK fusion advanced NSCLC. Consequently, ALK-positive advanced NSCLC is increasingly being viewed as a controllable chronic condition.

2.1.3 ROS1

ROS1 gene is localized in the 2q2 band of the long arm of chromosome 6. This gene encodes a transmembrane tyrosine kinase receptor, which is notably expressed in various tumor cell lines. ROS1 can activate critical signaling pathways involved in cell differentiation, proliferation, growth, and survival. In NSCLC, ROS1 gene mutations occur in about 1–2% of cases. These mutations are typically commonly seen in nonsmokers or occasional smokers, especially in adenocarcinomas. Notably, NSCLC with ROS1 fusion exhibits a higher risk of venous thromboembolism compared to those without ROS1 fusion or those with other oncogenic drivers.

The ROS1 gene shares homology with the v-Ros sequence found in the Manchester University tumor virus type 2 (UR2) sarcoma virus. Despite extensive research, the ligand for ROS1 remains under investigation. In 1987, a fusion of the ROS1 gene known as FIG-ROS, which now referred to as GOPC-ROS1, was first identified in the U118MG glioblastoma cell line. Soon after, researchers elucidated the role of GOPC-ROS1 in glioma formation and its associated signaling pathways [9]. The ROS1 protein comprises three main components: the intracellular kinase domain, the transmembrane region, and the extracellular region. As a crucial component of many cell surface receptors, the ROS1 protein's extracellular region binds to specific ligands. This binding activates the intracellular kinase domain through the transmembrane region, leading to autophosphorylation of specific tyrosine residues in the cell. These residues act as anchor points for various adaptor proteins.

The subsequent recruitment of SH2 domains and other characteristic adaptor proteins triggers signaling cascades, like RAS-RAF-MEK-ERK, PI3K-AKT-mTOR, and JAK-STAT3, which play vital roles in regulating cell survival, growth, and proliferation.

Crizotinib presents as the inaugural US FDA-approved inhibitor targeting ROS1. Its validation is primarily on ALK-rearranged patients, given the amino acid sequence homology and analogous conformations between ROS1 and ALK. The phase I PROFILE 1001 trial, which focused on NSCLC patients with ROS1 rearrangements, underscored crizotinib's efficacy against ROS1-positive NSCLC. Subsequently, entrectinib secured approval for treating metastatic NSCLC bearing ROS1 fusion in Japan on June 19, 2019, and from the US FDA on August 15, 2019. According to the NCCN guidelines for NSCLC (Version 5, 2021), advanced NSCLC patients with ROS1 fusion positivity are recommended to undergo first-line treatment with either crizotinib or entrectinib as preferred choices, with ceritinib presented as an alternative. Lorlatinib and entrectinib are suggested for subsequent treatment after disease progression. Furthermore, several potential ROS1 inhibitors, including brigatinib, cabozantinib, and repotrectinib, are in the clinical trial phase and have demonstrated promising results in ROS1-positive NSCLC patients [10].

2.1.4 KRAS

KRAS is a gene that encodes a guanosine triphosphatase (GTPase) anchored to the cell membrane. Mutations in this gene can promote tumor growth. The most frequent occurrences of these mutations are seen in pancreatic, colorectal, and lung cancers [11]. The KRAS gene belongs to the RAS gene family and is situated on human chromosome 12. It encodes two proteins: KRAS4A and KRAS4B, which arise from distinct transcripts of the KRAS gene. Additionally, this gene encodes a GTPase anchored to the cell membrane, having a sequence identical to the initial 165 amino acids of proteins encoded by other family members. Due to its molecular weight of 12 kDa, it's also referred to as the P12 protein.

The KRAS protein functions primarily as a small GTPase. It remains inactive when bound to GDP but becomes active upon binding to GTP, influencing several downstream signaling pathways, like MAPK, PI3K, and Ral-GEFs. The shift of the KRAS protein from its inactive to active state is orchestrated by two kinds of factors: GEF and GAP. GEF factors, such as the SOS protein, facilitate the KRAS protein's binding to GTP, leading to its activation. Conversely, GAP aids in the conversion of GTP, bound to the KRAS protein, back to GDP, resulting in its deactivation. As a result, the KRAS protein plays a pivotal role in governing cell growth, proliferation, differentiation, and apoptosis.

In 1964, Dr. Jennifer Harvey made a significant observation: rats infected with the *Moloney leukemia virus* (MLV) swiftly developed tumors. A few years later, in 1967, Professor Werner Kirsten discovered that rats exposed to the erythroid hyperplasia virus underwent a similar transformation. These groundbreaking findings led to the identification of two retroviral transformation genes, which were subsequently named Ha-ras and Ki-ras. The term "ras" is an acronym for "rat sarcoma." By 1983, a third member of the ras gene family, NRAS, was identified in human neuroblastomas [12]. A year later, researchers identified the first activated KRAS mutation, G12R, in the tumor tissue of a 66-year-old man diagnosed with squamous cell lung cancer. These pioneering studies underscored the intricate and unique link between the activation of the KRAS oncogene and the onset of human cancers [13].

For years, KRAS has remained at the forefront of precision medicine efforts. These efforts encompass targeting the KRAS protein itself, its posttranslational modifications, membrane localization, protein-protein interactions, and the downstream signaling pathways of RAS. Despite this concentrated focus, many compounds developed based on RAS gene strategies encountered roadblocks. However, the recent US FDA approval of the first KRAS G12C inhibitor marks a pivotal breakthrough. This achievement has reignited immense interest in advancing KRAS inhibitors. Moving forward, it's imperative to delve deeper into the understanding of drug resistance mechanisms and potential off-target effects. Moreover, the pressing need to develop additional drugs that specifically target KRAS mutations.

2.1.5 BRAF

The BRAF is an oncogene located on chromosome 7q34. It encodes a serine/threonine protein kinase and belongs to RAF protein kinase family [14]. The BRAF protein plays a pivotal role in the MAP kinase cascade. Together with the KRAS protein, it serves as an upstream regulator in the RAS-RAF-MEK-ERK signaling pathway. This pathway orchestrates the sequential phosphorylation of MEK and ERK proteins, which in turn activates genes crucial for cell proliferation and survival. Notably, cancer-associated BRAF mutations have been detected in roughly 8% of cancer cases. These are primarily somatic activating mutations, leading to enhanced kinase activity in the mutated BRAF protein [15].

2.1.5.1 Mutation Types of BRAF

2.1.5.1.1 Class I Mutation

The V600 mutation activates the kinase monomer and is considered the most oncogenic and therapeutically significant mutation. Common V600 mutations in BRAF are V600D, V600E, V600K, and V600R. These mutations lead to a robust activation of BRAF kinase activity and exhibit sensitivity to both BRAF and MEK inhibitors. It is worth noting that BRAF mutations typically occur in a mutually exclusive manner, which means they are not found concurrently with mutations in EGFR, KRAS, or other genes. The co-occurrence of these mutations is rare.

2.1.5.1.2 Class II Mutation

The kinases, including the BRAF mutations like K601, L597, G464, and G469, are activated as dimers. These mutations are localized in the activating segment or site. They function as RAS-independent dimers and are classified as class II mutations. Importantly, they may not benefit from EGFR-targeted drugs.

2.1.5.1.3 Class III Mutation

The kinase is inactivated when it forms a heterodimer, which includes the BRAF mutations G466, N581, D594, and D596. These mutations are localized in the folded catalytic loop or the DGF motif of the binding site. The kinase activity of these mutations is either lower than that of the wild-type BRAF or completely lacks kinase activity. Notably, class III mutations might benefit from EGFR-targeted drug therapy.

BRAF has over 200 identified mutation sites. Interestingly, some BRAF mutations, despite lacking kinase activity, possess a stronger binding ability to RAS activation bodies (RAS-GTP) compared to the wild-type BRAF. This enhanced binding ability facilitates the assembly into activated dimers, which in turn reactivates ERK, playing a role in the onset of lung adenocarcinoma. In contrast to the wild-type BRAF, these mutations are sensitive to ERK negative feedback. Their activation is RAS-dependent, which leads to the effective activation of RAS. Furthermore, they bind to RAS-GTP more tenaciously than the wild-type BRAF, amplifying the activation of CRAF and subsequently intensifying the ERK pathway. Clinical studies have shed light on the fact that melanomas harboring such BRAF mutations typically also present with RAS mutations or NF1 deletions, suggesting that cancer development might arise due to both BRAF and RAS anomalies.

According to the NCCN guidelines, the most common BRAF mutation in NSCLC is BRAF V600E. Per the NCCN guidelines, BRAF V600E is the most common BRAF mutation found in NSCLC. While the incidence of other BRAF mutations is similar to that of BRAF V600E, only BRAF V600E has a dedicated targeted drug currently available. For NSCLC patients with the BRAF V600E mutation, the first-line treatment recommendation is "dual targeting." This strategy involves inhibiting the upstream BRAF V600E mutation with dabrafenib, coupled with downstream MEK inhibition using trametinib. If patients are unable to tolerate the dual-targeting regimen, they can be prescribed BRAF inhibitors like vemurafenib or dabrafenib as monotherapy. However, in such cases, the MEK inhibitor trametinib is not recommended. Furthermore, for lung cancer patients bearing the BRAF V600E mutation, BRAF V600E inhibitor monotherapy can trigger CRAF self-aggregation, potentially leading to the development of benign tumors. Therefore, this monotherapy is not recommended.

2.1.6 MET

The MET is located on the long arm of chromosome 7, specifically at 7q21-31, and comprises 21 exons. Beyond encoding the MET protein, the MET gene plays a role in cell cycle regulation. The protein c-MET, synthesized by the MET gene, is a receptor tyrosine kinase (RPTK) present on the cell surface. It has the ability to bind to the hepatocyte growth factor (HGF). When the c-MET pathway is normally expressed, it can promote tissue differentiation and repair. In its typical expression or regulation, the c-MET pathway fosters tissue differentiation and repair. Conversely, deregulated expression of this gene promotes tumor cell proliferation and metastasis. Aberrant activation of the MET pathway can arise through non-HGF-dependent mechanisms. Predominantly, these mechanisms include MET exon 14 skipping mutation, MET amplification, rearrangement, and MET protein overexpression.

2.1.6.1 MET Amplification

2.1.6.1.1 Primary MET Amplification

In NSCLC, tumors that are highly amplified and predominantly MET-driven tend to have a worse prognosis compared to those with a combined oncogenic drive or those with moderate-to-low MET amplification.

2.1.6.1.2 Secondary MET Amplification

When EGFR inhibitors, such as the first-generation drug gefitinib, inhibits the PI3K pathway, crafty cancer cells recognize the obstructed EGFR route. In response, they devise alternative strategies, specifically activating the MET pathway. The same to EGFR, MET is also an RPTK receptor, leading to secondary MET amplification when these cells adapt.

When the original inhibitor fails to block the MET signal pathway from paving the way for cancer progression, the efficacy of the inhibitor is diminished. This phenomenon represents the resistance mechanism known as bypass activation.

2.1.6.2 MET Gene Mutation

Exon14 mutation is observed in 3–4% of NSCLC patients. When this mutation occurs in the exon14, the MET receptor is unable to initiate its degradation process. As a result, the MET signaling pathway remains persistently activated. This continuously open gate incessantly stimulates downstream cells, leading to their malignant transformation. Notably, the exon 14 mutation often coexists with MET amplification.

2.1.6.3 MET Gene Rearrangement/Fusion

MET gene rearrangements or fusion events are relatively uncommon. However, fusion events involving the MET gene with other genes, such as TPR, PTPRZ1, and KIF5B, have been observed. The exon 15 of the MET gene is particularly prone to fusion, which can activate the MET protein without the requirement of the HGF ligand. In the context of NSCLC, a MET rearrangement can either serve as the primary driver of tumorigenesis or act as a contributor to targeted drug resistance.

2.1.6.4 MET Protein Overexpression

The proportion of cases with MET protein overexpression is high, but this overexpression is not sensitive to current MET inhibitors.

In NSCLC patients, the three most crucial mutations in the MET pathway are MET exon 14 mutation, MET amplification, and MET protein overexpression. These mutations are currently targeted by specific drugs and yield promising clinical outcomes. MET high-level amplification and exon 14 skipping mutation is treatable mutations and found in approximately 5% of NSCLC patients. In clinical practice, MET inhibitors are divided into two main categories: small-molecule kinase inhibitors and monoclonal antibodies. The small-molecule tyrosine kinase inhibitors category includes cabozantinib, crizotinib, and savolitinib, alongside several multi-target kinase inhibitors. The US FDA has approved highly selective MET kinase inhibitors, including tepotinib and capmatinib. These drugs are primarily used to treat NSCLC with MET exon 14 skipping mutation. Furthermore, the bispecific antibody amivantamab, which targets both c-MET/HGFR and EGFR, has exhibited remarkable efficacy in NSCLC patients with MET amplification compared to those with TKI-resistant EGFR mutations. Apart from treating MET amplification, amivantamab is also employed to treat NSCLC patients harboring EGFR exon 20 insertion mutations.

2.1.7 RET

The RET gene, also known as the proto-oncogene tyrosine-protein kinase receptor Ret, is located on the long arm of chromosome 10 at position 10q11.2. It spans a length of 60 kb and comprises 21 exons. This gene encodes the RET protein, a receptor tyrosine kinase of the tyrosine kinase receptor superfamily, which composed of 1100 amino acids [16]. The RET gene plays a crucial role in organogenesis and neural development. Its protein product, the RET protein, is a receptor tyrosine kinase that can activate downstream signaling pathways, such as RAS, PI3K, and STAT, promoting cell proliferation. Occasionally, the RET undergoes breakage and fusion with other genes, resulting in the creation of a new gene that is self-phosphorylated and perpetually active. In the context of NSCLC, RET fusion genes, like KIF5B-RET, CCDC6-RET, TRIM33-RET, and NCOA4-RET, have been identified. These fusions rank as the third most common gene fusions in lung cancer, following ALK and ROS1.

In 1985, three scientists from Harvard Medical School employed DNA transfection to introduce human T-cell lymphoma DNA into NIH-3T3 cells in mice. The formation of novel "colonies" post-transfection, which had not been previously observed, suggested the activation of a new oncogene. Several genes from the Ras family were identified in this manner [17]. Later studies confirmed the RET gene as a proto-oncogene that fosters cancer cell proliferation and survival [18]. It was not until 2011 that a Korean research team reported NSCLC patients with a KIF5B-RET fusion [19]. When the RET gene undergoes mutations that triggers cancer initiating, such as fusion sites or point mutations, the resulting RET protein can become abnormally overactivated without a need for a ligand. For instance, RET missense mutations typically observed in MEN2A often arise in the cysteine-rich extracellular domains. It leads the RET protein to form a homodimer and activate without requiring ligand binding. Point mutations can also appear in the kinase domain within the cell, such as the frequently observed M918T mutation in MEN2B. This mutation increases the affinity between the RET protein and ATP, stabilizes the activated RET monomer, and triggers downstream signaling pathways that encourage cancer development [20]. In the context of RET fusion, even though the extracellular domains of the RET gene are lost, coiled-coil domains often remain in partner genes, like KIF5B and CCDC6. These domains drive homodimerization in the newly formed protein, allowing the RET kinase domain to remain continuously activated without ligand binding, thus propelling cancer [21]. RET fusion mutations are predominant in NSCLC and papillary thyroid carcinoma (PTC). In contrast, point mutations in somatic and germ cells are more frequently observed in medullary thyroid carcinoma (MTC) and MEN2.

While RET fusion occurs as a rare driver gene mutation in NSCLC, affecting only about 1–2% of patients, the primary treatment for these patients varies based on their pathological type and disease stage [22]. Those in the early stages may undergo surgery to completely remove tumor lesions. In contrast, patients with locally advanced or metastatic disease might need targeted therapy or chemotherapy.

2.1.8 *PD-1/PD-L1*

PD-1 is an immune checkpoint receptor found on activated T cells. It plays a role in regulating the immune system's response to the body's own cells by dampening the immune response. By inhibiting T-cell inflammatory activity, PD-1 promotes self-tolerance, helping prevent autoimmune diseases. However, this also means it can hinder the immune system from targeting and eliminating cancer cells. PD-L1, the ligand for PD-1, is implicated in immune suppression as it conveys inhibitory signals. Tumor cells can also express PD-L1. When PD-1 and PD-L1 bind together, they send inhibitory signals to T cells, rendering these T cells incapable of recognizing and attacking cancer cells. This mechanism allows tumor cells to achieve "immune escape."

In 1992, Tasuku Honjo from Kyoto University in Japan identified the PD-1 receptor while researching important genes involved in apoptosis. He utilized LyD9 hematopoietic progenitor cells and T-cell hybridoma 2B4.11 cells for subtractive hybridization analysis. Despite the significance of this discovery, it did not garner much attention at the time. The importance of PD-1 in immune regulation became evident only in 1999 when the first PD-1-deficient mouse model was developed. In the same year, Chinese scientist Professor Chen Leping discovered another member of the B7 family, B7-H1, which was later renamed PD-L1. Regrettably, Professor Chen did not recognize B7-H1 as the ligand for PD-1, assuming it was merely a new costimulatory molecule for T cells [23]. It was in 2000 that Tasuku Honjo and Gordon Freeman identified the B7 family protein, PD-L1, as the ligand for PD-1. They demonstrated that PD-L1 inhibited T-cell proliferation and cytokine secretion by binding to PD-1, a pivotal discovery that began to draw more attention to the field [24]. Once PD-1 and PD-L1 bind, they create an inhibitory pathway that suppresses T-cell proliferation and expansion. Normally, the binding of PD-1 to PD-L1 tempers the immune response of T cells to adjacent tissue, mitigating the risk of immune-related diseases. However, certain tumor cells also express PD-L1, leading to immune escape. This expression diminishes the immune response, allowing T cells in the tumor microenvironment to thrive. By interrupting the PD-1/PD-L1 signaling pathway, the antitumor activity of T cells can be revived, enhancing their ability to target and destroy tumor cells [25].

Currently, more than 10 monoclonal antibody drugs targeting the PD-1/PD-L1 pathway have been approved for global marketing. Out of these, seven are specifically used in the treatment of lung cancer.

2.1.8.1 PD-1 Drugs

2.1.8.1.1 Pembrolizumab

Pembrolizumab, when combined with pemetrexed and platinum-based chemotherapy, is indicated for several patient categories. It serves as a first-line treatment for metastatic non-squamous NSCLC patients who test negative for both EGFR gene mutation and ALK rearrangement. Additionally, pembrolizumab can be used as a monotherapy for locally advanced or metastatic NSCLC patients who test negative for the EGFR gene mutation and ALK rearrangement and have a PD-L1 tumor proportion score (TPS) of 1% or higher. Lastly, it is recommended as a first-line treatment in combination with carboplatin and paclitaxel for patients with metastatic squamous NSCLC.

2.1.8.1.2 Nivolumab

Nivolumab is approved for treating adults with locally advanced or metastatic NSCLC who test negative for both EGFR gene mutation and ALK rearrangement and who have experienced disease progression or intolerance after undergoing platinum-based chemotherapy.

2.1.8.1.3 Atezolizumab

Atezolizumab, when combined with pemetrexed and platinum-based chemotherapy, is recommended as a first-line treatment for locally advanced or metastatic non-squamous NSCLC patients who test negative for both EGFR gene mutation and ALK rearrangement and are not candidates for surgical resection.

2.1.8.1.4 Carilizumab

Carilizumab, when combined with pemetrexed and carboplatin, is indicated as a first-line treatment for advanced or metastatic non-squamous NSCLC.

2.1.8.1.5 Sintilimab

Sintilimab, when combined with gemcitabine and platinum-based chemotherapy, is recommended as a first-line treatment for unresectable advanced or recurrent squamous cell NSCLC.

2.1.8.2 PD-L1 Drugs

2.1.8.2.1 Durvalumab

Durvalumab is used as consolidation therapy for NSCLC patients that is inoperable following concurrent chemoradiotherapy.

2.1.8.2.2 Atezolizumab

Atezolizumab, when combined with chemotherapy, is recommended as a first-line treatment for extensive-stage small-cell lung cancer. Tumor resistance can generally be divided into two categories: primary and acquired resistance. Primary resistance refers to the inherent lack of response to molecularly targeted drugs, while acquired resistance emerges over time, even after an initial positive response to treatment. Despite the availability of these targeted treatments, patients may still face challenges, including resistance to these targets and side effects like vomiting and rashes. However, with ongoing advancements in detection technology and drug development, it's anticipated that more therapeutic targets will be identified, further enhancing treatment outcomes for lung cancer patients.

2.2 Target Identification to Targeted Therapies

With the evolution of biomedical technologies, the discovery of molecular targets for tumor treatment can be realized through a myriad of methods. However, regardless of technological advancements, the core principles of molecular target identification have remained steadfast. The goal is to exploit the molecular biological differences between tumor and normal cells, preventing the growth and multiplication of tumor cells, culminating in their death. Such differences can include varying gene characteristics, enzymes, and signal transduction pathways, among others. The journey from pinpointing a molecular target, through the identification of targeted inhibitors, to clinical trials, and ultimately securing approval for patient treatment is extensive.

In the history of targeted cancer therapy, the unearthing of the epidermal growth factor receptor (EGFR) has significantly propelled the fight against lung cancer. This renowned anticancer target was initially identified by Cohen in the 1970s. Carpenter et al. ascertained that EGF formed a complex with plasma membrane receptors in cells, leading to augmented cell growth both in vitro and in vivo [26]. This pivotal discovery invigorated the burgeoning exploration of targeted therapy, spurring the evolution of drugs targeting the EGFR pathway specifically for lung cancer [27]. However, during this period, the intricate molecular mechanism through which EGFR stimulated tumor growth remained an enigma. Over the subsequent decades, relentless collaborative endeavors were aimed at discerning small-molecule inhibitors that targeted the kinase domain of EGFR to curb tumor growth. This eventually bore fruit with the US FDA approval of two small-molecule EGFR inhibitors: gefitinib in 2004 and erlotinib in 2005 [28, 29]. Notwithstanding their promising clinical trial results, the real-world clinical efficacy of these drugs was unexpectedly subpar. Despite the rampant overexpression of EGFR in lung cancer, the efficacy of anti-EGFR medications was disproportionately low. In light of these puzzling outcomes, two independent research groups revealed that patients harboring specific mutations in either the 19th or 21st exon of the EGFR gene exhibited enhanced responsiveness to targeted medications. Intriguingly, these mutations were found to be more prevalent in Asian patients. Hence, anti-EGFR therapy has, over the years, immensely improved the prognosis of lung cancer, especially for Asian patients. The saga of anti-EGFR epitomizes the trajectory of targeted cancer therapy development. From target discernment and the conception of molecule inhibitors to the elucidation of clinical efficacy biomarkers, it encapsulates the evolution of a target from rudimentary research to clinical implementation. In subsequent sections, we will delve into the preclinical identification of targets, the design of targeted inhibitors, the discovery of clinical biomarkers, as well as the underlying antitumor mechanisms and potential drug resistance.

2.2.1 Screening and Identification of Molecular Targets

The initial wave of genetically targeted therapies for cancer therapies zeroed in on drugging gene products recurrently mutated in specific cancer types. Notably, the renowned targets, ALK and ROS1, were identified in this manner. These discoveries have dramatically enhanced the prognosis of patients with ALK- or ROS1-rearranged lung cancer [30–33]. Genomic analysis has been pivotal in pinpointing genes and signaling pathways linked with distinct cancer types. Further validation of these discoveries has been achieved using molecular biology and bioinformatics techniques. This strategy has been instrumental in uncovering targetable molecules and propelling drug development for lung cancer. However, the exclusive reliance on genomic analysis for identifying new druggable cancer targets has reached its limits. Some established genetic drivers of cancer elude targeting due to their molecular makeup, making them undruggable oncogenes, or because they result in a functional loss, as seen in tumor suppressor genes. Presently, most oncology researchers leverage the confluence of multi-omics analysis with bioinformatics [34–37]. Through the analysis of multi-omics data, researchers can pinpoint disease-associated proteins and signaling pathways, as well as uncover potential targets and therapeutics. Bioinformatics aims to uncover disease-related biomarkers and targets. It involves harnessing computer algorithms and statistical techniques to dissect and compare biological data across varying scenarios, such as genetic mutations, transcriptional changes, protein expression and structural shifts, and alterations in metabolites. Over recent decades, researchers, utilizing multi-omics and bioinformatics, have unraveled the biological variances of distinct molecular tumor subtypes and identified therapeutic targets for tumors with various molecular foundations [38]. The evolution of omics technologies, inclusive of spatial omics and single-cell omics, has profoundly expanded our understanding of tumor heterogeneity, proving instrumental in the creation of innovative targeted drugs tailored to this tumor trait.

Beyond the application of genomics and bioinformatics techniques for the identification of therapeutic molecular targets—akin to searching for a needle in a haystack and heavily contingent on biotechnological progress—researchers can also delve into targets anchored in their comprehension of tumor biology. This approach involves probing known biological molecular pathways and tumor behaviors to spotlight potential targets. For instance, functional genomic screening, grounded in the genetic principle of synthetic lethality, offers a route to unearth drug targets in cancers [39]. Fusing contemporary biotechnologies with high-throughput screening, notably CRISPR/Cas-based gene perturbation screening, has become a formidable instrument for identifying new targets for cancer immunotherapy. A spectrum of CRISPR screening strategies have been used for the identification of molecular targets. The CRISPR/Cas framework targets genomic sequences ranging from coding sequences to non-coding RNA/DNA, including miRNA, lncRNA, circRNA, promoters, and enhancers, which may be potential drug targets [40]. Through the integration of CRISPR screening with complementary approaches, scientists have successfully painted a panoramic picture of potential tumor treatment targets.

2.2.2 Drug Development Based on the Targets

In addition to identifying molecular targets with therapeutic significance, developing effective drugs that target these molecules is pivotal in preclinical oncology research. Currently, there are several commonly used methods for discovering drugs that inhibit these targets:

High-throughput screening: This method is prevalent in drug discovery. It involves testing thousands to millions of compounds with the goal of identifying those that bind to the target and either activate or inhibit its function. This technique facilitates the swift identification of novel drug targets in a limited time span. High-throughput screening utilizes robotic systems and automated equipment designed for rapid screening of vast compound arrays.

Structure-based drug design: This approach focuses on creating drugs informed by the structure of the target molecule. Using techniques like X-ray crystallography or NMR spectroscopy, the three-dimensional structure of the target molecule is determined. This structural information guides the design of drugs that can specifically interact with the target.

Ligand-based drug design: This approach centers on developing drugs informed by the structure of a known ligand—a molecule that binds to the desired target molecule. In ligand-based drug design, the structure of the ligand serves as a blueprint to develop new drugs that can mimic its binding characteristics, ensuring effective interaction with the target molecule [41–43].

Fragment-based drug design: This approach involves screening small molecular fragments against the target molecule. These fragments are subsequently built up into larger molecules that can effectively interact with the target molecule.

Virtual screening: This method utilizes computer-based techniques to sift through extensive databases of compounds, identifying potential binders to the target molecule. This process leverages various techniques, such as molecular docking, molecular dynamics simulations, and machine learning algorithms, facilitating the prediction and assessment of compound interactions with the target molecule.

Phenotypic screening: This approach involves testing compounds against whole cells or organisms to pinpoint those that produce a desired biological outcome. It proves particularly beneficial when the target molecule is not thoroughly characterized or when a disease involves multiple targets.

Cell-based screening methods: This technique employs cell culture systems to identify compounds with specific pharmacological effects, subsequently verifying their targets through molecular biology and complementary methods.

We've outlined some commonly used methods for drug discovery against targets above. Typically, a blend of these methods is employed to pinpoint and fine-tune lead compounds for drug development, as each approach has its strengths and weaknesses. For instance, high-throughput screening can sift through a vast array of compounds in a relatively condensed timeframe, even without prior insight into the target's structure or function. This allows for the identification of lead compounds with robust potency against the target. However, this technique can yield false positives or negatives and might overlook compounds that differ significantly from known ligands. On the other hand, a structure-based drug design strategy can refine drug properties, such as solubility and bioavailability, enhancing the specificity and affinity of the drug design for its target. Nonetheless, this strategy hinges on having knowledge of the target's structure, which might not always be accessible. Moreover, it might fail to detect compounds that bind to allosteric sites or other unconventional binding locations.

2.2.3 Therapeutic Targets Test in Preclinical Settings

Before therapeutic target inhibitors can advance to clinical trials, their efficacy must be validated through a series of animal model experiments. To best replicate the potential therapeutic effects of a drug in humans, it's vital to employ appropriate preclinical tumor models during this stage. The choice of these models is determined on the factors, such as research goals, necessary data, and available resources. Currently, a plethora of tumor models are at researchers' disposal, broadly categorized into in vitro and in vivo types. Within the in vitro category, cell lines and primary cells stand out as the most prevalent and convenient models for tumor research [44, 45]. Cell lines are collections of tumor cells isolated from tumors and subsequently cultivated and propagated in a culture medium. In contrast, primary cells are directly harvested from a patient's tumor and then cultivated and propagated in vitro. These cell lines and primary cells are instrumental in studying aspects of tumors, including cell growth, proliferation, invasion, and drug resistance. Virtually all drugs undergo initial studies using cell lines. Owing to their robust utility, cell lines are a well-established tool for investigating molecular mechanisms, having made significant contributions to oncological research. Beyond evaluating drug efficacy, tumor cell lines are frequently used for high-throughput target screening, attributed to their ease of manipulation and straightforward culture and detection attributes. As previously mentioned, employing cell lines to screen targets via the CRISPR-Cas9 system has been pivotal in understanding tumors of various origins and molecular subtypes [46, 47].

In vivo tumor models are essential for assessing drug efficacy. Animal models, as is widely acknowledged, provide insights into tumor formation, progression, and therapeutic responses [48]. Xenograft tumor models, for instance, involve transplanting tumor cells or tissues into an animal to observe tumor growth and treatment outcomes. These models are prevalent in tumor biology, drug screening, and evaluation studies [49]. Depending on the research objectives and specific tumor types, researchers can select appropriate tumor cell lines for implantation, either subcutaneously or orthotopically. Xenograft models are notable for their consistency, ease of creation, and their ability to mimic human tumor growth and progression. Their high relevance to tumor biology and therapeutic research makes them a staple for drug screening and evaluation. However, it's worth noting that xenograft models typically involve transplanting tumor cells into mice or other animals, which don'' entirely replicate the human microenvironment. Moreover, the suitability of xenograft tumor models is contingent upon the origin of the tumor cells. Cells from varied sources possess distinct characteristics and biological behaviors that can impact the accuracy of experimental outcomes. Researchers must weigh these factors during both the preliminary experimental design and subsequent result analysis.

A genetically modified animal model refers to an experimental animal that has had exogenous genes introduced into its genome, leading to the expression of specific proteins or the emergence of distinct phenotypes [50, 51]. Four prevalent methods are employed to create genetically modified animal models:

Pronuclear injection: This method is the most widely adopted approach for creating genetically modified animal models. It entails introducing a plasmid, which carries the desired exogenous genes, into the fluid surrounding the nucleus of a fertilized egg. This modified egg is then implanted into a female animal. Once the offspring matures, researchers observe the expression of the introduced genes or the manifestation of specific phenotypes.

Gene knockout: The gene knockout technique involves deleting or substituting a specific segment of the target gene with an exogenous DNA sequence. This alteration interrupts or nullifies the standard regulation of the target gene. Researchers use the gene knockout approach to delve into the function and underlying mechanisms of the targeted gene.

Gene knock-in: The gene knock-in technique entails introducing an exogenous DNA sequence from a specific gene into a designated site within the target gene. This incorporation can regulate the expression of the target gene or result in an altered protein structure. Researchers employ the gene knock-in approach to investigate the relationship and mechanisms linking the target gene to particular diseases.

Gene mutation: This technique involves integrating exogenous DNA sequences into the genome, leading to point mutations or targeted gene knockouts. It allows for the emulation of human genetic disorders or the study of specific gene functions. Furthermore, this approach can be employed for drug screening or to identify novel therapeutic targets for disease management [52, 53].

Transgenic animal models provide invaluable insights for simulating human tumors in vivo, enhancing our comprehension of disease mechanisms and drug discovery. By inducing specific gene mutations or manipulating gene expression, these models can emulate a variety of tumors, aiding in dissecting gene roles. Transgenic techniques can also expedite tumor onset and progression, offering cost and time efficiencies. Additionally, these transgenic animals are pivotal for gauging the efficacy and potential side effects of new drugs, thereby informing clinical interventions. However, there are inherent uncertainties in transgenic technology, which might produce unexpected outcomes, like unforeseen phenotypes or irreversible changes. It's also worth noting that human tumors' complexity and heterogeneity may not be entirely replicated by these models. Moreover, creating and maintaining transgenic tumor models can be costly and requires specialized skills and equipment. Such challenges might restrict their broader application.

Furthermore, it's worth noting a particular tumor model that has surged in prominence recently due to its ability to more closely replicate the genuine conditions of patient tumors [54–56]. Known as the patient-derived xenograft model (PDX), this approach involves extracting tumor cells directly from patient tissues and transplanting them into animal models, typically mice. These in vivo experiments are crucial for evaluating both the therapeutic impacts and potential side effects of drugs on tumors. The PDX model provides a more precise representation of individual tumor attributes and drug sensitivities, cementing its role as a crucial instrument in the development and preclinical screening of innovative antitumor drugs. Numerous studies have validated the model's capability to precisely forecast patient drug responses, positioning it as a pivotal tool for clinical drug sensitivity assessment.

Apart from the PDX model, the tumor organoid model stands out as another representation that more accurately mirrors the preclinical drug efficacy [57–60]. Developed through three-dimensional cell culture techniques, this model replicates intricate tumor growth and development processes in vitro. It captures essential features like cell-cell interactions, cell-matrix connections, and angiogenesis, closely mirroring conditions within the human body. In contrast to the conventional 2D cell culture models, tumor organoid models more closely align with in vivo tumor growth and development. These models can be derived from patient-derived tumor cells or established tumor cell lines. The creation process can incorporate various advanced techniques, such as cryopreservation, microfluidics, and bioprinting. The tumor organoid model is an invaluable resource for delving into tumor biology, facilitating drug screening, and advancing personalized medicine. The tumor organoid model has many advantages. Primarily, it closely mirrors the specific characteristics and drug sensitivities of an individual's tumor, paving the way for tailored treatments. Furthermore, it offers deeper insights into the mechanisms underpinning tumor growth and development, enriching our comprehension of tumor biology. Notably, this model presents an ethical alternative, potentially reducing the need for animal testing. However, this model is not without its challenges. Constructing the organoid is intricate, and streamlining the process for high throughput remains a hurdle. Ensuring the sustained growth of organoids demands specialized culture environments, which can escalate costs. Lastly, more rigorous validation is essential to confirm its practical value in cancer therapy.

Overall, each tumor model offers unique strengths and limitations. Their usage should be selective, based on specific research objectives. The choice of model should be tailored to the research goals at hand. While PDX and organoid models are favored for assessing drug sensitivity, cell lines and transgenic animals excel in elucidating molecular mechanisms and target biology.

2.3 Challenges in Clinical Trials

Before a drug can be approved for the market, it must undergo clinical trials. However, the outcome of these clinical trials can be influenced by a myriad of factors [61]. Although a drug might demonstrate potential in preclinical studies, it doesn't always translate to similar efficacy in clinical trials. Challenges like tumor heterogeneity and the lack of reliable biomarkers can hinder a drug's transition into clinical evaluation [62]. A multitude of factors determine whether a drug will prevail in clinical trials.

From a clinical trial design standpoint, patient recruitment emerges as a predominant challenge. The inability to enlist a sufficient number of appropriate patients can thwart the trial's primary objectives. Moreover, challenges like patient dropouts and lost follow-ups during the trial phase can compromise the integrity and reliability of the outcomes. Patient-related factors, such as genotype, lifestyle, diet, and disease severity, can affect the reliability of trial results. Therefore, incorporating a diverse range of patients is essential for results that better represent the larger population. Executing clinical trials is not only a lengthy process but also requires substantial funding. Every phase—from designing the trial, implementation, and data analysis to presenting the results—demands rigorous cost and time management while upholding the quality and credibility of the trial. Furthermore, clinical trials are bound by stringent ethical and regulatory stipulations. This includes aspects like informed consent, maintaining confidentiality, ensuring data security, and more—all of which are vital to safeguarding patient rights and safety. Interpreting and applying the outcomes of clinical trials is intricate, necessitating a thorough analysis of various components, such as trial design, presented data, involved patient demographics, and other pertinent factors. This ensures that the conclusions drawn are both scientifically valid and reliable, ultimately offering valuable insights for clinical practices [63].

Beyond these tangible factors, the crux of many clinical trial failures, especially for new cancer drugs, often hinges on tumor heterogeneity and the absence of reliable efficacy biomarkers before commencing clinical trials [64]. This unpredictability can cast doubt on the therapeutic potential of the drug in question. Hence, it's crucial to delve deep into the research on target mechanisms. A comprehensive understanding of the target's mode of action might enable predictions about which specific patient subgroups might benefit from target inhibitors, thereby bolstering the likelihood of successful clinical trials. Furthermore, besides acquired drug resistance, some patients manifest primary drug resistance. The underlying mechanisms of such primary resistance in tumors might remain elusive, underscoring the intricate nature of tumor biology.

2.4 Antitumor Mechanism and Discovery of Biomarkers

In addition to highlighting the role of a target in promoting tumors, it's equally crucial to understand the molecular mechanism through which the target functions. Presently, the action mechanisms of approved targeted drugs can be grouped into three primary categories: inhibition of tumor-enhancing signaling within cancer cells, halting angiogenesis, and modulating antitumor immune responses. Take, for instance, the frequently employed targeted therapy for lung cancer: anti-EGFR treatment. EGFR, a protein, plays a role in fostering cell growth and division [65]. Overexpression or mutations in EGFR can result in rampant cell growth, leading to cancer initiation. From a mechanical perspective, EGFR gets activated upon binding to its specific ligands, encompassing growth factors like EGF and TGF-α. This binding instigates a cascade of intracellular signaling events, notably the PI3K/Akt and MAPK/ERK pathways, facilitating heightened cell growth and division [66, 67]. Moreover, EGFR signaling is pivotal in angiogenesis, the formation of new blood vessels [68, 69]. This process is critical for the advancement of cancer, providing the necessary nutrients and oxygen for the unchecked growth and division of cancer cells. While apoptosis, a form of programmed cell death, serves as a pivotal system for eliminating harmful or aberrant cells, EGFR signaling can bolster cell survival and impart resistance against apoptosis. This enables cancer cells to sidestep this cell death mechanism. Considering the profound influence of EGFR signaling on these processes, therapies targeting EGFR have demonstrated remarkable efficacy, especially in lung cancer patients where EGFR signaling is hyperactivated. Furthermore, given that EGFR primarily promotes tumor growth via the PI3K/Akt and MAPK/ERK pathways, the secondary activation of these pathways emerges as a resistance mechanism against anti-EGFR treatments [70].

Understanding how a drug inhibits tumor growth is fundamental, offering insights into its interplay with cancer cells and the implicated pathways. Indeed, this is invaluable in designing effective drugs or optimizing the utilization of existing ones. Moreover, discerning the precise drug mechanisms ensures that specific patient populations, most likely to respond positively, are identified. This precision medicine approach promises enhanced therapeutic outcomes [71]. Moreover, many tumors develop resistance to standalone drugs. However, combination drugs with varied action mechanisms can potentially bypass such resistance. The recognition of a drug's antitumor mechanisms empowers researchers to pinpoint synergistic drug combinations that might be more effective against cancer [72, 73]. While some antitumor drugs might present pronounced side effects, understanding their operational mechanisms helps in formulating strategies to either alleviate these unwanted reactions or to pivot to alternative drugs with milder side effects. In essence, probing the mechanisms of antitumor drugs not only offers therapeutic advantages but also deepens our grasp of cancer biology. This, in turn, lights the way to uncovering fresh targets for drug discovery.

The presence of efficient clinical biomarkers has significantly enhanced the efficacy of some drugs, especially those targeting specific mutations. Nonetheless, there's a pressing need for effective biomarkers for certain medications, such as immune checkpoint inhibitors [74, 75]. The discovery and application of efficacy biomarkers hold immense value in oncology. Primarily, these biomarkers can predict patient responses to specific cancer treatments, paving the way for individualized care and shielding patients from unwarranted toxicity and undue expenses. Furthermore, recognizing drug-response-related biomarkers is instrumental in unveiling novel drug targets. This accelerates the drug innovation trajectory, diminishing both the time and financial investment essential for new drug introductions. Leveraging efficacy biomarkers refines optimizing both efficacy and efficiency in gauging treatment responses. For instance, enrolling patients based on particular biomarker profiles amplifies the chances of noting a discernible therapeutic effect and concurrently minimizes the sample size required. As treatment progresses, continuous monitoring through biomarkers offers a more immediate insight into treatment success or early signs of relapse, in comparison to conventional diagnostic tools like imaging. Such timely insights allow for prompt remedial measures, potentially elevating the prognosis for patients. To encapsulate, the hunt for and application of efficacy biomarkers in cancer therapeutics is not just beneficial—it's pivotal. It promises enhanced patient experiences, swift drug innovation, and streamlined clinical trial designs.

References

1. Siegel RL, Miller KD, Fuchs HE, et al. Cancer statistics, 2022. CA Cancer J Clin. 2022;72:7–33.
2. Broderick SR. Adjuvant and neoadjuvant immunotherapy in non-small cell lung cancer. Thorac Surg Clin. 2020;30:215–20.
3. Alexander M, Kim SY, Cheng H. Update 2020: management of non-small cell lung cancer. Lung. 2020;198:897–907.
4. Hendler FJ, Ozanne BW. Human squamous cell lung cancers express increased epidermal growth factor receptors. J Clin Invest. 1984;74:647–51.

5. Fang W, Huang Y, Hong S, et al. EGFR exon 20 insertion mutations and response to osimertinib in non-small-cell lung cancer. BMC Cancer. 2019;19:595.
6. Zhou C, Ramalingam SS, Kim TM, et al. Treatment outcomes and safety of mobocertinib in platinum-pretreated patients with EGFR Exon 20 insertion-positive metastatic non-small cell lung cancer: a phase 1/2 open-label nonrandomized clinical trial. JAMA Oncol. 2021;7:e214761.
7. Siordia-Reyes AG, Ferman-Cano F, Rodriguez-Velasco A. [ALK-1 positive anaplastic large cell lymphoma of the lung. Report of a pediatric case]. Gac Med Mex. 2005;141:531–4.
8. Soda M, Choi YL, Enomoto M, et al. Identification of the transforming EML4-ALK fusion gene in non-small-cell lung cancer. Nature. 2007;448:561–6.
9. Yu ZQ, Wang M, Zhou W, et al. ROS1-positive non-small cell lung cancer (NSCLC): biology, diagnostics, therapeutics and resistance. J Drug Target. 2022;30:845–57.
10. Drilon A, Jenkins C, Iyer S, et al. ROS1-dependent cancers—biology, diagnostics and therapeutics. Nat Rev Clin Oncol. 2021;18:35–55.
11. Drosten M, Barbacid M. Targeting the MAPK pathway in KRAS-driven tumors. Cancer Cell. 2020;37:543–50.
12. McKay IA, Paterson H, Brown R, et al. N-RAS and human cancer. Anticancer Res. 1986;6:483–90.
13. Parikh K, Banna G, Liu SV, et al. Drugging KRAS: current perspectives and state-of-art review. J Hematol Oncol. 2022;15:152.
14. Lavoie H, Therrien M. Regulation of RAF protein kinases in ERK signalling. Nat Rev Mol Cell Biol. 2015;16:281–98.
15. Santarpia L, El-Naggar AK, Cote GJ, et al. Phosphatidylinositol 3-kinase/Akt and Ras/Raf-mitogen-activated protein kinase pathway mutations in anaplastic thyroid cancer. J Clin Endocrinol Metab. 2008;93:278–84.
16. Pachnis V, Durbec P, Taraviras S, et al. III. Role of the RET signal transduction pathway in development of the mammalian enteric nervous system. Am J Phys. 1998;275:G183–6.
17. Cox AD, Der CJ. Ras history: the saga continues. Small GTPases. 2010;1:2–27.
18. Jhiang SM. The RET proto-oncogene in human cancers. Oncogene. 2000;19:5590–7.
19. Ju YS, Lee WC, Shin JY, et al. A transforming KIF5B and RET gene fusion in lung adenocarcinoma revealed from whole-genome and transcriptome sequencing. Genome Res. 2012;22:436–45.
20. Wagner SM, Zhu S, Nicolescu AC, et al. Molecular mechanisms of RET receptor-mediated oncogenesis in multiple endocrine neoplasia 2. Clinics (Sao Paulo). 2012;67(Suppl 1):77–84.
21. Osta BE, Ramalingam SS. RET fusion: joining the ranks of targetable molecular drivers in NSCLC. JTO Clin Res Rep. 2020;1:100050.
22. Sung H, Ferlay J, Siegel RL, et al. Global cancer statistics 2020: GLOBOCAN estimates of incidence and mortality worldwide for 36 cancers in 185 countries. CA Cancer J Clin. 2021;71:209–49.
23. Wang J, Yuan R, Song W, et al. PD-1, PD-L1 (B7-H1) and tumor-site immune modulation therapy: the historical perspective. J Hematol Oncol. 2017;10:34.
24. Carter L, Fouser LA, Jussif J, et al. PD-1:PD-L inhibitory pathway affects both CD4(+) and CD8(+) T cells and is overcome by IL-2. Eur J Immunol. 2002;32:634–43.
25. Tang Q, Chen Y, Li X, et al. The role of PD-1/PD-L1 and application of immune-checkpoint inhibitors in human cancers. Front Immunol. 2022;13:964442.
26. Carpenter G, King L Jr, Cohen S. Epidermal growth factor stimulates phosphorylation in membrane preparations in vitro. Nature. 1978;276:409–10.
27. Voldborg BR, Damstrup L, Spang-Thomsen M, et al. Epidermal growth factor receptor (EGFR) and EGFR mutations, function and possible role in clinical trials. Ann Oncol. 1997;8:1197–206.
28. Roskoski R Jr. Small molecule inhibitors targeting the EGFR/ErbB family of protein-tyrosine kinases in human cancers. Pharmacol Res. 2019;139:395–411.
29. da Cunha SG, Shepherd FA, Tsao MS. EGFR mutations and lung cancer. Annu Rev Pathol. 2011;6:49–69.

30. Schneider JL, Lin JJ, Shaw AT. ALK-positive lung cancer: a moving target. Nat Cancer. 2023;4:330–43.
31. Remon J, Pignataro D, Novello S, et al. Current treatment and future challenges in ROS1- and ALK-rearranged advanced non-small cell lung cancer. Cancer Treat Rev. 2021;95:102178.
32. Camidge DR, Doebele RC. Treating ALK-positive lung cancer—early successes and future challenges. Nat Rev Clin Oncol. 2012;9:268–77.
33. Tan AC, Tan DSW. Targeted therapies for lung cancer patients with oncogenic driver molecular alterations. J Clin Oncol. 2022;40:611–25.
34. Sammut SJ, Crispin-Ortuzar M, Chin SF, et al. Multi-omic machine learning predictor of breast cancer therapy response. Nature. 2022;601:623–9.
35. Gong Y, Ji P, Yang YS, et al. Metabolic-pathway-based subtyping of triple-negative breast cancer reveals potential therapeutic targets. Cell Metab. 2021;33:51–64 e9.
36. Chen K, Bai J, Reuben A, et al. Multiomics analysis reveals distinct immunogenomic features of lung cancer with ground-glass opacity. Am J Respir Crit Care Med. 2021;204:1180–92.
37. Foster DS, Januszyk M, Delitto D, et al. Multiomic analysis reveals conservation of cancer-associated fibroblast phenotypes across species and tissue of origin. Cancer Cell. 2022;40:1392–1406 e7.
38. Hicks MA, Hou CYC, Iranmehr A, et al. Target discovery using biobanks and human genetics. Drug Discov Today. 2020;25:438–45.
39. Huang A, Garraway LA, Ashworth A, et al. Synthetic lethality as an engine for cancer drug target discovery. Nat Rev Drug Discov. 2020;19:23–38.
40. Zhou Y, Zhang Y, Lian X, et al. Therapeutic target database update 2022: facilitating drug discovery with enriched comparative data of targeted agents. Nucleic Acids Res. 2022;50:D1398–407.
41. Wang M, Wang Z, Sun H, et al. Deep learning approaches for de novo drug design: an overview. Curr Opin Struct Biol. 2022;72:135–44.
42. Xie W, Wang F, Li Y, et al. Advances and challenges in de novo drug design using three-dimensional deep generative models. J Chem Inf Model. 2022;62:2269–79.
43. Zhou SF, Zhong WZ. Drug design and discovery: principles and applications. Molecules. 2017;22:279.
44. Dumont J, Euwart D, Mei B, et al. Human cell lines for biopharmaceutical manufacturing: history, status, and future perspectives. Crit Rev Biotechnol. 2016;36:1110–22.
45. Gazdar AF, Gao B, Minna JD. Lung cancer cell lines: useless artifacts or invaluable tools for medical science? Lung Cancer. 2010;68:309–18.
46. Wang SW, Gao C, Zheng YM, et al. Current applications and future perspective of CRISPR/Cas9 gene editing in cancer. Mol Cancer. 2022;21:57.
47. Chan YT, Lu Y, Wu J, et al. CRISPR-Cas9 library screening approach for anti-cancer drug discovery: overview and perspectives. Theranostics. 2022;12:3329–44.
48. Rebecca VW, Somasundaram R, Herlyn M. Pre-clinical modeling of cutaneous melanoma. Nat Commun. 2020;11:2858.
49. Rudin CM, Poirier JT, Byers LA, et al. Molecular subtypes of small cell lung cancer: a synthesis of human and mouse model data. Nat Rev Cancer. 2019;19:289–97.
50. Zitvogel L, Pitt JM, Daillere R, et al. Mouse models in oncoimmunology. Nat Rev Cancer. 2016;16:759–73.
51. Cheon DJ, Orsulic S. Mouse models of cancer. Annu Rev Pathol. 2011;6:95–119.
52. Sander JD, Joung JK. CRISPR-Cas systems for editing, regulating and targeting genomes. Nat Biotechnol. 2014;32:347–55.
53. Kos CH. Cre/loxP system for generating tissue-specific knockout mouse models. Nutr Rev. 2004;62:243–6.
54. Yoshida GJ. Applications of patient-derived tumor xenograft models and tumor organoids. J Hematol Oncol. 2020;13:4.
55. Hidalgo M, Amant F, Biankin AV, et al. Patient-derived xenograft models: an emerging platform for translational cancer research. Cancer Discov. 2014;4:998–1013.

56. Shi J, Li Y, Jia R, et al. The fidelity of cancer cells in PDX models: characteristics, mechanism and clinical significance. Int J Cancer. 2020;146:2078–88.
57. Sun CP, Lan HR, Fang XL, et al. Organoid models for precision cancer immunotherapy. Front Immunol. 2022;13:770465.
58. Semertzidou A, Brosens JJ, McNeish I, et al. Organoid models in gynaecological oncology research. Cancer Treat Rev. 2020;90:102103.
59. Yang L, Yang S, Li X, et al. Tumor organoids: from inception to future in cancer research. Cancer Lett. 2019;454:120–33.
60. Weeber F, Ooft SN, Dijkstra KK, et al. Tumor organoids as a pre-clinical cancer model for drug discovery. Cell Chem Biol. 2017;24:1092–100.
61. Bhatt DL, Mehta C. Adaptive designs for clinical trials. N Engl J Med. 2016;375:65–74.
62. Le-Rademacher J, Dahlberg S, Lee JJ, et al. Biomarker clinical trials in lung cancer: design, logistics, challenges, and practical considerations. J Thorac Oncol. 2018;13:1625–37.
63. Verweij J, Hendriks HR, Zwierzina H, et al. Innovation in oncology clinical trial design. Cancer Treat Rev. 2019;74:15–20.
64. Liu Y, deSouza NM, Shankar LK, et al. A risk management approach for imaging biomarker-driven clinical trials in oncology. Lancet Oncol. 2015;16:e622–8.
65. Levantini E, Maroni G, Del Re M, et al. EGFR signaling pathway as therapeutic target in human cancers. Semin Cancer Biol. 2022;85:253–75.
66. Tomas A, Futter CE, Eden ER. EGF receptor trafficking: consequences for signaling and cancer. Trends Cell Biol. 2014;24:26–34.
67. Zaryouh H, De Pauw I, Baysal H, et al. Recent insights in the PI3K/Akt pathway as a promising therapeutic target in combination with EGFR-targeting agents to treat head and neck squamous cell carcinoma. Med Res Rev. 2022;42:112–55.
68. Le X, Nilsson M, Goldman J, et al. Dual EGFR-VEGF pathway inhibition: a promising strategy for patients with EGFR-mutant NSCLC. J Thorac Oncol. 2021;16:205–15.
69. Cascone T, Herynk MH, Xu L, et al. Upregulated stromal EGFR and vascular remodeling in mouse xenograft models of angiogenesis inhibitor-resistant human lung adenocarcinoma. J Clin Invest. 2011;121:1313–28.
70. Wu SG, Shih JY. Management of acquired resistance to EGFR TKI-targeted therapy in advanced non-small cell lung cancer. Mol Cancer. 2018;17:38.
71. Wheeler DL, Dunn EF, Harari PM. Understanding resistance to EGFR inhibitors-impact on future treatment strategies. Nat Rev Clin Oncol. 2010;7:493–507.
72. Palmer AC, Sorger PK. Combination cancer therapy can confer benefit via patient-to-patient variability without drug additivity or synergy. Cell. 2017;171:1678–91.
73. Wang L, Wang H, Song D, et al. New strategies for targeting drug combinations to overcome mutation-driven drug resistance. Semin Cancer Biol. 2017;42:44–51.
74. Park S, Ock CY, Kim H, et al. Artificial intelligence-powered spatial analysis of tumor-infiltrating lymphocytes as complementary biomarker for immune checkpoint inhibition in non-small-cell lung cancer. J Clin Oncol. 2022;40:1916–28.
75. Jardim DL, Goodman A, de Melo GD, et al. The challenges of tumor mutational burden as an immunotherapy biomarker. Cancer Cell. 2021;39:154–73.

Chapter 3
Preclinical and Translational Study Design

Liang Zeng, Xing Zhang, and Hongzhi Ma

Abstract The urgent need for new antitumor medications, driven by high cancer mortality rates and limited success of current treatments, necessitates a robust drug development process divided into preclinical and clinical phases. Preclinical research, fundamental in this process, involves pharmaceutical studies, drug formulation, and extensive pharmacological and toxicological analyses to establish safety and effective dosing. Guided by regulatory frameworks like those from the National Medical Products Administration and the International Council for Harmonisation, these studies are crucial for transitioning to clinical trials. Preclinical evaluation determines a drug's safety profile, including safe starting doses and target organ identification, with an emphasis on quality and adaptability to novel drug properties. The outcomes of preclinical research significantly influence the design of clinical trials, with accurate documentation being vital for regulatory approval. This intricate blend of preclinical and clinical studies, aligned with global standards, is essential for developing effective antitumor medications.

Keywords Preclinical study · Clinical evaluation · Antitumor medication

The escalating mortality rates and limited success of current therapeutic strategies underscore the pressing need for the development of new and more effective antitumor medications. The process of drug development is bifurcated into preclinical and clinical research phases. The preclinical stage encompasses pharmaceutical

L. Zeng (✉) · H. Ma
Hunan Cancer Hospital, The Affiliated Cancer Hospital of Xiangya School of Medicine, Central South University, Changsha, China
e-mail: zengliang@hnca.org.cn

Department of Medical Oncology, Lung Cancer and Gastrointestinal Unit, Changsha, China
e-mail: mahongzhi@hnca.org.cn

X. Zhang
Department of Medical Oncology, Lung Cancer and Gastrointestinal Unit, University of South China, Changsha, China

© The Author(s), under exclusive license to Springer Nature Singapore Pte Ltd. 2024

Y. Zhang, N. Yang (eds.), *New Anti-cancer Drug Development and Evaluation*,
https://doi.org/10.1007/978-981-97-7274-2_3

studies, drug formulation strategies, and comprehensive pharmacological and toxicological analyses. The clinical research phase comprises phase I, II, and III clinical trials, followed by post-marketing surveillance (phase IV). It's worth noting that preclinical studies play a pivotal role in paving the way for the clinical trials of antitumor agents (Fig. 3.1). However, the design and execution guidelines for these trials vary across different global jurisdictions [1–3].

In China, the nonclinical evaluation of pharmaceuticals is steered by guidelines from the National Medical Products Administration (NMPA). The guidelines provided by the International Council for Harmonisation (ICH) of Technical Requirements for Pharmaceuticals for Human Use serve as an instrumental reference. The ICH stands as a global entity, championing the formulation and advocacy of standards for the life cycle of pharmaceutical products. Its overarching mission is to unify technical requirements for the registration of pharmaceutical products across diverse regions, thereby catalyzing global drug development and ensuring patients have access to top-tier medications [2, 4–6].

Preclinical evaluation is a cornerstone in drug development, aiming to delineate a drug's pharmacological and toxicological profiles, which includes determining a safe starting dose and identifying target organs. Adherence to quality practices in preclinical safety studies is pivotal. Yet, traditional preclinical trial protocols might require modifications to cater to novel properties or specificities associated with the drug or its intended population.

During the research and development (R&D) process, alterations in the production process might present. Nonetheless, the active ingredients used in preclinical studies must be clearly defined in terms of their characteristics and should accurately represent those intended for use in clinical trials. The outcomes of preclinical results influence the design of clinical trials. Therefore, it's imperative to present these findings with precision to regulatory authorities to support drug approval [7].

The journey to develop innovative and effective antitumor medications involves an intricate blend of both preclinical and clinical studies [8]. Regulatory guidelines set forth by entities such as the ICH are instrumental in ensuring the safety and efficacy of these new drugs. Preclinical assessments are pivotal in mapping out the drug's pharmacological and toxicological attributes, and their results act as a foundation for clinical trial designs. Accurate documentation and presentation of preclinical findings are essential for obtaining drug authorization.

3.1 Preclinical Evaluation

Preclinical evaluation is fundamental in the drug development process. This preliminary phase involves studies to understand the drug's mechanism of action, dosage dependence, and antitumor efficacy. Typically conducted before phase I clinical trials, it is vital to ascertain the drug's safety and effectiveness prior to its introduction to human subjects [2, 6, 9].

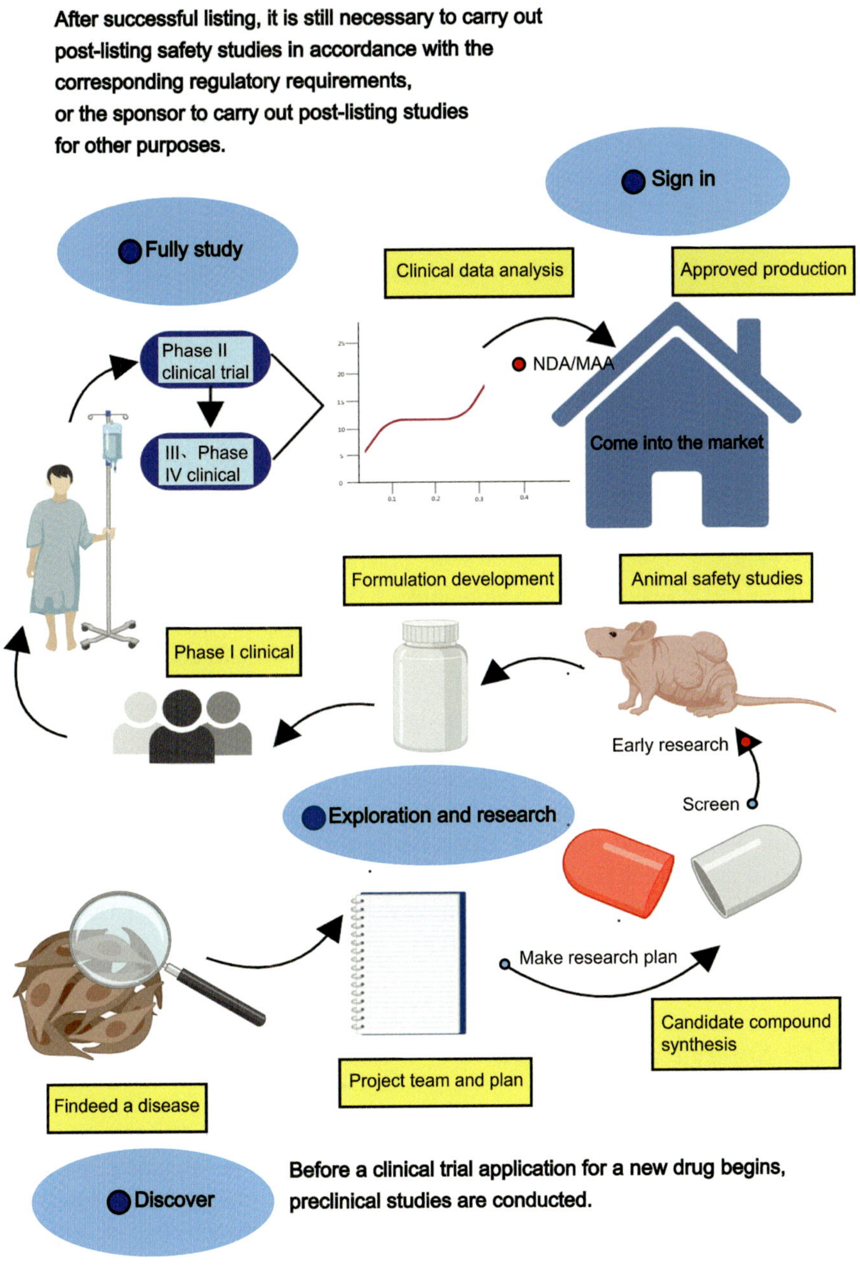

Fig. 3.1 Procedure for drug evaluation

In preclinical evaluation, the initial step is choosing suitable models based on the drug's target and mechanism of action. Although it's not mandatory to use the exact tumor types assessed in clinical trials, selecting models that closely replicate the clinical scenarios faced by cancer patients is vital. This method not only reduces developmental risks but also furnishes nonclinical evidence concerning the drug's mode of action. Nonetheless, it's crucial to note that current preclinical efficacy studies for anticancer drugs don't always precisely forecast the clinical efficacy of the substance under examination. This discrepancy stems from the constraints in research methodologies and the intricate dynamics of cancer biology. Consequently, efficacy studies should prioritize understanding mechanisms of action. Additionally, the selected models ought to closely mirror real-world clinical scenarios faced by cancer patients to mitigate developmental risks.

An essential facet of preclinical evaluation is determining the appropriate dosing schedules and devising a dose escalation plan [3, 10]. This is pivotal for structuring clinical trials and safeguarding human participants. Moreover, preclinical studies aid in selecting suitable biomarkers to track drug response and, when necessary, validate the logic behind drug combinations.

Choosing the right animal species for preclinical evaluation is of paramount importance and demands meticulous scrutiny. It is crucial to ensure that the selected animal models closely mirror the human demographic in question. Such an approach bolsters the relevance of preclinical study outcomes to humans and provides an in-depth grasp of the drug's associated risks.

Therefore, preclinical evaluation aimed at understanding the drug's mechanism of action, dosage requirements, and antitumor potential. While preclinical efficacy studies for anticancer drugs may not always accurately forecast clinical outcomes, they provide invaluable guidance on dosing schedules, dose escalation strategies, biomarker choices, and the logic behind drug combinations. Through judicious selection of appropriate models, test animal species, and study methodologies, preclinical evaluation can substantially diminish developmental risks, ensuring the safety and effectiveness of anticancer drugs.

3.1.1 Safety Pharmacology

Safety pharmacology is an integral part of drug development, centered on assessing a drug's impact on crucial organ functions, including the cardiovascular, respiratory, and central nervous systems. Prior to initiating clinical trials, gathering data on these organ systems is imperative to confirm the drug's safety and effectiveness [10, 11]. General toxicology testing is a prevalent method used to assess organ functions. This approach evaluates the impact of a drug on multiple organs in animals prior to human clinical trials. This testing helps to identify potential safety concerns and determine the appropriate dosage and administration methods [11, 12]. Detailed clinical symptom observations coupled with relevant electrocardiogram (ECG) assessments are typically deemed adequate for evaluating organ functions in non-rodents. Such observations are pivotal in pinpointing potential adverse reactions, thereby providing critical insights into the drug's safety landscape [13]. While standalone safety pharmacology studies aren't always requisite for clinical trials with patients bearing advanced tumors, there are scenarios where supplementary safety evaluations become essential to ascertain the drug's overall safety and efficacy [12, 14].

In essence, safety pharmacology strives to guarantee the safety and efficacy of drugs intended for human administration. By assessing crucial organ functions and pinpointing potential safety hazards, it plays a pivotal role in reducing risks and enhancing patient results. It is an integral component of the drug development process, providing valuable insights that contribute to the overall safety profile of the drug and its suitability for human use.

3.1.2 Pharmacokinetics

Pharmacokinetics plays a pivotal role in discerning how drugs interact within living organisms. Pharmacokinetics sheds light on the absorption, distribution, metabolism, and expulsion of drugs from the body. By leveraging nonclinical studies in animals, we can glean valuable insights into the pharmacokinetics parameters. This, in turn, facilitates the structuring of clinical trials and the determination of doses that are both safe and efficacious [15].

A pivotal pharmacokinetic parameter is the peak blood concentration, denoting the apex of a drug's concentration in the bloodstream post-administration. This metric is instrumental in determining both the maximum tolerated dose (MTD) and the ideal dosing interval. Another crucial parameter is the area under the curve, or AUC, which encapsulates the drug's total exposure to the body over a given period. The AUC assists in pinpointing the apt dose for specific patient groups and in gauging the drug's duration of action. The half-life is another key pharmacokinetic parameter, denoting the time it takes for half of the drug to be cleared from the body. This metric offers insights into the drug's duration of action, dosing intervals, and the likelihood of drug build-up in the body over prolonged periods [16].

Though nonclinical studies offer significant insights into pharmacokinetic parameters, it's crucial to supplement this data with parallel studies during clinical trials. These trials yield information on the absorption, distribution, metabolism, and elimination of drugs specific to humans, which can differ from animal models. Furthermore, clinical trials are pivotal in detecting any potential safety issues or adverse reactions associated with drug administration in humans [17]. Overall, assessing pharmacokinetic parameters through animal studies assists in choosing safe doses, determining dosing intervals, and gauging drug action duration. Yet, it remains essential to complement this with parallel studies in clinical trials for a more holistic understanding of drug pharmacokinetics in humans.

3.1.3 General Toxicology

Phase I clinical trials often serve as the inaugural stage in assessing a new drug's safety and tolerability in humans, particularly for patients with advanced cancer. The primary aim of phase I trials is to ascertain the drug's MTD and its dose-limiting toxicity (DLT). Evaluating toxicity is pivotal when gauging the safety of a new drug, with the dosing regimen playing a substantial role in its effects [18].

Toxicity testing for anticancer drugs often aims to identify the no-observed-adverse-effect level (NOAEL) or the no-observed-effect level (NOEL)—doses at which adverse reactions aren't evident. Yet, such testing isn't invariably required to endorse the clinical use of anticancer medications. For pinpointing and managing potential toxicities, it's crucial to review toxicology studies that utilize dosing regimens mirroring those in clinical settings [19].

Evaluating the potential for toxicity recovery is vital to ascertain if severe adverse effects are reversible. When serious toxicities emerge at or close to the clinical exposure level, and predicting recovery becomes challenging via scientific evaluation, general toxicology studies should incorporate a recovery phase at their end. If a study demands a recovery period, its results should precede the clinical study. Complete recovery is typically not deemed mandator [20].

For small-molecule drugs, general toxicology studies typically include tests on both rodents and non-rodent animals. Such testing is vital for evaluating toxicity potential and setting the correct dose range for clinical trials. Depending on the issue at hand, alternative test methodologies might be fitting in specific instances. For instance, drugs with genetic toxicity aimed at swiftly dividing cells might necessitate repeat-dose toxicity testing in a single rodent species. This could be deemed adequate if the species in question is pertinent [21].

In summary, toxicity testing is pivotal in assessing the safety and tolerability of novel drugs for human use, particularly for patients with advanced cancer. Phase I clinical trials play a key role in establishing the drug's MTD and DLT. It's essential for toxicology studies to mirror clinical dosing regimens, gauge the potential for toxicity recovery, and employ alternative testing methods when suitable. The overarching objective remains to confirm that new drugs are safe and effective for humans.

3.1.4 Reproductive Toxicity

Testing for embryonal-fetal toxicity in antineoplastic drugs should be completed before marketing. However, it isn't a prerequisite for clinical trials in patients with advanced cancer. Developmental toxicity tests are also not mandated at the marketing stage for agents that show genotoxicity, target rapidly dividing cells (like crypt cells and bone marrow) during general toxicology assessments, or belong to drug classes known to cause developmental toxicity. Likewise, testing for fertility and early embryonic developmental toxicity, and typically, perinatal toxicity, isn't required either for clinical trials or marketing when the drugs are intended for patients with advanced tumors.

3.1.5 Genetic Toxicity

Genotoxicity studies are not required to support clinical trials for drugs in patients with advanced cancer. However, genotoxicity testing should be undertaken to support marketing efforts. Biologic drugs should follow the principles outlined in ICH S6. If in vitro test results prove positive, then in vivo testing might be deemed unnecessary.

3.1.6 Carcinogenicity

The ICH S1A guidelines outline the relevance of carcinogenicity evaluation for antineoplastic agents. Generally, carcinogenicity testing is not considered necessary for agents that are marketed to treat patients with advanced cancer.

3.1.7 Immunotoxicity

For the majority of antineoplastic drugs, the content outlined in a general toxicology trial is sufficient to evaluate immunotoxic potential and to support marketing. However, for immunomodulatory drugs, the trial design might incorporate additional end points, such as immunophenotyping via flow cytometry.

3.1.8 Light Safety

Before initiating phase I clinical trials, an initial evaluation of the drug's phototoxic potential should be conducted, taking into account its photochemical properties and data from other drugs within the same chemical class. If these data indicate potential risks, suitable precautions must be established for outpatient trials. When the light safety risk isn't conclusively determined from nonclinical data or clinical experiences, a light safety evaluation aligned with the principles laid out in ICH M3 should be presented before the drug's marketing.

3.2 Nonclinical Data Supporting Clinical Trial Design and Marketing

3.2.1 Determining the Initial Dose of Medication for Humans

The primary objective when selecting a starting dose is to identify a dose anticipated to produce a pharmacological effect while maintaining an acceptable safety profile. This starting dose must be rooted in rigorous scientific rationale, drawing from all pertinent nonclinical data, including pharmacokinetics, pharmacodynamics, and toxicity evaluations. The dose selection should be informed by various methodologies. For the majority of small-molecule drugs delivered systemically, converting animal doses to human equivalents should, in most cases, rely on a standardized method that considers human surface area. For both small molecules and biologic drugs, it is feasible to perform interspecies conversion utilizing body weight, AUC, or other exposure metrics. Notably, when dealing with biologic drugs exhibiting immunoagonist properties, the choice of starting dose should take the lowest expected biological effect level into consideration.

3.2.2 Dose Escalation and Maximum Dose in Clinical Trials

Typically, the dose escalation or the highest dose examined in clinical trials for cancer patients shouldn't be confined by the maximum dose or exposure observed in nonclinical studies. However, if severe toxicity emerges in nonclinical toxicology studies, especially with pronounced dose-response or exposure-response curves, or if there's an absence of early indicators of severe toxicity, it might be prudent to consider smaller increments for dose escalation. Instead of the usual multiplicative increases, fractional multiples might be more appropriate.

3.2.3 Toxicological Study Duration and Protocol to Support Early Clinical Trials

In phase I clinical trials, treatment continuation may be based on the patient's response. If this is the case, a subsequent toxicity trial with a longer administration period than the previously completed trial isn't necessary to support prolonged clinical treatment. Given the potential for varied dosing regimens in early clinical trials, selecting the right nonclinical study design becomes essential. While toxicity studies may not always align precisely with clinical protocols, the information they provide should adequately support clinical doses, methodologies, and the identification of potential toxicities.

Table 3.1 Commonly used nonclinical trial dosing regimens

Clinical schedule	Example of nonclinical treatment schedule
Once every 3–4 weeks	Single dose
Daily for 5 days every 3 weeks	Daily for 5 days
Daily for 5–7 days, alternating weeks	Daily for 5–7 days, alternating weeks (two-dose cycles)
Once a week for 3 weeks, 1 week off	Once a week for 3 weeks
Two or three times a week	Two or three times a week for 4 weeks
Daily	Daily for 4 weeks
Weekly	Once a week for 4–5 doses

Table 3.1 presents commonly used nonclinical trial dosing regimens for antineoplastic drugs, applicable to both small-molecule and biologic drugs. If existing toxicity data doesn't justify adjustments to clinical dosing regimens, further toxicological testing in just one animal species is typically adequate.

3.2.4 Duration of Toxicological Studies to Support Subsequent Clinical Trials and Marketing

Nonclinical data and phase I results that support phase I clinical trials are adequate to support phase II clinical trials and to back second- or first-line treatments for patients with advanced tumors. Before the commencement of phase III trials for the further development of antineoplastic agents intended for patients with advanced tumors, results from repeated administration toxicity tests, which align with the clinical development protocol, should be available. For the majority of drugs designed for patients with advanced tumors, a 3-month nonclinical toxicity trial is typically sufficient to support their marketing.

3.2.5 Combined Use of Drugs

Drugs intended for combined use should undergo thorough individual toxicological evaluations. Before embarking on clinical studies, it's essential to provide data supporting the rationale behind the combination. Typically, a safety toxicology study of a combination drug designed for patients with advanced cancer is not required. If a drug's human toxicity profile is well-established, conducting nonclinical studies for drug combinations is usually deemed unnecessary. However, when it comes to combination studies involving compounds in the early stages of development, where the human toxicity profile remains uncharacterized, a pharmacological study validating the combination becomes crucial. This study should evidence an enhancement in activity without a marked increase in toxicity, focusing on limited safety endpoints like mortality, clinical symptoms, and body weight changes. The decision on the need for a toxicology study of the combination should hinge on the information available.

3.2.6 *Support Nonclinical Studies in Pediatric Populations*

A typical approach for most antineoplastic drug studies targeting pediatric patients is to first ascertain a reasonably safe dose in adults, and then to administer a proportionately reduced dose in an initial pediatric clinical trial. Recommendations for nonclinical trials delineated in this guideline are also pertinent to the pediatric population. Generally, studies involving young animals aren't conducted to justify including pediatric oncology patients in cancer treatment trials. Only consider studies on young animals if the human safety data and extant animal test data aren't deemed adequate to back the safety evaluation in children within the relevant age bracket.

3.2.7 *Binding Drugs*

Binding drugs refer to those that covalently attach to carrier molecules like proteins, lipids, or sugars. The safety of the resulting compound is of paramount concern. For components that aren't bonded, such as linkers, the safety assessments might be more restricted. Nonetheless, it's crucial to furnish details concerning the stability of the binding drug in the plasma of test animals, across different species, and in humans. Toxicokinetics necessitates the evaluation of both the conjugated and the free compounds post-administration.

3.2.7.1 Antibody Drug Conjugate (ADC)

The concept of ADCs dates back a long time. As early as 1913, Professor Paul Ehrlich, the father of chemotherapy and a Nobel Prize laureate, introduced the idea of the "magic bullet." This involved tethering cytotoxic drugs to specific monoclonal antibodies, thereby enabling targeted destruction of tumor cells. Modern ADC drugs on the market are grounded in this principle. They connect cytotoxic drugs to monoclonal antibodies, utilizing these antibodies as carriers to efficiently deliver the cytotoxic agents to target tumor cells in a precise manner.

ADCs are typically composed of three primary components: antibodies, linkers, and cytotoxic small molecules. Once introduced into the bloodstream, the antibody component of the ADC identifies and binds to tumor cells exhibiting high levels of specific surface antigens. Upon binding, the tumor cells internalize the ADC-antigen complex through endocytosis. Within the lysosome of the cell, this complex is broken down, releasing the cytotoxic payload. This payload then acts either by damaging the DNA or by disrupting the tumor cell's division process, consequently leading to the cell's demise.

The inaugural attempt to develop ADC drugs dates back to 1958 when researchers combined anti-mouse leukocyte immunoglobulin with methotrexate in hopes of treating leukemia. The first ADC drug to achieve market approval was Mylotarg, greenlit by the FDA in 2000 as a treatment for acute myeloid leukemia (AML). However, concerns over severe and, in some cases, fatal liver damage combined with an unclear survival benefit led to its withdrawal from the market [22]. Key limitations of these first-generation ADCs included the use of antibodies derived from mice, the employment of non-cleavable linkers, suboptimal cytotoxins, and targeting antigens with low expression.

The second-generation of ADC drugs was ushered in with the approval of trastuzumab emtansine, which was specifically developed for targeting breast cancer [23, 24]. Brentuximab vedotin emerged as a standout in the treatment of hematologic malignancies, notably in its use for treating classical Hodgkin's lymphoma and anaplastic large-cell lymphoma [25]. These second-generation ADCs offered multiple benefits like a broader scope in target antigen development, the use of humanized antibodies, and the integration of cleavable linker technology. However, they also had shortcomings, such as inconsistent drug loading rates, a limited therapeutic range, and diminished efficacy. The third-generation of ADCs is epitomized by enfortumab vedotin. This ADC specifically targets solid tumors and caters to patients who haven't responded to PD-1/PD-L1 antibody treatments. The advantages accompanying this generation encompass site-specific conjugation technology involving small molecules and monoclonal antibodies, the inception of bispecific antibodies, and enhanced specificity achieved through nucleic acid splice inhibitors [26]. Nevertheless, challenges persist, including the complexity of replicating conjugation technology and a resistance to microtubule inhibitors.

By the end of 2022, the FDA had given its approval to 13 ADC drugs, with a notable 10 of these approvals granted post-2017. Phase III clinical trials primarily targeted HER2, Trop2, and BCMA, encompassing a variety of cancers, including breast, gastric, lung, and multiple myeloma. In China, six ADC drugs had received approval and entered the market. The standout moment of 2022 was the approval of T-DXd (DS-8201), which revolutionized the treatment approach for HER2+ advanced breast cancer. This was based on the significant findings from the DESTINY-Breast03 and DESTINY-Breast04 studies. On February 21, 2023, T-DXd secured approval from China's NMPA [27]. Previously, in June 2021, China celebrated the approval of its first indigenous antibody-conjugated drug: vadastuximab monotherapy. This drug is indicated for HER2+ locally advanced or metastatic gastric cancer (including gastroesophageal junction adenocarcinoma) patients who have previously undergone at least two systemic chemotherapy regimens. Vadastuximab's approval marked the end of the absence of original domestic ADC drugs in the arena and filled a global treatment gap for HER2+ gastric cancer patients. This achievement represents a significant milestone in the evolution of China's biopharmaceutical innovation. Till now, more than 170 ADC investigational drugs were being developed by domestic manufacturers in China. However, apart from vadastuximab monotherapy, none have successfully gained approval yet.

3.3 Preclinical Study Results of Vedolizumab Monoclonal Antibody

Pharmacological action: Vedolizumab monoclonal antibody is a novel antibody-drug conjugate targeting HER2. It comprises a recombinant humanized HER2 IgG1 monoclonal antibody linked to the microtubule inhibitor monomethyl auristatin E (MMAE) via a linker. Upon binding of the antibody portion of vedolizumab to the extracellular domain of HER2 on the cell surface, the complex is internalized and shuttled to lysosomes. Here, the linker undergoes cleavage, releasing MMAE. This inhibitor disrupts the intracellular microtubule network, inducing cell cycle arrest and apoptosis in mitotic cells. Moreover, in vitro studies indicate that vedolizumab can suppress HER2 receptor signaling and demonstrate antibody-dependent cellular cytotoxicity (ADCC) [28, 29].

Genotoxicity: The microtubule inhibitor MMAE serves as the small-molecule component of the vedolizumab monoclonal antibody. In vitro assessments, including the Ames test and the L5178Y mouse lymphoma mutation assay, demonstrated negative results for MMAE, indicating it lacks mutagenic potential. However, the in vivo rat bone marrow micronucleus assay yielded a positive outcome, suggesting that MMAE possesses genotoxic activity [30, 31].

Reproductive toxicity: Fertility and embryo-fetal development studies have not been conducted for vedolizumab. However, in a 12-week repeated dose toxicity study involving rats, vedolizumab monoclonal antibody was administered every 2 weeks via intravenous injection. At doses of ≥6 mg/kg, both testicular and epididymal atrophy were observed, and no full recovery was noted even after a 6-week recovery period. Furthermore, literature on ADCs with MMAE as the small-molecule component revealed embryo-fetal toxicity in pregnant rats administered with CD30-MMAE. This toxicity manifested as increased early resorptions, post-implantation losses, and external malformations, specifically umbilical hernia and hindlimb deformity [32]. There have been no studies conducted on the carcinogenicity of vedolizumab or MMAE [33].

3.3.1 Immune Checkpoint Inhibitors

Immune checkpoint inhibitors (ICIs) are cancer immunotherapies designed to bolster anticancer immune responses by targeting immunologic receptors on the surface of T-lymphocytes. ICIs emerged as a groundbreaking treatment option in 2011 with the approval of ipilimumab, transforming the landscape of cancer therapy.

These drugs have the potential to produce durable responses with, in some cases, a more favorable toxicity profile compared to traditional treatments. Unlike conventional therapeutic strategies, ICIs act by rejuvenating the host's immune system to combat tumor cells. Immune checkpoints help maintain a balance between pro-inflammatory and anti-inflammatory signals under normal conditions. These checkpoints encompass both inhibitory and stimulatory pathways that modulate immune cell function. In the past decade, antibodies targeting immune inhibitory receptors, such as CTLA-4, PD-1, and PD-L1, have been the predominant immunotherapeutic agents. However, several antibodies and small molecules aimed at various immune checkpoint proteins, including B7H3, CD39, CD73, the adenosine A2A receptor, and CD47, are currently under clinical investigation. Recent research has identified additional potential immune checkpoint targets, such as lymphocyte activation gene-3 (LAG-3), T-cell immunoglobulin and mucin-domain containing-3 (TIM-3), and T-cell immunoglobulin and ITIM domain (TIGIT). In this era of tumor immunotherapy, Chinese pharmaceutical companies have rapidly advanced their efforts, conducting numerous studies on different mechanisms of immune checkpoint inhibition, yielding many promising preclinical and clinical results.

3.3.1.1 PD-1/PD-L1 Inhibitors

PD-1 is an inhibitory receptor that plays a pivotal role in programmed death signaling, regulating T-cell-mediated responses. When engaged, PD-1 can suppress cytokine secretion, including IL-2, IFN-γ, and TNF-α, by disrupting the CD28-costimulatory signaling pathway. PD-1 expression has been identified on various immune cells within the tumor microenvironment (TME), such as activated monocytes, dendritic cells (DCs), natural killer (NK) cells, T cells, and even B cells. PD-1 has two primary ligands: PD-L1 and PD-L2. Both tumor cells and immune cells can express PD-L1, which serves as a valuable biomarker for predicting responses to anti-PD-1/PD-L1 antibodies in certain cancer patients. PD-L1, also referred to as B7-H1 or CD274, contributes to the inhibition of the cancer-immunity cycle by binding to negative regulators of T-cell activation, namely, PD-1 and B7.1 (CD80). Consequently, PD-L1 engagement is known to inhibit the migration and proliferation of T cells, ultimately reducing tumor cell destruction.

At present, China has approved 13 PD-1/PD-L1 drugs, comprising 9 PD-1 inhibitors (7 domestic and 2 imported) and 4 PD-L1 inhibitors (2 domestic and 2 imported). Among these, camrelizumab boasts approvals for eight indications, spanning five major types of malignant tumors, making it the domestic PD-1 product with the most approved indications and the broadest tumor coverage. Toripalimab is the world's pioneering immune checkpoint inhibitor sanctioned for nasopharyngeal carcinoma treatment, marking a significant milestone in this field. Envafolimab is China's premier self-developed PD-L1 antibody and the world's first PD-L1 drug capable of subcutaneous injection, deliverable in just 30 s. The objective response rates of tislelizumab in melanoma and sintilizumab in Hodgkin's lymphoma have been outstanding. Beyond the approved PD-1/PD-L1 inhibitors, over 20 PD-1/

PD-L1 monoclonal antibodies are in development in China. These include Penpulimab (Akeso Biopharma), HLX-10 (Shanghai Henlius Biotech, Inc.), CS1003 (Siqi Pharmaceutical), cemiplimab (Sanofi), and many others.

Nevertheless, the response rate for single-agent PD-1 treatment averages between 10% and 20%. Some patients don't achieve optimal response durations, while others discontinue therapy due to immune-related adverse events (irAEs). Given these challenges, numerous pharmaceutical companies are keen on exploring combination therapies.

AK112, developed entirely by Akeso Biopharma, is the world's first PD-1/VEGF bispecific antibody drug. It not only inhibits PD-1-mediated immunosuppression but also blocks angiogenesis in the TME. The tetravalent structure of AK112 enables it to form a large complex with dimeric VEGF, thereby enhancing its affinity and functional activity toward PD-1. This results in potent antitumor effects, as observed in preclinical studies. It has been revealed that AK112 could bind to human VEGF and PD-1 with affinities comparable to or better than bevacizumab and nivolumab, respectively. Size-exclusion high-performance liquid chromatography (SEC-HPLC) confirmed that AK112 forms a soluble complex with VEGF, further intensifying its affinity for PD-1. Furthermore, in the presence of VEGF, its binding activity to PD-1 is enhanced. This VEGF-facilitated binding promotes PD-1 internalization and amplifies the blockade of PD-1/PD-L1 signaling. To assess its in vivo pharmacological effects, AK112's antitumor activity was examined in SCID/beige mice implanted with HCC827 cells. In this mouse model, AK112 demonstrated more pronounced antitumor effects than bevacizumab.

IBI319 is a cutting-edge bispecific antibody that simultaneously targets both PD-1 and CD137. Besides the combined advantages of an immune checkpoint inhibitor and a CD137 agonist, IBI319 offers unique characteristics: ① The PD-1 terminus of IBI319 has a considerably higher affinity than its CD137 terminus. This results in the antibody predominantly accumulating in tumor-infiltrating T/NK lymphocytes with high PD-1 expression, minimizing its presence in the systemic circulation. ② The trimerization of CD137 and the initiation of its downstream signaling are wholly reliant on the PD-1 terminus anchoring, mitigating potential toxic side effects that could arise from systemic circulation. In both CT26 and MC38 mouse models, IBI319 exhibited a synergistic effect. It not only amplified PD-1 pharmacologic activity but also activated CD137 signaling, promoting T- and NK-cell tumor infiltration. Importantly, this was achieved without the hepatotoxicity observed when combining PD-1 and CD137. Furthermore, toxicological testing in cynomolgus monkeys indicated that IBI319 has a favorable safety profile, without notable side effects like liver toxicity. The drug's efficacy and safety will be further assessed in upcoming clinical trials.

KN052 is a PD-L1/OX40 bispecific antibody independently developed by Corning & Jer. It has the ability to simultaneously recognize PD-L1 and OX40, effectively inhibiting the interaction between PD-L1 and PD-1 while also activating the OX40 signaling pathway. Preclinical studies have demonstrated that KN052 possesses favorable pharmacokinetics and safety profiles. Notably, its antitumor efficacy is significantly superior to that of either single-targeted control antibodies used individually or in tandem. In February 2022, the NMPA of China granted KN052 an Investigational New Drug (IND) approval.

3.3.1.2 CTLA-4 Inhibitors

CTLA-4 was identified as a protein within the immunoglobulin superfamily, primarily expressed by activated T cells in a cytotoxic T lymphocyte cDNA library. Unique to T cells, CTLA-4 modulates the magnitude of T-cell activation during the initial stages. It primarily counteracts the function of CD28, a T-cell co-stimulatory receptor. Although CTLA-4 and its homolog, CD28, both bind to the B7 ligand, activation via CTLA-4 results in T cell-mediated suppression of antibody production and averts allograft rejection. In addition, the kinetics of CTLA-4 expression significantly differed from that of CD28. After TCR/CD3-mediated T-cell activation, CTLA-4 expression peaks at 2–3 days, starting around 24 h post-TCR triggering, while CD28 is already expressed in naive T cells. This discovery indicated CTLA-4's pivotal role in controlling activated T cells; its absence leads to unrestrained T-cell proliferation. With this deeper understanding of CTLA-4's function, scientists began to explore if inhibiting CTLA-4 could enhance antitumor immune responses. Presently, 23 drugs are undergoing clinical trials, and another 13 are in the preclinical research phase. Cadonillimab, developed by Akeso Biopharma, is a domestic CTLA-4 drug approved in China, alongside others like QL-1706 (by Qilu Pharma), KD6001 (by Shanghai Kangdai Bio), SHR-8068 (by Suzhou Shengda Bio), JS-007 (by Shanghai Junshi Bio), and IBI310 (by Suzhou Xinda Bio).

3.3.1.3 LAG-3 Inhibitors

LAG-3 is an immune checkpoint protein prominently displayed on effector T cells and regulatory T cells (Tregs). Within adaptive immunity, it modulates signaling pathways of T lymphocytes and antigen-presenting cells (APCs). Unlike PD-1 and CTLA-4, naive T cells don't express LAG-3. However, upon antigenic stimulation, its presence is induced on both CD4+ and CD8+ T cells. The inhibitory function of LAG-3 is proportional to its cell surface expression, highlighting the importance of its regulation. Chronic infections by viruses, bacteria, and parasites result in persistent antigen exposure, causing T cells to maintain high expression of LAG-3. Consequently, these T cells, termed "exhausted," diminish in their effector functions. This reduction leads to compromised tumor cytotoxicity, enhanced Treg immunosuppressive roles, and reduced response rates. It has been demonstrated that LAG-3 inhibition can rejuvenate T-cell cytotoxic capabilities and diminish Treg-mediated immune suppression, amplifying tumor-killing effects. Simultaneously inhibiting LAG-3 and PD-1 or PD-L1 on tumor cells offers multiple therapeutic advantages, from impeding Treg activity to boosting DC maturation and rehabilitating dysfunctional CD4+/CD8+ T cells.

Following the trials of CTLA-4/PD-1/PD-L1, LAG-3 has emerged as a novel target for tumor immunotherapy. Currently, nearly ten Chinese companies, including Cinda Bio, Zai Lab, Jiangsu Hengrui Pharmaceuticals, and Weilizhibo Biotechnology, have delved into LAG-3 inhibitors. Six of these are in preclinical trials, with most products centered on the LAG-3/PD-(L)1 dual antibody, targeting advanced malignancies like malignant melanoma. Beyond oncology, potential indications span autoimmune and inflammatory disorders.

As a nascent inhibitory checkpoint, LAG-3's therapeutic promise is intriguing. However, its molecular mechanisms remain not fully elucidated, and its therapeutic potency is yet to be ascertained. Current clinical data hints that LAG-3 monotherapy might not meet expectations. Consequently, the research emphasis has shifted to combined LAG-3 and PD-1 therapies, with bifunctional monoclonal antibodies, such as the LAG-3 and PD-1 dual antibodies, coming into focus. Domestic enterprises spearheading this approach include Anmai Biotech (EMB-02), Akeso Biopharma Bio-Tech (AK-129), and Zidong Pharmaceutical (MGD013).

3.3.1.4 TIM-3 Inhibitors

The TIM-3 protein, a member of the TIM family, was identified in 2002 [34]. Initially, it was observed to be expressed on the surface of Th1 cells. Subsequent research revealed its presence on Th17 cells, monocytes, and macrophages as well. TIM-3 has garnered significant attention due to its efficacy in various cancer models. Multiple studies have confirmed that TIM-3 acts as a negative regulator by binding to its ligand, galectin-9 (Gal-9), which results in the depletion of Th1 cells. This interaction between TIM-3 and its ligand can also induce peripheral immune tolerance. Notably, blocking TIM-3 has been shown to prevent the development of tolerance in Th1 cells.

In preclinical colon cancer models, the concurrent administration of TIM-3 and PD-1 inhibitors has proven more effective in tumor regression than using blockers for either TIM-3 or PD-1 pathways in isolation [35, 36]. Parallel findings were observed in mouse models for AML, where a combined blockade of the TIM-3/PD-1 pathway extended the survival duration of the mice. Notably, research has highlighted that in AML patients, there's an observed upregulation of PD-1 and TIM-3 in depleted CD4+ and CD8+ T cells. This upregulation potentially contributes to immunosuppression within the microenvironment. Thus, a combined blockade of both PD-1/PD-L1 and TIM-3/Gal-9 signaling pathways could offer a strategy to prevent T-cell dysfunction in hematological malignancy patients. Furthermore, in AML patients, NK cells that express TIM-3 have shown enhanced cytotoxicity, which affects the disease's prognosis [37, 38]. There's supporting evidence that both CD4+ and CD8+ T cells in the peripheral blood of patients with diffuse large B cell lymphoma upregulate TIM-3, particularly in those with bone marrow involvement. The significant increase in TIM-3 expression on these T cells underscores its pivotal role in the progression of diffuse large B cell lymphoma, offering a foundation for potential treatments [39, 40]. Lastly, the heterogeneity of TIM-3+ T cells in multiple myeloma patients reveals a nuanced immunosuppressive landscape. The interaction between TIM-3 and its primary ligand, Gal9, triggers apoptosis in helper T cells (Th1/Th17).

Within the TME, TIM3 expressed on tumor-associated dendritic cells interacts with high-mobility group box 1 (HMGB1), which is released by apoptotic tumor cells. This interaction impedes the transport of nucleic acids to dendritic cell endosomes, subsequently inhibiting the innate immune response to tumor-derived nucleic acids typically mediated by dendritic cells. Notably, when TIM3 is upregulated in mature NK cells, it prompts the release of cytokines such as IL-12, IL-15, and IL-18, thereby enhancing the cytotoxicity against tumor cells. Furthermore, TIM3, along with other inhibitory immune checkpoint molecules like PD-1 and CD160, is expressed in CD8+ T cells. Molecules like 2B4 and LAG3 are suggested to be involved in T-cell differentiation and activation. Their presence is associated with elevated levels of IFN-γ and TNF-α. Targeting the TIM3 pathway could potentially inhibit the activation of Tregs. TIM-3 represents a focal point in immunotherapy research. However, no drugs targeting this molecule have received approval. Within China, Baiji Shenzhou is advancing its phase II clinical trials, while both Henrui and Zhikang Hongyi are in phase I trials. Additionally, Shanghai Henlius Biotech, Vanenshi, Zhao derivative, and Zhiren Meibo are all in the preclinical developmental stages.

3.3.1.5 TIGIT Inhibitors

TIGIT, also known as V-set and immunoglobulin domain-containing protein 9 (VSIG9), V-set and transmembrane domain-containing protein 3 (VSTM3), or Washington University cell adhesion molecule (WUCAM), is a co-inhibitory molecule within the immunoglobulin superfamily. It was first identified in 2009 [15–17]. Structurally, TIGIT comprises an extracellular immunoglobulin variable (IgV) domain, a type I transmembrane domain, and an intracellular domain, featuring both an immunoreceptor tyrosine-based inhibitory motif (ITIM) and an immunoglobulin tail tyrosine (ITT)-like motif [18]. TIGIT expression is exclusive to NK cells and various T cells, encompassing CD8+ T cells, CD4+ T cells, and Tregs.

In China, BeiGene leads in the R&D of the TIGIT monoclonal antibody, ociperlimab. Data indicates that TIGIT possesses full Fc function and can efficiently bind to C1q and Fcγ receptors. This results in antibody-dependent cytotoxicity. Furthermore, when combined with anti-PD-1/PD-L1 antibodies, it exhibits a synergistic antitumor effect.

Cinda Biologics has the distinction of being the first company in China to undertake clinical research on TIGIT drugs. During the 2022 ESMO IO conference, Cinda Biologics unveiled the clinical data for the TIGIT monoclonal antibody IBI939 when combined with sintilimab in the first-line treatment of non-small cell lung cancer (NSCLC). The study demonstrated prolonged progression-free survival with promising efficacy. The combined treatment was generally well-tolerated.

In October 2021, the phase I clinical trial of the TIGIT inhibitor AK127, combined with the PD-1/CTLA-4 dual antibody AK104 for the treatment of advanced or metastatic solid tumors, was completed in Australia, with the first patient receiving the treatment.

Nonclinical data indicate that AK127 possesses potent biological activity, effectively blocking the TIGIT/PVR interaction. PVR serves as the physiological ligand for TIGIT, and its binding with TIGIT can suppress the functions of T cells and NK cells. This suggests that AK127 can counteract the inhibition of immune cell activity and restore their regular immune functions. Beyond the aforementioned pharmaceutical companies, several others, including Jiangsu Xiansheng, Akeso Biopharma, and Huabo Biological, have also made their mark in this area.

3.3.1.5.1 E.g., 1. Pharmacokinetics of Almonertinib

Pharmacology

Almonertinib is an irreversible EGFR-TKI that demonstrates strong inhibitory activity against common EGFR sensitizing mutations (ex19del and L858R) as well as T790M-resistant mutations. In contrast, its inhibitory activity against the EGFR wild type is weak [41]. Preclinical biochemical kinase inhibition studies reveal that the inhibitory concentration (IC_{50}) values of almonertinib for T790M, L858R, and ex19del are 0.37 ± 0.04 nmol/L, 0.29 ± 0.10 nmol/L, and 0.21 ± 0.10 nmol/L, respectively. However, the IC_{50} for EGFR WT stands at about 3.39 nmol/L. Highlighting its selectivity, the IC_{50} values of almonertinib for resistant or sensitizing mutations are approximately 2–16 times lower than for the wild-type enzymes [42].

Toxicology

General toxicity: In studies assessing general toxicity, rats were administered almonertinib orally for durations of 13 and 26 weeks. The main toxic reactions observed included liver damage, lung inflammation, skin reactions, gastrointestinal toxicity, and abnormal eye examinations. The MTD for these durations were 60 mg/kg and 30 mg/kg, respectively, with plasma exposure ranging from 0.4 to 1.9 times the recommended human dose of 110 mg. In parallel studies with dogs, oral administration was carried out for 13 and 39 weeks. The primary toxic reactions identified in dogs were skin reactions, oral mucosal inflammation, mucosal hyperplasia, and abnormal eye examinations. The maximum non-severe toxicity dose for dogs was 10 mg/kg, and the plasma exposure was approximately 4.5 times the recommended human dose of 110 mg.

Genotoxicity: Almonertinib mesylate tested negative in the Ames test, the Chinese hamster lung fibroblast chromosomal aberration test, and the mouse micronucleus test.

Reproductive toxicity: In male rats, almonertinib mesylate administered at a dose of 100 mg/kg showed no discernible adverse effects on fertility. However, in female rats, the compound impacted early embryonic development, leading to a decrease in the number of corpus luteum, implantations, and live births during pregnancy. Additionally, there was an increase in postimplantation loss and fetal absorption rates. These effects were not observed at a dose of 30 mg/kg, which is approximately twice the recommended human dose of 110 mg when measured in mg/m [2]. When pregnant rats were given oral doses of almonertinib mesylate at a maximum dose of 100 mg/kg, equivalent to three times the human dose of 110 mg, from pre-implantation to the hard palate closure phase (days 6–16 of pregnancy), no abnormalities in embryo-fetal development were detected. However, in reproductive toxicity tests on New Zealand rabbits, oral administration of almonertinib mesylate at doses of 30 mg/kg and ≥15 mg/kg during days 6–19 of pregnancy resulted in miscarriages, premature births, and fetal growth retardation, attributed to maternal toxicity. Despite this, no teratogenic effects were identified. No studies on perinatal toxicity have been conducted.

Carcinogenicity: No carcinogenicity related studies have been conducted.

Pharmacodynamics

In cell proliferation assays, almonertinib displayed potent inhibitory activity against human lung cancer cell lines, specifically H1975 and PC9-GR, which harbor EGFR-resistant mutations, as well as HCC827 and PC9 with EGFR activating mutations. In contrast, its inhibitory effect was minimal against the wild-type EGFR human epidermoid carcinoma cell line A431 [42]. Moreover, the antitumor efficacy of almonertinib was validated using patient-derived xenograft (PDX) models from NSCLC patients. Almonertinib effectively curtailed the growth of xenograft tumors possessing both the EGFR T790M-resistant mutation and the Del19-sensitive mutation. However, its suppressive effect on EGFR wild-type A431 xenograft tumors was notably modest [43]. Rat brain metastasis models have also revealed that almonertinib's brain exposure is over seven times greater than its plasma exposure, resulting in a pronounced reduction in brain metastases. In vivo investigations in mice demonstrated that almonertinib penetrates the blood-brain barrier effectively, inhibiting advanced NSCLC brain and spinal cord metastasis. In contrast, its metabolite, HAS-719, exhibited limited blood-brain barrier penetration capabilities [44].

Pharmacokinetics

Ametinib has a half-life of 30–35 h. Within the dose range of 55–220 mg, both the maximum plasma concentration and the area under the curve rise linearly in a dose-dependent fashion, reaching saturation at 260 mg [42]. The primary active metabolite of ametinib is HAS-719. Interestingly, the pharmacokinetic parameters of both ametinib and HAS-719 are not significantly impacted by food intake. In vitro studies indicate that their plasma protein binding rate in humans exceeds 99.5%. Ametinib is extensively distributed in the body, with an apparent volume of distribution equating to 554 L. In plasma, ametinib predominantly exists in its original form and undergoes metabolism to HAS-719 via the CYP3A4 enzyme in the liver. The primary metabolic routes involve N-dimethylacetamide and demethylation, while secondary pathways entail oxidation [45]. The average plasma elimination half-lives for ametinib and HAS-719 stand at 30.62 and 55.36 h, respectively. Most of the drug is excreted through feces (85%), with a minor fraction (5%) being excreted in urine. It's notable that ametinib is a moderately sensitive substrate of the CYP3A4 enzyme. When coadministered with a potent CYP3A4 inhibitor like itraconazole or an inducer such as rifampicin, there can be a significant alteration in ametinib exposure. Based on concentrations observed in brain tissue and plasma, ametinib can penetrate the blood-brain barrier post-oral administration in a mouse brain metastases xenograft model. However, the presence of its active metabolite HAS-719 in brain tissue is trivial compared to its plasma concentration [44]. Furthermore, ametinib effectively curbed the growth of intracranial and spinal tumors in mouse models, and an equivalent osimertinib exposure was recorded in mouse brain tissue after a singular 5 mg/kg dosage of either medication.

3.3.1.5.2 Eg 2. Pharmacokinetics of Ensartinib

Pharmacology of Ensartinib

Ensartinib stands as a pioneering ALK inhibitor in China. On a molecular scale, its IC_{50} for ALK tyrosine kinase is pegged at 0.16 nmol/L. When mapped against the wild-type ALK and 17 ALK mutants, ensartinib hydrochloride demonstrated notable inhibition across all evaluated ALK mutants, with an IC_{50} less than 4 nmol/L. Specifically, it showed pronounced inhibitory effects on wild-type ALK fusion and secondary mutations, such as F1174, C1156Y, L1196M, S1206R, and T1151, registering an IC_{50} less than 0.4 nmol/L. However, its inhibitory prowess against the G1202 mutant was comparatively subdued, with an IC_{50} of 3.8 nmol/L. Beyond ALK, ensartinib also effectively inhibits targets like ROS1 and tropomyosin receptor kinase (TRK) with an IC_{50} under 1 nmol/L.

At the cellular level, particularly in the EML4-ALK fusion gene-positive lung cancer cell line H3122, ensartinib curtails ALK phosphorylation, which in turn leads to a corresponding suppression of downstream targets such as the extracellular regulated protein kinase (ERK) and protein kinase B (PKB). When examining its impact on tumor cell growth, ensartinib showcased potent anti-proliferation activity across tumor cells housing varied ALK fusion proteins. Notably, its inhibitory action surpasses that of crizotinib by over tenfold in certain contexts. For instance, in the H3122 lung cancer cell line, ensartinib and crizotinib's IC_{50} were recorded at 15 nmol/L and 180 nmol/L, respectively. Nevertheless, ensartinib's growth-inhibitory effect on MKN-45 gastric cancer cells, which carry the MET mutation, lagged behind crizotinib, underscoring its heightened selectivity and inhibitory action on ALK [46].

Furthermore, ensartinib displayed certain inhibitory effects on crizotinib-resistant cell lines, like Ba/F3-EML4-ALK L1196M and Ba/F3-EML4-ALK C1156Y. Their respective IC_{50} values were 106 and 48 nmol/L, hinting at ensartinib hydrochloride's potential in counteracting crizotinib-resistant mutations. In relation to brain metastasis, ensartinib hydrochloride revealed a noteworthy intracranial drug concentration in SH-SY5Y mouse models. Specifically, its concentration was over five times the required level to inhibit EML4-ALK-positive tumor growth. It's worth highlighting that ensartinib functions as a multi-target inhibitor of ALK, MET, ROS1, and AXL, and in vitro tests have affirmed its ALK inhibitory activity to be between 3 and 10 times stronger than that of crizotinib [46].

Toxicology

In a 10-day repeated dose toxicity trial conducted on rats, there were no observed drug-related toxicities in the groups receiving doses of 20 mg/kg, 40 mg/kg, and 80 mg/kg. Consequently, the non-severe toxic dose (NST) of ensartinib was determined to be 80 mg/kg. At this NST dose, the only noticeable effects were elevations in alanine aminotransferase (ALT) and aspartate transaminase (AST), both of which increased by less than 50% [46].

Pharmacodynamics

In various animal models, ensartinib exhibited strong antitumor efficacy, especially against ALK-driven central nervous system metastases [46]. Upon oral administration, ensartinib hydrochloride notably inhibited the growth of xenografted tumors in nude mice that carried the EML4-ALK-positive human NSCLC and human neuroblastoma with the EML4-ALK F1174L drug-resistant mutation. Compared to crizotinib, ensartinib hydrochloride demonstrated significantly enhanced antitumor activity at equivalent dose levels. Paolo et al. [47] indicated that ensartinib hydrochloride significantly prolonged the average survival time of human neuroblastoma-bearing nude mice with the EML4-ALKF1174L drug-resistant mutation, while crizotinib did not exhibit such an effect. Notably, the intracranial concentration of ensartinib hydrochloride was over five times the concentration needed to suppress the growth of EML4-ALK-positive tumors. In contrast, crizotinib achieved only 44% of that concentration. This suggests that ensartinib hydrochloride can effectively penetrate the blood-brain barrier and exert its tumor-inhibiting properties.

Pharmacokinetics

Ensartinib's time to reach maximum plasma concentration (Tmax) ranged between 0.5 and 4 h. After administration, the plasma elimination half-life (T1/2) was between 2.8 and 7.8 h. With the repeated dosing of ensartinib, accumulation within the system was observed. Tissue distribution tests revealed that 2 and 8 h post-administration of 25–100 mg ensartinib to mice, intracerebral concentrations stood at 13% and between 20% and 34% of plasma concentration, respectively. The intratumoral concentration was between 17 and 32 times that of plasma [46, 47]. From a US phase I clinical study, following once-daily oral intake of ensartinib (ranging from 50 to 225 mg), both the peak serum concentration (C_{max}) and area under the curve (AUC) increased in proportion to the dosage. However, for dosages >225 mg once-daily (QD), pharmacokinetics parameters displayed a faint linearity. There was accumulation with multiple dosing. About 12 h after a single dose, the average drug concentration in the skin was roughly nine times that in plasma. In the 225 mg dosage group, T1/2 was between 33.2 and 37.7 h, while Tmax was from 3.1 to 3.6 h. Food intake didn't significantly affect ensartinib's absorption [46]. During the phase I clinical trial in China, participants was administrated ensartinib orally without food. Within the 150–250 mg dose range, regardless of whether it was a single dose or multiple doses, the average Tmax for each dosage group was between 2.67 and 5 h. The average T1/2 spanned from 21.0 to 36.4 h. Steady-state drug concentration was achieved around the 8–15 days of continual administration. These findings supported that a QD dosing regimen for ensartinib was appropriate.

References

1. Wong KM, Capasso A, Eckhardt SG. The changing landscape of phase I trials in oncology. Nat Rev Clin Oncol. 2016;13:106–17.
2. Le Tourneau C, Lee JJ, Siu LL. Dose escalation methods in phase I cancer clinical trials. J Natl Cancer Inst. 2009;101:708–20.
3. Araujo D, Greystoke A, Bates S, et al. Oncology phase I trial design and conduct: time for a change-MDICT guidelines 2022. Ann Oncol. 2023;34:48–60.
4. Bransford P, Cook J, Gupta M, et al. ICH M9 guideline in development on biopharmaceutics classification system-based biowaivers: an industrial perspective from the IQ Consortium. Mol Pharm. 2020;17:361–72.
5. Bhatt A. International council for harmonisation E6(R2) addendum: challenges of implementation. Perspect Clin Res. 2017;8:162–6.
6. Iasonos A, O'Quigley J. Adaptive dose-finding studies: a review of model-guided phase I clinical trials. J Clin Oncol. 2014;32:2505–11.
7. Tabata M, Ganapathi R. NF-kappa B activation in topoisomerase I inhibitor-induced apoptotic cell death in human non-small cell lung cancer. Ann N Y Acad Sci. 2000;922:343–4.
8. Kim HS, Kim JH, Jang HJ. Pathologic and prognostic impacts of FGFR2 amplification in gastric cancer: a meta-analysis and systemic review. J Cancer. 2019;10:2560–7.
9. Jaki T, Burdon A, Chen X, et al. Early phase clinical trials in oncology: realising the potential of seamless designs. Eur J Cancer. 2023;189:112916.
10. He C, Wan H. Drug metabolism and metabolite safety assessment in drug discovery and development. Expert Opin Drug Metab Toxicol. 2018;14:1071–85.
11. Redfern WS, Wakefield ID, Prior H, et al. Safety pharmacology—a progressive approach. Fundam Clin Pharmacol. 2002;16:161–73.
12. Singh S, Loke YK. Drug safety assessment in clinical trials: methodological challenges and opportunities. Trials. 2012;13:138.
13. Dubrot J, Lane-Reticker SK, Kessler EA, et al. In vivo screens using a selective CRISPR antigen removal lentiviral vector system reveal immune dependencies in renal cell carcinoma. Immunity. 2021;54:571–85.
14. Naci H, Ioannidis JP. How good is "evidence" from clinical studies of drug effects and why might such evidence fail in the prediction of the clinical utility of drugs? Annu Rev Pharmacol Toxicol. 2015;55:169–89.
15. Andrade EL, Bento AF, Cavalli J, et al. Non-clinical studies in the process of new drug development-part II: good laboratory practice, metabolism, pharmacokinetics, safety and dose translation to clinical studies. Braz J Med Biol Res. 2016;49:e5646.

16. Pritchard JF, Jurima-Romet M, Reimer ML, et al. Making better drugs: decision gates in non-clinical drug development. Nat Rev Drug Discov. 2003;2:542–53.
17. Aliyu UM, Okwonna CO. Delayed hypersensitivity to oxaliplatin in a nigerian patient with colorectal cancer-a case report. J Oncol Pharm Pract. 2021;27:1258–60.
18. Dent SF, Eisenhauer EA. Phase I trial design: are new methodologies being put into practice? Ann Oncol. 1996;7:561–6.
19. Maliepaard M, Carree W, van Bussel MTJ. Dose selection and tolerability of anticancer agents evaluated by the European Medicines Agency in the period 2015–2020. ESMO Open. 2021;6:100301.
20. Wong WW, Woo G, Heathcote EJ, et al. Disease burden of chronic hepatitis B among immigrants in Canada. Can J Gastroenterol. 2013;27:137–47.
21. Kotiw M, Johnson M, Pandey M, et al. Immunological response to parenteral vaccination with recombinant hepatitis B virus surface antigen virus-like particles expressing Helicobacter pylori KatA epitopes in a murine H. pylori challenge model. Clin Vaccine Immunol. 2012;19:268–76.
22. Milly PC, Wetherald RT, Dunne KA, et al. Increasing risk of great floods in a changing climate. Nature. 2002;415:514–7.
23. Zolot RS, Basu S, Million RP. Antibody-drug conjugates. Nat Rev Drug Discov. 2013;12:259–60.
24. Shen X, Yang Y, Xu Y, et al. [Protective effect of TGF-beta-Smads signal-based oxymatrine on myocardial fibrosis induced by acute myocardial infarction in rats]. Zhongguo Zhong Yao Za Zhi. 2012;37:632–6.
25. Moskowitz CH, Nademanee A, Masszi T, et al. Brentuximab vedotin as consolidation therapy after autologous stem-cell transplantation in patients with Hodgkin's lymphoma at risk of relapse or progression (AETHERA): a randomised, double-blind, placebo-controlled, phase 3 trial. Lancet. 2015;385:1853–62.
26. Tarantino P, Carmagnani Pestana R, Corti C, et al. Antibody-drug conjugates: smart chemotherapy delivery across tumor histologies. CA Cancer J Clin. 2022;72:165–82.
27. Ilana Schlam , Sara M Tolaney, Paolo Tarantino .How I treat HER2-low advanced breast cancer.Breast. 2023 Feb:67:116-123.
28. Wyant T, Fedyk E, Abhyankar B. An overview of the mechanism of action of the monoclonal antibody vedolizumab. J Crohns Colitis. 2016;10:1437–44.
29. Colombel JF, Sands BE, Rutgeerts P, et al. The safety of vedolizumab for ulcerative colitis and Crohn's disease. Gut. 2017;66:839–51.
30. Li L, Xu MZ, Wang L, et al. Conjugating MMAE to a novel anti-HER2 antibody for selective targeted delivery. Eur Rev Med Pharmacol Sci. 2020;24:12929–37.
31. Best RL, LaPointe NE, Azarenko O, et al. Microtubule and tubulin binding and regulation of microtubule dynamics by the antibody drug conjugate (ADC) payload, monomethyl auristatin E (MMAE): mechanistic insights into MMAE ADC peripheral neuropathy. Toxicol Appl Pharmacol. 2021;421:115534.
32. Rosario M, Dirks NL, Milch C, et al. A review of the clinical pharmacokinetics, pharmacodynamics, and immunogenicity of vedolizumab. Clin Pharmacokinet. 2017;56:1287–301.
33. Bye WA, Jairath V, Travis SPL. Systematic review: the safety of vedolizumab for the treatment of inflammatory bowel disease. Aliment Pharmacol Ther. 2017;46:3–15.
34. Monney L, Sabatos CA, Gaglia JL, et al. Th1-specific cell surface protein Tim-3 regulates macrophage activation and severity of an autoimmune disease. Nature. 2002;415:536–41.
35. Haanen JB, Thienen H, Blank CU. Toxicity patterns with immunomodulating antibodies and their combinations. Semin Oncol. 2015;42:423–8.
36. Koyama S, Akbay EA, Li YY, et al. Adaptive resistance to therapeutic PD-1 blockade is associated with upregulation of alternative immune checkpoints. Nat Commun. 2016;7:10501.
37. Huang S, Zhao Y, Lai W, et al. Higher PD-1/Tim-3 expression on IFN-γ+ T cells is associated with poor prognosis in patients with acute myeloid leukemia. Cancer Biol Ther. 2023;24:2278229.

38. Rakova J, Truxova I, Holicek P, et al. TIM-3 levels correlate with enhanced NK cell cytotoxicity and improved clinical outcome in AML patients. Onco Targets Ther. 2021;10:1889822.
39. Zhang L, Du H, Xiao TW, et al. Prognostic value of PD-1 and TIM-3 on CD3+ T cells from diffuse large B-cell lymphoma. Biomed Pharmacother. 2015;75:83–7.
40. Zhang T, Ren T, Song Z, et al. Genetic mutations of Tim-3 ligand and exhausted Tim-3(+) CD8(+) T cells and survival in diffuse large B cell lymphoma. J Immunol Res. 2020;2020:6968595.
41. Nagasaka M, Zhu VW, Lim SM, et al. Beyond osimertinib: the development of third-generation EGFR tyrosine kinase inhibitors for advanced EGFR+ NSCLC. J Thorac Oncol. 2021;16:740–63.
42. Yang JC, Camidge DR, Yang CT, et al. Safety, efficacy, and pharmacokinetics of almonertinib (HS-10296) in pretreated patients with EGFR-mutated advanced NSCLC: a multicenter, open-label, phase 1 trial. J Thorac Oncol. 2020;15:1907–18.
43. Shirley M, Keam SJ. Aumolertinib: a review in non-small cell lung cancer. Drugs. 2022;82:577–84.
44. Zhang Y, Zhang Y, Niu W, et al. Experimental study of almonertinib crossing the blood-brain barrier in EGFR-mutant NSCLC brain metastasis and spinal cord metastasis models. Front Pharmacol. 2021;12:750031.
45. Zhou C, Xie L, Liu W, et al. Absorption, metabolism, excretion, and safety of [(14)C] almonertinib in healthy Chinese subjects. Ann Transl Med. 2021;9:867.
46. Lovly CM, Heuckmann JM, de Stanchina E, et al. Insights into ALK-driven cancers revealed through development of novel ALK tyrosine kinase inhibitors. Cancer Res. 2011;71:4920–31.
47. Di Paolo D, Yang D, Pastorino F, et al. New therapeutic strategies in neuroblastoma: combined targeting of a novel tyrosine kinase inhibitor and liposomal siRNAs against ALK. Oncotarget. 2015;6:28774–89.

Chapter 4
Clinical Trials

Huan Yan, Ting Li, and Lianxi Song

Abstract Clinical trials are essential for evaluating new medical treatments, structured into four phases to assess safety, efficacy, and optimal usage. Phase I trials, involving a small number of participants, primarily focus on safety and dosage. Phase II expands the pool to evaluate efficacy and further assess safety. Phase III trials, conducted on a larger scale, confirm efficacy, monitor side effects, and compare against standard treatments, pivotal for regulatory approval. Following approval, phase IV trials continue to evaluate effectiveness and long-term impacts in diverse populations. These trials, adhering to strict ethical and regulatory standards, employ methods like randomization and blinding to ensure credible results, playing a crucial role in advancing medical knowledge and patient care.

Keywords Clinical trial · Safety · Efficacy · Optimal usage

H. Yan (✉)
Department of Medical Oncology, Lung Cancer and
Gastrointestinal Unit, Hunan Cancer Hospital/The Affiliated Cancer Hospital of Xiangya School of Medicine, Central South University, Changsha, China
e-mail: yanhuan@hnca.org.cn

T. Li
Department of Medical Oncology, Lung Cancer and Gastrointestinal Unit, Hunan Cancer Hospital/The Affiliated Cancer Hospital of Xiangya School of Medicine, Central South University, Changsha, China
e-mail: liting2761@hnca.org.cn

L. Song
Department of Medical Oncology, Yiyang Central Hospital, Yiyang, China
e-mail: Songlianxi@hnca.org.cn

© The Author(s), under exclusive license to Springer Nature Singapore Pte Ltd. 2024

Y. Zhang, N. Yang (eds.), *New Anti-cancer Drug Development and Evaluation*,
https://doi.org/10.1007/978-981-97-7274-2_4

4.1 Definition of Clinical Trials

According to the National Institutes of Health (NIH), a clinical trial is characterized by several key components: it includes one or more human participants; these participants are assigned to specific interventions in a prospective manner; the effect of the interventions is then evaluated; and the trial aims to yield a health-related biomedical or behavioral outcome. Clinical trials encompass a broad spectrum of research areas and can address various questions through multiple approaches, such as mechanistic, exploratory/developmental, pilot/feasibility studies, interventional methods, or behavioral techniques.

4.1.1 Clinical Trial Monitor

Data Safety Monitoring Board: An Independent Data Monitoring Committee (IDMC), also known as a *Data Monitoring Committee* (DMC) or *Data Safety Monitoring Board* (DSMB), is a panel of experts with pertinent expertise and experience. This independent body is tasked with the ongoing review of cumulative data from one or multiple active clinical trials. Its primary roles are to safeguard the welfare of trial participants, ensure the integrity of the trial, and validate the credibility of its results. The DSMB is integral to upholding the safety and ethical standards of randomized clinical trials, fulfilling a variety of essential functions. The *New England Journal of Medicine* (NEJM) has published a series titled "Data and Safety Monitoring Board: Protecting Patients and Scientific Credibility," which delves into four principal justifications for the premature termination of a trial: efficacy, harm, futility, and a shifting therapeutic landscape. These considerations bear upon the principle of clinical equipoise—the balance of benefits and risks the trial is predicated upon—as well as the trial's overall significance.

The DSMB is comprised of a compact team that meticulously scrutinizes the data collected from each segment of a clinical trial. This part is pivotal for monitoring patient safety and the effectiveness of the treatment, upholding the validity and reliability of the trial, and performing thorough benefit-risk evaluations. The DSMB's paramount duty is to shield participants from excessive or inequitable harm, which could stem either from the administration of active treatment or the denial of an efficacious one. This committee enhances the scientific trustworthiness of a trial, as it is uniquely positioned to examine the aggregated trial data without bias, a process essential for a comprehensive appraisal of the new treatment's effects, whether beneficial or adverse. Such unblinded oversight by the DSMB enables the trial sponsor and research personnel to preserve the blinding of the study's outcomes, maintaining the trial's integrity. The DSMB's autonomy is crucial; its members, unaffiliated with other facets of the trial and free from conflicts of interest, must be granted unimpeded access to all unmasked data, encompassing safety and efficacy metrics. This unrestricted access facilitates their capability to make well-informed decisions about the advantages and possible dangers of the treatments being tested.

4.1.2 Ethics Committee

An ethics committee is an independent group comprising medical, scientific, and nonscientific members, responsible for the protection of human subjects in clinical trials, ensuring their rights, safety, and well-being [1]. The committee should include at least five members, with at least one being from a nonscientific background and one independent of the trial site. It conducts reviews to ensure ethical standards are upheld, particularly in studies involving vulnerable populations such as those with mental disorders, children, and pregnant women. The committee's duties involve initial, ongoing, and repeated evaluations of research projects, and they are also tasked with organizing ethical training sessions. The existence of an ethics committee within an institution symbolizes the institution's commitment to research management and fulfills a regulatory obligation. These committees are entrusted with protecting the interests and dignity of participants, ensuring standardized biomedical research, maintaining records of all ethical reviews, and promoting integrity in scientific research, with all records being preserved for at least 10 years after the clinical trial's end.

4.1.3 The Start a Clinical Trial

The initial phase of organizing a clinical trial is critical and can present significant challenges if not meticulously planned. The cornerstone of this phase is the development of the research question. Crafting this question involves a thorough literature review and examination of existing registered clinical trials to ensure the question is novel and relevant. The formulation of this question is foundational, as it underpins the rationale for the trial and should be compelling enough to garner interest and support from various stakeholders, such as funding bodies, pharmaceutical companies, and other potential sponsors. It's this central inquiry that drives the trial's purpose and is a key factor in engaging both financial and academic backers.

4.1.4 Data Management

The effectiveness and safety of new medical treatments can vary among patient populations due to factors such as sex, race, age, and lifestyle. Recognizing and understanding these variations necessitates conducting clinical trials that include a diverse range of participants. In the context of China, the management of clinical trial data has seen significant evolution. Prior to 2015, data from clinical trials were predominantly recorded on paper case-report forms, leading to inefficiencies in review processes and delays in application approvals. This changed in August 2016 when the China Food and Drug Administration (CFDA) released technical guidelines for the use of electronic data capture (EDC) systems in clinical trials. With this announcement, EDC became the preferred method for managing clinical trial data in China, streamlining the process and potentially enhancing the speed and accuracy of data handling and approvals [2].

4.1.5 Power Analysis and Sample Size Calculation

Power analysis is a critical step that should be taken before initiating a clinical trial, and its results need to be included when the trial's findings are published. This statistical method is used to determine the required sample size to detect an anticipated effect of the treatment, while also considering acceptable thresholds for type I and type II errors [3]. In simpler terms, a type I error occurs when a study incorrectly attributes a difference in outcomes to the treatment rather than to chance, while a type II error happens when a study incorrectly concludes there is no treatment effect when, in fact, there is. Typically, clinical trials are designed to limit the probability of a type I error to 5% and a type II error to 20%. Power, which is defined as the probability of correctly identifying a true treatment effect, is calculated as one minus the type II error rate.

4.1.6 Statistical Analysis Plan

While there are notable instances of treatments for serious illnesses that have shown remarkable efficacy, the majority of claims proposing substantial improvements often prove to be fleeting. Holding unrealistic expectations for discovering large treatment effects can be misleading, leading to the erroneous belief that evidence from small-scale randomized trials or observational studies is sufficient. The accurate determination of moderate treatment effects, which is the most feasible outcome to expect from most interventions for common serious conditions, necessitates studies designed to minimize bias through proper randomization and appropriate analysis, without overemphasizing selective parts of the data. Such studies must also control random errors, typically necessitating large sample sizes to observe a significant number of outcomes, such as deaths. Previous lapses in generating robust evidence and interpreting it correctly have unfortunately resulted in numerous premature fatalities and widespread unnecessary suffering [4].

The formulation of a clear and comprehensive statistical analysis plan (SAP) is vital for ensuring the reproducibility of clinical trials. This sentiment is echoed by leading organizations and funding bodies, which advocate data sharing as the best practice. It is recommended that SAPs be accessible to the public, a practice further reinforced by the NIH Final Rule for Clinical Trials Registration and Results Information Submission. This rule mandates that SAPs be posted on ClinicalTrials.gov, unless they are already included within the study's protocol. The public discussion on this Final Rule highlighted the value reviewers place on the statistical analysis component of the protocol, underlining the role of SAPs in mitigating and identifying bias, particularly concerning selective analysis and reporting [5, 6]. Notably, medical journals such as *The Journal of the American Medical Association* (JAMA) have made it mandatory for SAPs to be submitted with clinical trial reports during the peer-review process, and they are often published as supplementary material or as independent articles. This movement toward transparency is promising; however, the actual benefit of SAPs is contingent on the quality of their content, and currently, there is no standardized guidance on how they should be leveraged or appraised [7].

4.1.7 Ethical Consideration

When an acceptable treatment with low toxicity is available, ethical considerations may preclude testing against a new treatment with uncertain benefits and high toxicity. Key considerations include the potential impact of the study on clinical practice, the meaningful advancements it may offer to the field, and the direct benefits to patients. Furthermore, the risk to patients from an ineffective treatment must be weighed carefully. It's essential to verify if there's substantial evidence of the treatment's effect on the disease. Ethical ambiguities within the clinical trials could negatively affect not only the current study but future research as well. Ethical oversight also extends to the use of animals in research. All personnel should possess the requisite human, animal, and laboratory training as stipulated by their institutions and regulatory authorities. Engaging an ethicist during the planning phase when ethical questions arise could prove invaluable.

4.1.8 Overview of Conducting a Clinical Trial

Designing a clinical trial is a crucial phase in clinical research, as the findings directly influence clinical practice. Any deficiencies in the trial's design, data gathering, analytical methods, or reporting can compromise the validity of the results, leading to misinterpretation of the outcomes. Therefore, a solid understanding of clinical trial design is imperative for accurately interpreting the results and assessing their validity and applicability. In the following sections, we will provide a concise overview of clinical trials, covering fundamental principles, design strategies, and recent advancements in the field of oncology clinical trials.

4.1.9 Basic Concepts of Clinical Trials

Clinical trial design typically originates from questions that arise during clinical care. These research questions should embody innovation and feasibility. An exhaustive review of both domestic and international literature is conducted to identify issues that have not been thoroughly explored. The goal is to design studies that are both innovative and feasible. Research questions must clearly articulate the population, intervention, comparator, and outcomes (PICO) [8].

4.1.9.1 Study Population

The characteristics of a study population in clinical trials should be defined based on age, sex, physical condition, disease stage, and the presence of specific biomarkers [8]. The selection of participants should adhere to uniform and recognized diagnostic criteria. However, not all cases with a clear diagnosis will be suitable for the study, necessitating carefully crafted inclusion criteria tailored to the study's goals and specific conditions. Implementing narrow inclusion and exclusion criteria enhances the homogeneity of the study population, which in turn diminishes the variability of participant characteristics that could influence the effectiveness of the treatment. While this approach can lead to more precise estimations of treatment effects, it may also limit the broader applicability of the study findings to the general population. For instance, in designing clinical trials related to tumor immunity, including multiple biomarker conditions such as PD-L1 expression, tumor mutational burden (TMB), and microsatellite instability (MSI) status as part of the inclusion criteria could increase the variability of the outcomes.

4.1.9.2 Intervention

Interventions in clinical trials can encompass medical products like drugs or devices, treatment procedures, or modifications to participant behaviors, such as dietary changes. Clinical trials often assess new medical treatments against established standards, placebos lacking active ingredients, or the absence of any intervention. These interventions must have demonstrated efficacy and safety in humans prior to trial commencement and should be explicitly detailed in the trial protocol, specifying aspects such as the drug's formulation, dosage, administration route, and treatment duration.

4.1.9.3 Comparator

In clinical trials, a comparator drug, which can either be an investigational or marketed product (active control), or a placebo (inactive control), serves as a reference to evaluate the efficacy of the investigational drug against an existing treatment. While placebo-controlled trials are not conducted due to inherent effectiveness, they are often utilized because they make it simpler to demonstrate an effect, facilitating claims of efficacy to regulatory bodies. Trials that compare new drugs against placebos are still considered the gold standard for assessing drug efficacy, as they yield valid and reliable results that regulatory authorities widely accept.

4.1.9.4 Blinding

Blinding is a crucial component of clinical trial design, utilized to prevent both participants and researchers from knowing the group assignments. This method is key in mitigating placebo effects and curbing potential biases that could affect the trial's outcomes. By obviating conscious or subconscious biases stemming from treatment awareness, blinding contributes to the accuracy and reliability of the study's results.

4.1.9.5 Randomization

Randomization in clinical trials is used to ensure that the assignment of participants to either the intervention or comparator groups is not influenced by factors that could affect the outcomes. Participants are typically assigned in equal numbers to either the intervention or control arms through a process that includes a random element, often generated by computer algorithms. While the overall probability of being allocated to a particular group is predetermined, each individual assignment is randomized. Randomization helps to minimize the risk of selection bias and confounding in the study [9].

4.1.9.5.1 Endpoints

An endpoint in a clinical trial is a specific event or condition that the study aims to measure, such as the incidence of a disease, the presence of symptoms or signs, or changes in laboratory test results. These endpoints must be clearly defined and relevant to the conditions under investigation. Clinical studies may designate several types of endpoints: primary, secondary, and exploratory. The primary endpoint is crucial, as it determines the success of the study's objectives and, in interventional trials, serves as the primary measure for regulatory approval. Secondary endpoints provide additional insights into the primary endpoint's effects or reveal further impacts on the disease. Exploratory endpoints are included to investigate potential outcomes that may occur too rarely to demonstrate a significant treatment effect or to test new hypotheses, even though they may be less likely to yield a discernible effect.

4.1.9.6 Sample Size

The sample size in clinical trials refers to the number of participants involved. Various stages of clinical trials require different sample sizes, reflecting the distinct objectives of each phase. To calculate the appropriate sample size, several statistical considerations must be taken into account: the anticipated effect size (delta), the acceptable probability of making a type I error, and the desired power of the study, which is the probability of correctly rejecting the null hypothesis when it is false. These elements are critical for determining a sample size that is sufficiently large to detect the intended effect while also being statistically efficient [10].

4.1.9.7 Statistical Analysis

Statistical analysis is pivotal in ascertaining the significance of results derived from a clinical trial. This analysis must be delineated in advance within the trial protocol, tailored to the study's design and its specified endpoints. It is crucial that such analyses are carried out by a biostatistician with the requisite expertise to ensure the validity and reliability of the trial's conclusions [11]. The process of clinical trials is depicted in Fig. 4.1.

4.1.10 Phases of Clinical Trials

Clinical trials are methodically structured studies that evaluate the efficacy and safety of new treatments in human subjects, typically progressing through four distinct phases. Each phase is designed to build upon the findings of the previous one, thereby providing a comprehensive assessment of the treatment's effects.

4.1.10.1 Preclinical Studies

Preclinical studies, commonly referred to as laboratory studies, encompass both in vitro and in vivo experiments. These studies primarily investigate the safety profile of a drug at doses that mirror human exposure, elucidate the drug's mechanism of action, examine the effects of varying doses on clinical outcomes, and study the drug's pharmacokinetics—how it is absorbed, distributed, metabolized, excreted, and how it interacts with other drugs within the body. While preclinical research yields valuable data, not all findings are directly translatable to human medicine due to physiological differences between humans and animal models. A drug that is effective in treating cancer in mice, for example, may not necessarily have the same success in humans. Additionally, side effects and adverse reactions can differ significantly when a treatment is transitioned from animal models to human subjects.

4.1.10.2 Phase I Trials

Phase I clinical trials are the initial step in testing a new drug or treatment in humans, focusing on safety. Conducted with a small number of participants, these trials aim to establish the safe dosage range, identify the best mode of administration (oral, intravenous, etc.), and observe any side effects. The volunteers may receive

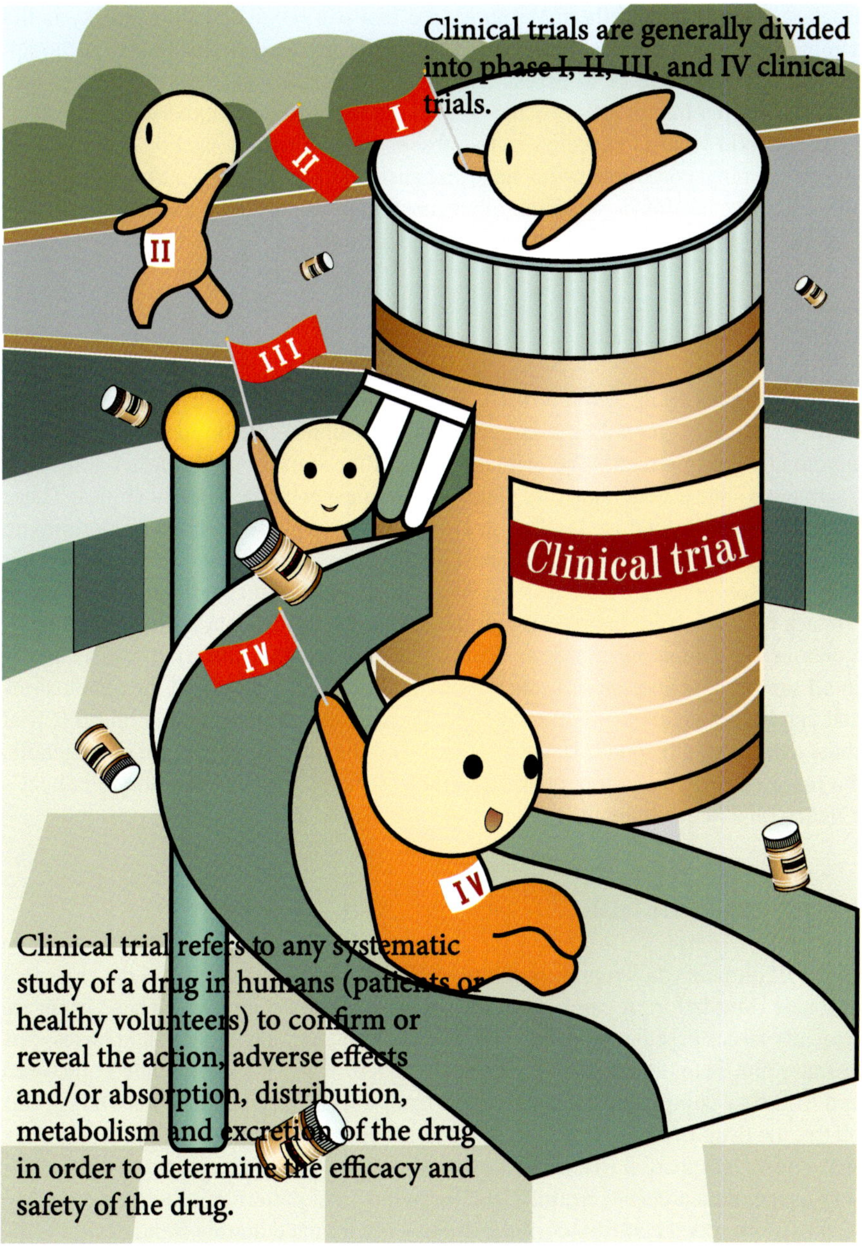
Clinical trials are generally divided into phase I, II, III, and IV clinical trials.
I
II
II
III
IV
IV
Clinical trial
Clinical trial refers to any systematic study of a drug in humans (patients or healthy volunteers) to confirm or reveal the action, adverse effects and/or absorption, distribution, metabolism and excretion of the drug in order to determine the efficacy and safety of the drug.

Fig. 4.1 Phases for clinical trials

escalating doses to find the maximum dose that can be given safely. Safety is the paramount concern; hence, placebos are typically not used in this phase. Although the primary objective is to assess safety, phase I trials also provide preliminary insights into the treatment's efficacy, especially if participants experience improvements beyond what is expected in the absence of the treatment. For patients with life-threatening conditions who have exhausted other options, participating in a phase I trial can offer a potential, albeit uncertain, opportunity for benefit, always considering the balance of possible risks and advantages.

4.1.10.3 Phase II Trials

Phase II clinical trials, often termed "therapeutic exploratory' trials, expand upon phase I studies by including a larger cohort of volunteers who have the condition targeted by the treatment. The primary goals of these trials are to further assess the treatment's safety, understand its pharmacokinetics, and pharmacodynamics. These studies are also crucial for laying the groundwork for phase III trials by optimizing dosing regimens, determining the best routes of administration, and establishing endpoints for more extensive testing. While phase II trials do begin to gather data on efficacy by comparing the investigational drug to historical data from existing treatments or by evaluating different dosing schedules within the trial, the relatively small sample size and the continued focus on safety generally limit the conclusions that can be drawn about the treatment's effectiveness. If patients in a phase II trial show a promising response to the treatment and the adverse effects are manageable, the research progresses to a phase III trial to conclusively evaluate the treatment's efficacy on a larger scale.

4.1.10.4 Phase III Trials

Phase III clinical trials represent the pivotal phase in the research and development of a new drug before it can be considered for regulatory approval. These trials are typically larger in scale, more expensive, and more complex than earlier phases. The primary aim is to definitively assess the drug's efficacy for the intended outcomes and to gather comprehensive safety data from a large participant pool. During this phase, the drug is administered to a broad group to confirm its effectiveness, track side effects, compare it to standard treatments, and obtain information essential for safe usage. Researchers scrutinize the frequency and pattern of adverse events and may explore specific attributes of the drug. A randomized double-blind design is the gold standard for these trials, though other methodologies may be employed, such as open-label or single-blind designs, especially for long-term safety evaluations. The data collected from phase III trials are critical to support the submission of a new drug application to regulatory bodies. The duration of phase III trials can span several years to ensure the reliability of the results, which is vital for regulatory approval. This meticulous approach is necessary for the approval process but also contributes to the length and cost of this phase, making it one of the most resource-intensive stages in the drug development pipeline.

4.1.10.5 Phase IV Trials

After a drug receives approval, the agency may mandate that the sponsor conduct phase IV trials as a condition of the drug's approval. However, it has been reported that less than half of these required studies are either completed or initiated by the sponsors [12]. Phase IV trials, also known as "therapeutic use" or "post-marketing" studies, are conducted on drugs that have already been approved by the agency. The objectives of these trials are twofold: firstly, to detect less common adverse reactions that may not have been apparent in premarketing trials due to the limited size and diversity of the study population, and, secondly, to assess the cost-effectiveness and overall effectiveness of the drug in conditions, populations, or dosages that are either similar to or different from those used in initial trials. The limitations of pre-marketing studies, typically phase III trials, often come to light through post-marketing surveillance statistics; roughly 20% of drugs receive new black box warnings after being marketed, and about 4% are withdrawn from the market due to safety concerns. These statistics underscore the importance of phase IV trials in ensuring the ongoing evaluation of drug safety and efficacy in a broader, more diverse patient population over a longer period [13].

4.1.11 Clinical Trial Design

The design of a clinical trial is paramount to its success and hinges on the trial's specific goals. It must be rooted in the research question at hand and tailored to the population under study. A robust clinical trial design is characterized by a clear and focused research question, a precisely defined population, an appropriate intervention and control group, and well-chosen outcome measures. Common clinical trial designs include:

4.1.11.1 Randomized Controlled Trials (RCTs)

RCTs are considered the gold standard in clinical research for determining the efficacy of interventions [14]. This stature is attributed to the randomization process, which aims to balance group characteristics, thereby providing the most definitive evidence of the effects of an intervention on outcomes [15]. In RCTs, participants are randomly allocated to either the intervention group, which receives the new treatment, or the control group, which receives a placebo or the standard treatment. The impact of the intervention is assessed by comparing the outcomes of these two groups, with the goal of ascertaining any statistically significant effects that the intervention may have. The strength of RCTs lies in their ability to infer causality between an intervention and its outcomes, a feat achieved through the random assignment of participants that mitigates the influence of confounding variables. Furthermore, blinding methods can be employed to shield both the allocation process and outcome assessment from bias. However, despite their critical role in clinical research, RCTs come with their own set of limitations. They can be costly, require substantial time to conduct, and may not be practical or ethical for all types of research queries. Additionally, the results of RCTs may not be universally applicable due to often stringent participant selection criteria and the controlled conditions under which the trials are conducted. These factors may limit the generalizability of the trial findings to broader, more diverse real-world populations [16].

4.1.11.2 Non-randomized Trials (NRCTs)

NRCTs serve as an alternative research method for assessing the effectiveness and safety of interventions, especially when RCTs are not feasible. In NRCTs, the assignment of participants to the treatment or control groups is not random but is determined by other factors, such as the preferences of the clinician or patient or the availability of interventions. NRCTs can provide valuable insights into the intervention's effects under less stringent conditions and are particularly useful in scenarios where RCTs may be impractical, unethical, or too costly to implement. However, due to the nonrandom allocation of participants, NRCTs are more susceptible to biases and confounding factors, which can affect the validity of their conclusions.

4.2 Innovation in Oncology Clinical Trial Design

Nonetheless, the practicality of conducting RCTs can be limited by several factors, including the urgency of evidence generation, the high costs involved, challenges in designing trials for narrow populations which may limit the generalizability of the findings, ethical considerations, and the extensive duration required to perform these trials. As a result, there is a pressing need for traditional trial design models to evolve in tandem with the rapid progress in genomics, immunology, and precision medicine [13]. A pivotal innovation in clinical trial design is the advent of adaptive clinical trials, which provide flexibility to modify trial parameters in response to interim data. This dynamic approach can expedite the trial process, curtail expenses, and enhance the probability of trial success. Recent sophisticated designs, such as basket trials, umbrella trials, and platform trials, are tailored to maximize efficiency and focus on specific patient subpopulations. These novel methodologies allow for the simultaneous investigation of multiple therapies or targets within a single trial framework, streamlining the evaluation process and potentially bringing effective treatments to patients more quickly [17].

4.2.1 *Basket Trials*

Basket trials, a form of master protocol, are generally situated within the framework of phase II clinical trials. Their design is intended to assess the effectiveness and durability of responses in patients receiving treatments that target specific molecular alterations, irrespective of the tumor's histological type. This approach allows for the inclusion of various tumor types in one trial if they share a common molecular characteristic that the treatment is designed to act upon. However, basket trials do pose certain challenges, particularly in statistical design, patient enrollment, and results interpretation [18, 19].

4.2.2 *Umbrella Trials*

An umbrella trial is designed to evaluate multiple investigational drugs, administered either as single agents or in combination, within a single disease population. Patients receive targeted treatments that are matched to their specific genetic aberrations [20]. The advantages include relative homogeneity (as all participants have the same tumor type) and the ability to observe the benefits of the genetic mutations, especially when the sub-studies are randomized [17].

4.2.3 *Platform Trials*

Platform trials are innovative multi-arm, multi-stage study designs that allow for the simultaneous comparison of multiple interventions against a single control group under a unified master protocol [21]. These trials are structured to explore optimal treatment timings, combinations, and selections for a particular disease using a flexible protocol framework. The hallmark of platform trials is their broad scope and adaptability [22]. Platform trials are disease-centric, rather than intervention-centric, enabling them to continue indefinitely. New therapeutic arms can be added as emerging treatments become available, while ineffective or harmful ones can be discontinued promptly. Moreover, the standard control arm can be updated to reflect new evidence-based treatments. This continual evolution makes platform trials a dynamic tool in the advancement of medical research.

4.2.3.1 Interpreting the Results of Clinical Trials

Clinical trials are indeed more critical than preclinical studies for drug development because they provide essential verification of a drug's efficacy and safety in humans. These trials fulfill the regulatory requirements for the review and registration of new drugs. They also inform market development strategies for pharmaceutical companies and guide the appropriate use of new medications by clinicians and patients. Clinical trials must be underpinned by a clear, well-articulated purpose and a scientifically robust design. The methodologies and subjects chosen should ensure representativeness, randomness, and balanced comparison, enhancing the trial's credibility. Additionally, the reproducibility of the results is vital for the reliability of the findings. The data gathered from clinical trials should be analyzed with validated statistical techniques. Such careful and systematic analysis is essential to reach unbiased, accurate, and scientifically valid conclusions. Through objective and comprehensive deliberation, clinical research can then contribute meaningfully to medical science and patient care.

4.2.3.2 Outline of Clinical Trials

Clinical trial results are often distilled into a binary outcome: positive or negative. While this simplification is common, it's not entirely reasonable as it belies the complexity of the data. Researchers typically determine the positivity of a trial based on whether the primary endpoint has met the pre-established criteria and whether the *p*-value for the efficacy difference is less than 0.05. However, the *p*-value should be regarded as part of a continuum, with smaller values indicating stronger evidence of a treatment effect [23, 24]. Confidence intervals are also crucial as they provide a range of values within which the true treatment effect likely falls, reflecting the precision of the estimate. While statistical significance in the primary outcome is a key criterion for the success of a clinical study, it is not the sole determinant. A comprehensive interpretation of a trial incorporates the totality of evidence, including secondary endpoints, safety profiles, the characteristics of the study population, and the scale and rigor of the trial [25]. The results of a clinical trial are subject to evaluation by a wide array of stakeholders, each with their own perspective and interests. These include regulatory authorities, pharmaceutical companies, researchers, ethics committees, clinicians, and patients. Thus, the success and impact of a clinical trial hinge on a multifaceted analysis rather than a single metric of efficacy.

4.2.3.3 Interpretation Elements

To assess whether clinical trial results warrant changes in treatment approaches, a comprehensive analysis of the trial data and findings from earlier related trials is crucial. Interpreting clinical trial outcomes requires critical evaluation, not just acceptance of the results at face value. In the context of RCTs, understanding the PICO framework is essential. PICO stands for Patient (P), Intervention (I), Comparison (C), and Outcome (O), and it is the backbone of the trial's structure, guiding its objectives and clinical relevance [26, 27]. The PICO framework not only shapes the study's purpose but also its clinical significance. A limitation of this approach, however, is that it can confine the study's conclusions to a specific population, potentially limiting the generalizability of the findings. This constraint is among the most significant limitations of RCTs. In the development of new drugs, clinical trials primarily focus on assessing the drug's efficacy and safety [28]. The careful interpretation of these aspects, taking into account the nuances of the study design and population, ensures the responsible advancement of medical treatments.

4.2.3.3.1 Study Design and Population

The protocol design and the presentation of results stand out as the most critical elements in a clinical trial. An innovative design, whether it's for a prospective or an observational study, can greatly enhance the persuasiveness of the results [29]. RCTs are the gold standard in the context of new drug development because of their efficacy in demonstrating causal relationships. The selection of study subjects is pivotal for clinical trial integrity. Reliable subjects are those diagnosed with the disease under investigation, ensuring the trial's relevance. Representativeness, on the other hand, refers to the degree to which the study population reflects the broader spectrum of the disease, including symptoms, signs, and prognostic factors. Crafting the inclusion and exclusion criteria is a crucial step in achieving this. Participants should ideally stand to benefit from the study outcomes, thereby maximizing the potential effects of the clinical investigation. While the representativeness of the study population is essential, it is equally important to ensure balance. An overemphasis on representativeness can compromise balance, and the reverse is also true [30]. Balance pertains to the uniformity of baseline characteristics among the study population, encompassing factors like gender, age, physical condition, and the type and stage of the disease. In addition, ethical considerations are nonnegotiable. It's imperative that a study receives ethical approval from the appropriate bodies and that informed consent is obtained from all participants, ensuring that the rights and welfare of the subjects are protected throughout the research process [31].

4.2.3.3.2 Observational Indexes of the Study

In clinical trials, observational indicators directly reflect the effect of the study intervention on study subjects [32, 33]. Therefore, we can evaluate the observation indicators based on several factors: First, the selected observation indicators should be fundamentally connected to the purpose of the clinical trial and accurately reflect the effect of the intervention measures. Second, the observation indicators should reflect the study results and be minimally affected by subjective factors, such as time to disease progression, duration of remission, and objective remission rate. Third, the authenticity of the observation indicators reflects how closely the study results align with the actual situation. Fourth, the precision or stability of the observation indicators is indicated by how consistent the results are when repeated measurements of a single indicator are taken. Fifth, the sensitivity of the observational indicators determines whether they can accurately reflect the subtle effects of intervention measures on the study subjects. Lastly, the specificity of the observation indicators refers to the degree to which they can reveal the problem under study without being significantly influenced by other factors.

4.2.3.3.3 Side Effects and Adverse Events

In clinical trials, the term "adverse events" encompasses all unfavorable medical occurrences experienced by subjects after administration of an investigational drug. This includes both adverse reactions that are potentially linked to the drug and serious adverse events that may not necessarily be related. These events can appear as symptoms, signs, diseases, or atypical laboratory results. It is crucial, for the assessment of drug safety, to meticulously report and scrutinize both adverse reactions and adverse events in terms of their severity and frequency within the study report. The occurrence rate of adverse events is a critical factor in evaluating a drug's risk-benefit profile [34]. For example, with the identification of CD47 as a significant target for anti-cancer drugs following the success of programmed cell death protein 1 (PD-1) inhibitors, numerous domestic pharmaceutical companies have raced to develop agents targeting CD47. Nevertheless, the development of many of these agents has been impeded by adverse events, such as anemia, highlighting the need for a careful balance between therapeutic efficacy and the potential for harm.

4.2.3.3.4 Conclusion and Clinical Significance

Summarizing the outcomes of a clinical trial is an essential step in understanding the broader implications of the study. Efficacy, safety, dosage, and treatment duration must be carefully weighed, and the findings should be contextualized against the backdrop of current clinical practices and guidelines. The clinical relevance and potential value of the drug in question must be assessed based on these results. An illustrative example of such an impact is the case of adalimumab, an immune checkpoint inhibitor developed by domestic pharmaceutical companies. It has broken the monopoly of international PD-L1 inhibitors in treating small-cell lung cancer within China, underscoring the significance of the CAPATONE-1 study [35].

4.3 Highlight of Clinical Trial Results

Interpreting clinical trial results necessitates a multifaceted approach. Firstly, possessing relevant clinical medical knowledge is essential to appropriately interpret and evaluate the outcomes of clinical trials. Accurate judgment hinges on a deep foundational understanding of the medical field. Secondly, a thorough grasp of clinical study theory, coupled with extensive practical experience, is vital for the correct interpretation and assessment of clinical trial results. A comprehensive and intuitive grasp of the entire trial process and the nuances of each stage can only be achieved through mastery of clinical trial basics, such as experimental design and randomization techniques. Thirdly, the integrity of the clinical trial methodology is critical in determining the accuracy and trustworthiness of the results. During interpretation, particular attention must be paid to the scientific rigor and validity of the methodology employed. Finally, a complete and objective evaluation of the trial results requires an exhaustive review of the related literature to contextualize and understand the findings fully. In essence, interpreting clinical trial outcomes demands an objective analysis of the study design, population, and observational indicators, underpinned by substantial theoretical knowledge and rich clinical experience.

4.3.1 When the Results Are Positive

When evaluating the outcomes of new drug development trials, it is natural to hope for positive results. However, a *p*-value of less than 0.05, while conventionally accepted as statistically significant, should be approached with heightened scrutiny. In instances where clinical trials seek to provide definitive evidence for contentious issues, a more stringent *p*-value, typically less than 0.001, is often expected to support a stronger level of evidence [36]. Taking the AK105-302 study as an example, when the intention-to-treat population was assessed by the Independent Review Radiology Committee (IRRC) for progression-free survival (PFS), the combination of pembrolizumab and chemotherapy significantly extended the median time to disease progression for patients with locally advanced or metastatic first-line squamous non-small cell lung cancer, boasting a *p*-value of less than 0.00001. Beyond statistical significance, the clinical relevance of the findings is paramount. Benefits should be quantified in both relative terms, such as hazard ratios (HRs), and absolute measures, like event rates after a specified follow-up duration. The 95% confidence interval is vital for describing the precision of these benefits. If a prespecified secondary endpoint also demonstrates a benefit, confidence in the trial's positive outcome is bolstered. This was seen in the CAPATONE-1 study, where both the primary endpoint of overall survival and secondary endpoints such as PFS and objective response rate reached statistical significance, indicating a benefit for patients with extensive-stage small cell lung cancer receiving the adebrelimab combined with an EP regimen [35]. Conversely, if secondary endpoints fail to show benefit, this may spark debate. Additionally, the credibility of positive results is inherently linked to the sample size; only sufficiently large studies can provide trustworthy evidence. Overall, while positive results are promising, they must be carefully weighed against both statistical and clinical significance, and supported by a robust sample size, to truly affirm the credibility and relevance of the trial outcomes [37].

4.3.2 *When the Result Is Negative*

In both basic research and clinical trials, outcomes may not always align with expectations. It's not uncommon to anticipate positive results from a drug trial, only to find a p-value greater than 0.05 after statistical analysis, indicating what is typically classified as a "negative" result. Upon encountering such outcomes, researchers often question the validity of their work, pondering if the treatment truly lacks efficacy or if there were errors in their methodology. However, a p-value above 0.05 does not automatically render a trial result meaningless; the interpretation should be context-specific. Negative results can be genuine, but they can also be attributed to factors intrinsic to the study's design or execution. The appropriateness of the study population and the treatment protocol, potential procedural flaws during the implementation of the study, and whether there are any positive findings within subgroup analyses should be considered [38]. A negative result doesn't necessarily invalidate the research. It can also provide valuable insights and guide further inquiry, leading to a better understanding of the treatment's limitations and potentially refining future research directions.

4.3.2.1 Problems in Study Design or Implementation

The design and execution of a study are fundamental to its success. If these aspects are not well-conceived and executed, there's a risk that the actual efficacy of a drug might be underestimated or entirely missed. Factors such as unsuitable inclusion criteria for participants, a treatment regimen with dosages that are not optimal, subpar patient adherence to the treatment protocol, and an imprecise or misaligned definition of the primary outcome measure can all contribute to a failure to observe the primary outcome. Each of these elements needs careful consideration and rigorous oversight to ensure that the true effect of an intervention is accurately captured and reflected in the trial results [39].

4.3.2.2 Insufficient Sample Size

The design of a study is often based on the results of prior studies. When confronted with negative results, the initial step is to verify the rationale behind the sample size estimation and determine if the study was adequately powered based on the actual results obtained. If a study is underpowered, a negative result might not be a true reflection of the drug's efficacy; it could instead be a false negative, which could turn positive if the sample size were increased sufficiently. When a sample size is too small to reliably detect a treatment effect, the findings should be termed inconclusive rather than negative. To achieve statistical power, researchers may adopt various strategies, such as enrolling more eligible patients, prolonging the follow-up period, using composite endpoints rather than single ones, or employing surrogate endpoints in place of direct clinical endpoints. These methods may be combined to enhance statistical power [33]. Nonetheless, it is equally critical to discern whether a statistically significant treatment effect observed in large-scale trials translates into a meaningful clinical benefit.

4.3.2.3 Negative Primary Outcome and Positive Subgroup Analysis

Clinical trials often report negative primary outcomes accompanied by positive subgroup analyses. For instance, no significant difference might be observed between intervention and control groups across all enrolled subjects, yet a significant effect might emerge within certain subpopulations, such as those with specific genetic mutations, racial backgrounds, more severe disease states, or particular comorbidities. The question arises: Can subgroup analysis alter clinical decision-making? One possibility is that the results of the subgroup analysis are true positive, indicating that the intervention is not universally effective but beneficial for individuals with certain characteristics. However, more commonly, results from subgroup analyses are false positives. Subgroup analysis typically entails multiple comparisons, which inherently increases the risk of type I error. Consequently, even when subgroup analyses yield positive outcomes, these results should be considered hypothesis-generating rather than confirmatory. It is rare, but feasible, for subgroup analysis to uncover a positive result in a trial with a negative primary outcome, which may then be substantiated in follow-up studies.

Additionally, it's essential to assess any indications of potential benefit that may not be captured through conventional analysis methods. Could alternative statistical approaches yield insights? Is there a robust biological rationale underpinning the intervention's hypothesized effectiveness [40]? When a trial's primary outcome does not reach statistical significance, researchers should not immediately dismiss the therapeutic value of the intervention. Instead, they could engage in exploratory inquiries that may reveal the intervention's worth. Preferably, such situations should be preempted through meticulous planning. This includes validating that the new therapy aligns with the disease's pathophysiology and mechanisms, choosing suitable patients and endpoints, ensuring the sample size is ample to detect meaningful effects, being meticulous about dosage regimens, clearly defining the disease and outcomes, and conducting pilot studies to pinpoint potential pitfalls and address foreseeable objections.

References

1. Slowther A, Johnston C, Goodall J, et al. Development of clinical ethics committees. BMJ. 2004;328:950–2.
2. Zhou Q, Chen XY, Yang ZM, et al. The changing landscape of clinical trial and approval processes in China. Nat Rev Clin Oncol. 2017;14:577–83.

3. Sessler DI, Imrey PB. Clinical research methodology 1: study designs and methodologic sources of error. Anesth Analg. 2015;121:1034–42.
4. Finfer S, Bellomo R. Why publish statistical analysis plans? Crit Care Resusc. 2009;11:5–6.
5. Kirkham JJ, Dwan KM, Altman DG, et al. The impact of outcome reporting bias in randomised controlled trials on a cohort of systematic reviews. BMJ. 2010;340:c365.
6. Dwan K, Altman DG, Clarke M, et al. Evidence for the selective reporting of analyses and discrepancies in clinical trials: a systematic review of cohort studies of clinical trials. PLoS Med. 2014;11:e1001666.
7. Gamble C, Krishan A, Stocken D, et al. Guidelines for the content of statistical analysis plans in clinical trials. JAMA. 2017;318:2337–43.
8. Schiavenato M, Chu F. PICO: what it is and what it is not. Nurse Educ Pract. 2021;56:103194.
9. Altman DG, Bland JM. Statistics notes. Treatment allocation in controlled trials: why randomise? BMJ. 1999;318:1209.
10. Greene T. Randomized controlled trials 6: determining the sample size and power for clinical trials and cohort studies. Methods Mol Biol. 2021;2249:281–305.
11. Alosh M, Fritsch K, Soukup M, et al. Clinical trials and statistical analyses: what should dermatologists look for in a report? Dermatol Ther. 2009;22:199–203.
12. Fontanarosa PB, Rennie D, DeAngelis CD. Postmarketing surveillance—lack of vigilance, lack of trust. JAMA. 2004;292:2647–50.
13. Lasser KE, Allen PD, Woolhandler SJ, et al. Timing of new black box warnings and withdrawals for prescription medications. JAMA. 2002;287:2215–20.
14. Umscheid CA, Margolis DJ, Grossman CE. Key concepts of clinical trials: a narrative review. Postgrad Med. 2011;123:194–204.
15. Zabor EC, Kaizer AM, Hobbs BP. Randomized controlled trials. Chest. 2020;158:S79–87.
16. Bondemark L, Ruf S. Randomized controlled trial: the gold standard or an unobtainable fallacy? Eur J Orthod. 2015;37:457–61.
17. Verweij J, Hendriks HR, Zwierzina H, et al. Innovation in oncology clinical trial design. Cancer Treat Rev. 2019;74:15–20.
18. Renfro LA, Sargent DJ. Statistical controversies in clinical research: basket trials, umbrella trials, and other master protocols: a review and examples. Ann Oncol. 2017;28:34–43.
19. Billingham L, Malottki K, Steven N. Research methods to change clinical practice for patients with rare cancers. Lancet Oncol. 2016;17:e70–80.
20. Ouma LO, Wason JMS, Zheng H, et al. Design and analysis of umbrella trials: where do we stand? Front Med (Lausanne). 2022;9:1037439.
21. Subbiah V. The next generation of evidence-based medicine. Nat Med. 2023;29:49–58.
22. Burki T. Platform trials: the future of medical research? Lancet Respir Med. 2023;11:232–3.
23. Sterne JA, Smith GD. Sifting the evidence-what's wrong with significance tests? BMJ. 2001;322:226–31.
24. Pocock SJ, McMurray JJ, Collier TJ. Making sense of statistics in clinical trial reports: part 1 of a 4-part series on statistics for clinical trials. J Am Coll Cardiol. 2015;66:2536–49.
25. Stone GW, Pocock SJ. Randomized trials, statistics, and clinical inference. J Am Coll Cardiol. 2010;55:428–31.
26. Ilic D. Assessing competency in evidence based practice: strengths and limitations of current tools in practice. BMC Med Educ. 2009;9:53.
27. Richardson WS, Wilson MC, Nishikawa J, et al. The well-built clinical question: a key to evidence-based decisions. ACP J Club. 1995;123:A12–3.
28. Kim J, Hu C, Moufawad El Achkar C, et al. Patient-customized oligonucleotide therapy for a rare genetic disease. N Engl J Med. 2019;381:1644–52.
29. Brown SR, Gregory WM, Twelves CJ, et al. Designing phase II trials in cancer: a systematic review and guidance. Br J Cancer. 2011;105:194–9.
30. Horng S, Emanuel EJ, Wilfond B, et al. Descriptions of benefits and risks in consent forms for phase 1 oncology trials. N Engl J Med. 2002;347:2134–40.
31. Cheung WY, Pond GR, Heslegrave RJ, et al. The contents and readability of informed consent forms for oncology clinical trials. Am J Clin Oncol. 2010;33:387–92.

32. Fiore LD, D'Avolio LW. Detours on the road to personalized medicine: barriers to biomarker validation and implementation. JAMA. 2011;306:1914–5.
33. Fleming TR, DeMets DL. Surrogate end points in clinical trials: are we being misled? Ann Intern Med. 1996;125:605–13.
34. Horstmann E, McCabe MS, Grochow L, et al. Risks and benefits of phase 1 oncology trials, 1991 through 2002. N Engl J Med. 2005;352:895–904.
35. Wang J, Zhou C, Yao W, et al. Adebrelimab or placebo plus carboplatin and etoposide as first-line treatment for extensive-stage small-cell lung cancer (CAPSTONE-1): a multicentre, randomised, double-blind, placebo-controlled, phase 3 trial. Lancet Oncol. 2022;23:739–47.
36. Pocock SJ, Ware JH. Translating statistical findings into plain English. Lancet. 2009;373:1926–8.
37. Pocock SJ, Stone GW. The primary outcome is positive—is that good enough? N Engl J Med. 2016;375:971–9.
38. Pocock SJ, Stone GW. The primary outcome fails—what next? N Engl J Med. 2016;375:861–70.
39. Stewart DJ, Whitney SN, Kurzrock R. Equipoise lost: ethics, costs, and the regulation of cancer clinical research. J Clin Oncol. 2010;28:2925–35.
40. Zhao S, Lv C, Gong J, et al. Challenges in anticancer drug R&D in China. Lancet Oncol. 2019;20:183–6.

Chapter 5
Small-Molecule Compounds

Lingli Liu, Yuanze Sun, and Dan Yang

Abstract Small-molecule compounds provide a range of pharmacokinetic advantages over therapeutic antibodies, including oral administration convenience, improved tissue penetration, optimal half-lives, and the ability to cross cell membranes to interact with intracellular targets. Furthermore, they are generally less expensive to produce, contributing to their widespread adoption in clinical environments. This chapter presents the research and development processes, clinical applications, and potential side effects of small-molecule compounds, focusing on those that are currently available or under development.

Keywords Tyrosine kinase inhibitor · Small molecular compound · EGFR · PD-1 · PD-L1

5.1 Targeted Protein Kinase

In non-small-cell lung cancer (NSCLC), the identification of mutations within the epidermal growth factor receptor (EGFR) has been pivotal for the advancement of targeted tumor treatments. The breakthroughs in detecting EGFR mutations and the subsequent sanctioning of tyrosine kinase inhibitors (TKIs)—a class of small-molecule compounds that target protein kinases—represent landmark achievements in the evolution of NSCLC therapies.

The discovery of the epidermal growth factor (EGF) dates back to the 1960s, when Stanley Cohen at Vanderbilt University in the United States conducted

L. Liu (✉)
Medical college, Hunan University of Medicine, Huaihua, China
e-mail: liulingli@hnca.org.cn

Y. Sun · D. Yang
Department of Medical Oncology, Lung Cancer and Gastrointestinal Unit, Hunan Cancer Hospital/The Affiliated Cancer Hospital of Xiangya School of Medicine, Central South University, Changsha, China

© The Author(s), under exclusive license to Springer Nature Singapore Pte Ltd. 2024

Y. Zhang, N. Yang (eds.), *New Anti-cancer Drug Development and Evaluation*,
https://doi.org/10.1007/978-981-97-7274-2_5

groundbreaking research. His pivotal identification of EGF and its receptor earned him the prestigious Nobel Prize, recognizing his substantial contribution to the field of biological science. EGFR is one of the quartet that comprises the human epidermal growth factor receptor (HER) family, alongside HER2, HER3, and HER4, also known as erbB1, erbB2, erbB3, and erbB4, respectively. The HER family of growth factors consists of 11 species, broadly divided into those that specifically bind with EGFR (EGF, TGF-α, Amphiregulin), those that bind with both EGFR and HER4 (BTC, HB-EGF, epiregulins), and those that bind with HER3 and HER4 (neuregulins). Although HER2 does not have a corresponding ligand, it can form a dimer with other HER family members when activated by a ligand. EGFR is also a receptor tyrosine kinase, comprising a C-terminal intracellular region with kinase activity, an N-terminal extracellular ligand-binding site, and a hydrophobic transmembrane domain [1]. EGFR plays a crucial role in initiating numerous cellular signaling pathways that govern cell survival and proliferation, migration, angiogenesis, and apoptosis. The EGFR signaling network is essential for the maintenance and expansion of epithelial tissues. Active EGFR signaling is commonly observed in lung cancer, where elevated levels of EGFR are associated with advanced disease stages and poor prognoses [2]. The EGFR gene is known as an oncogene, with tyrosine kinase activity identified as a key driver [3]. In 2004, the discovery of EGFR mutations marked a watershed moment in lung cancer research, as these mutations were the first molecular alterations found to enhance sensitivity to targeted therapies. EGFR-TKIs work by inhibiting EGFR autophosphorylation and its subsequent signaling cascades, competing with adenosine triphosphate (ATP) for binding to the EGFR tyrosine kinase domain. To date, four generations of EGFR-TKIs have been designed and developed (Fig. 5.1).

5.1.1 First-Generation EGFR TKIs

First-generation EGFR TKIs, such as gefitinib, erlotinib, and icotinib, reversibly attach to the EGFR tyrosine kinase domain and obstruct ATP binding. This interference inhibits cellular proliferation and can lead to cell death [4]. Specific activating mutations in the EGFR gene, like the L858R point mutation in exon 21 and the exon 19 deletion (delE746-A750), have been identified to increase sensitivity to first-line treatments with gefitinib and erlotinib in NSCLC patients.

Gefitinib was granted accelerated approval by the US Food and Drug Administration (FDA) in May 2003 as a monotherapy for patients with advanced-stage NSCLC [5]. However, the approval was retracted in April 2012 due to unfavorable clinical trial outcomes [6, 7]. The IPASS study, which was pivotal in EGFR-TKI clinical research, targeted a specific demographic: East Asian patients with advanced lung adenocarcinoma who were non-smokers or light smokers. It found that those with positive EGFR mutations and treated with gefitinib had longer progression-free survival (PFS) than those who underwent chemotherapy [8]. Specifically, the median PFS in the gefitinib group was 9.5 months compared to 6.3 months in the

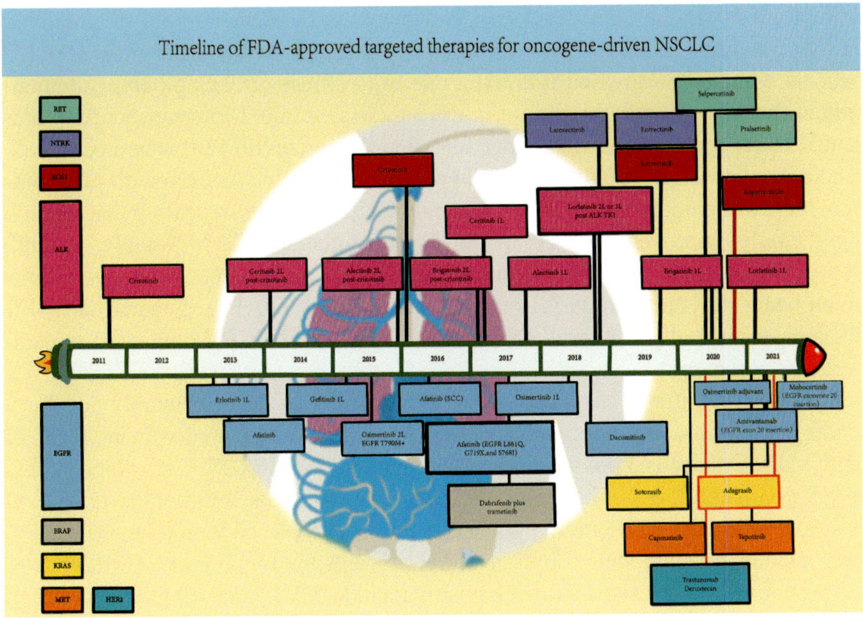

Fig. 5.1 EGFR-TKIs development

chemotherapy group, and the objective response rate was also higher (71.2% vs. 47.3%). Similar results were observed in two phase III Japanese studies, NEJ002 and WJTOG3405, conducted among NSCLC patients with EGFR mutations [9, 10]. These studies, along with IPASS, were crucial for the FDA and European Medicines Agency to approve gefitinib as a first-line treatment for EGFR-mutant NSCLC. In conclusion, the research and development of small-molecule compounds should consider specific patient populations to optimize therapeutic benefits.

Clinical trials initiated in China have indicated that patients with EGFR mutant NSCLC experience a significant overall survival (OS) benefit when treated with EGFR-TKIs, underscoring the role of these treatments in extending patient survival. The data suggest that erlotinib ought to be the standard first-line treatment for patients with EGFR mutations, and subsequent EGFR-TKI therapy following first-line treatment also confers considerable advantages [11–13]. Comparatively, no substantial differences have been observed between gefitinib and erlotinib in terms of progression-free survival, overall survival, overall response rate, and disease control rate [14]. Regarding side effects, gefitinib commonly causes rash, diarrhea, and liver damage. Erlotinib, on the other hand, has a higher rate of severe adverse events, particularly regarding diarrhea and rash, hence presenting with more significant side effects [8, 9, 15]. In preclinical studies, gefitinib exhibits limited brain penetration, with only a 1% rate [16], whereas erlotinib has been shown to permeate the cerebrospinal fluid (CSF) [17]. However, the distinctions between these two EGFR-TKIs in terms of efficacy for brain metastases have not been conclusively established in real-world studies [18, 19].

Icotinib hydrochloride, developed and patented by Beta Pharma in Zhejiang, China. The phase III ICOGEN trial, which compared icotinib to gefitinib in NSCLC patients who had progressed following one or two lines of chemotherapy, demonstrated that icotinib was equivalent in efficacy to gefitinib. Moreover, icotinib presented lower toxicity and was better tolerated than gefitinib [20]. The open-label, randomized phase III CONVINCE trial compared first-line icotinib with platinum-pemetrexed chemotherapy in EGFR-mutant NSCLC patients, revealing that icotinib significantly improved PFS compared to chemotherapy [21]. Notably, icotinib hydrochloride is the first independently developed small-molecule drug in China, and it bears structural similarities to erlotinib and gefitinib. First-generation EGFR TKIs have markedly enhanced PFS in EGFR-positive NSCLC compared to standard chemotherapy.

Despite the initial effectiveness of EGFR TKIs, resistance inevitably develops, leading to disease progression in nearly all patients. The predominant form of acquired resistance is a point mutation in exon 20, known as T790M, which occurs in approximately 50–60% of cases [22]. In this mutation, a threonine residue at position 790 in the ATP-binding pocket of EGFR is replaced with a larger methionine residue, creating steric hindrance that prevents the binding of EGFR TKIs to the receptor. Other resistance mechanisms include MET gene amplification [23], small cell transformation [24], and epithelial-mesenchymal transition [25], among others.

5.1.2 Second-Generation EGFR TKIs

Second-generation EGFR TKIs, which include afatinib, dacomitinib, neratinib, and canertinib, were developed to circumvent resistance to first-generation EGFR TKIs such as gefitinib and erlotinib. These second-generation TKIs possess enhanced potential to overcome or delay resistance to their predecessors and offer advancements in terms of target specificity, binding affinity, and overall efficacy [26].

Afatinib functions by covalently and irreversibly inhibiting the enzymatic activity of ErbB family receptor members [27]. It has been approved for first-line treatment of patients with EGFR-mutant NSCLC and for those with locally advanced or metastatic squamous-cell NSCLC who have progressed on platinum-based chemotherapy. In the phase II LUX-Lung 2 and phase III LUX-Lung 3 and LUX-Lung 6 studies, afatinib demonstrated effectiveness in patients with rare EGFR mutations that are not associated with resistance, as indicated by the objective response rate (ORR), duration of response, disease control, PFS, and OS [28, 29]. These studies included patients with uncommon EGFR mutations, including L861Q, G719X, or S768I. Based on this evidence, in January 2018, the FDA approved a supplemental New Drug Application for afatinib to treat patients with metastatic NSCLC harboring nonresistant EGFR mutations, specifically adding the mutations L861Q, G719X, and S768I. The most common adverse effects of afatinib are diarrhea and rash. In cases where adverse effects do not resolve, the dosage of afatinib can be adjusted downward without compromising its effectiveness.

Dacomitinib, a pan-HER inhibitor, has the capability to inhibit EGFR as well as HER2 and HER4 mutations [30]. In the ARCHER-1050 study, dacomitinib showed a significantly longer PFS compared to gefitinib, with 14.7 months versus 9.2 months. The study did not include patients with brain metastases, and the superiority of dacomitinib over gefitinib was more pronounced in Asian patients, with a hazard ratio (HR) of 0.51 (0.39–0.66), as opposed to a HR of 0.89 (0.57–1.39) in non-Asian patients [31]. The most common adverse reactions associated with dacomitinib are rashes, diarrhea, and stomatitis, with particularly high incidences of paronychia and dry skin, the highest among various EGFR TKIs. Reports of interstitial lung disease have also been associated with its use [31, 32].

5.1.3 Third-Generation EGFR-TKIs

The development of acquired resistance to EGFR-TKIs is an inevitable challenge, typically manifesting after 10–12 months of treatment. The T790M mutation in exon 20 is a common mechanism of such resistance, detected in 50–60% of patients who exhibit resistance to EGFR-TKIs [33]. In response to this issue, researchers have developed third-generation EGFR inhibitors that are mutant-selective and irreversible. These inhibitors are designed to form a covalent bond with the Cys797 residue, specifically targeting the ATP binding pocket of the T790M mutant EGFR, thereby overcoming resistance in patients with T790M-mutant NSCLC [34].

Osimertinib is the standard first-line treatment for advanced EGFR-mutant NSCLC due to its superiority in PFS and OS over first-generation EGFR TKIs, as evidenced by the FLAURA trial. It is also the treatment of choice for NSCLC with T790M mutations following therapy with first- or second-generation EGFR TKIs [35–37]. In China, the third-generation EGFR TKIs that have been approved include osimertinib, almonertinib, and alflutinib. Both almonertinib and alflutinib are drugs that have been independently developed in China.

In March 2020, almonertinib, a third-generation EGFR TKI developed in China, was approved for the treatment of EGFR T790M+ NSCLC, based on the results from the phase 2 extension study "APOLLO". Almonertinib is structurally characterized by a cyclopropyl group in place of the methyl group on the indole ring of osimertinib. Preclinical studies have revealed that almonertinib displays potent kinase inhibition, with low half maximal inhibitory concentration (IC_{50}) values against EGFR mutations associated with T790M, del19/T790M, and L858R/T790M, while having a higher IC_{50} for the wild type EGFR [38]. In cell-based assays, almonertinib has shown to inhibit EGFR phosphorylation effectively in mutant cell lines, with significantly reduced activity in wild type cells. The phase 1–2 dose escalation/expansion trial involving 120 patients determined the pharmacokinetics of almonertinib, establishing a half-life of 30.7 h at a daily dose of 110 mg and indicating a lower incidence of side effects such as creatinine phosphokinase elevation and diarrhea compared to higher doses. The 110 mg daily dose was thus established as the recommended phase 2 dose [38]. The efficacy and safety of almonertinib were further evaluated in a double-blind phase III trial against gefitinib as a first-line treatment for patients with locally advanced or metastatic EGFR-mutant NSCLC. The trial demonstrated a significant improvement in median PFS for patients treated with almonertinib. Although the ORR and disease control rate were similar for both treatments, almonertinib had a longer median duration of response and was associated with fewer grade ≥3 adverse events, rash, and diarrhea [39].

Alflutinib has a pyridyl ring replacing the phenyl ring and a trifluoroethyl group replacing the methyl group [40]. Detailed preclinical properties of alflutinib have not been formally published. A phase I dose escalation (NCT02973763) and phase I-II dose expansion study (NCT03127449) enrolled 130 patients across five dose levels. No maximum tolerated dose (MTD) was observed. The doses of 80 mg daily and 160 mg daily were explored in more patients in the phase I-II expansion. The Independent Review Committee (IRC)-assessed ORR at 80 mg daily and 160 mg daily were 77.8% (35/45) and 78.0% (39/50), respectively. The median progression-free survival (mPFS) at 80 mg daily and 160 mg daily was 11.1 months (95% CI: 8.2-not reached [NR]) with a 36% event rate, and NR (95% CI: 6.9-NR) with a 28% event rate. The most common treatment-related adverse events (TRAEs) for the 80 mg daily dose were decreased white blood cell count (21%), decreased neutrophil count (19%), diarrhea (17%), proteinuria (13%), and alanine aminotransferase (ALT) elevation (10%). Grade 3–4 TRAEs included decreased neutrophil count (4%) and at a rate of 2% each, diarrhea, decreased platelet count, hypertension, and hypokalemia. The TRAEs at the 160 mg daily dose were notably higher with decreased white blood cell count (27%), ALT elevation (26%), decreased neutrophil count (19%), anemia (17%), serum creatinine elevation (17%), and a spartate transaminase (AST) elevation (15%) [40]. Consequently, the recommended phase 2 dose (RP2D) of alflutinib was determined to be 80 mg daily. Alflutinib undergoes extensive metabolism mediated by CYP3A4, which also induces CYP3A4 activity. AST5902, the major metabolite of alflutinib, accounting for 52% of its metabolism, can also induce CYP3A4 activity [41]. The FURLONG study is a multicenter, double-blind, randomized, phase 3 study conducted in 55 hospitals across mainland China. It aimed to investigate the efficacy and safety of furmonertinib versus the first-generation EGFR TKI gefitinib as a first-line treatment for patients with EGFR mutation-positive locally advanced or metastatic NSCLC. A total of 750 patients were screened, with 358 patients being randomly assigned to receive either furmonertinib with a gefitinib-matching placebo or gefitinib with a furmonertinib-matching placebo. The median follow-up was 21.0 months (IQR 18.0–23.5) in both groups. The median IRC-assessed PFS was 20.8 months (95% CI 17.8–23.5) in the furmonertinib group compared to 11.1 months (9.7–12.5) in the gefitinib group (hazard ratio 0.44, 95% CI 0.34–0.58; $p < 0.0001$). TRAEs of grade 3 or higher occurred in 20 (11%) of the patients in the furmonertinib group and 32 (18%) in the gefitinib group. Treatment-related serious adverse events were reported in ten (6%) patients in the furmonertinib group and 11 (6%) in the gefitinib group. Adverse events led to death in ten (6%) patients in the furmonertinib group and three (2%) in the gefitinib group, which were all judged to be possibly unrelated to the study treatment by the investigators [42]. Some patients exhibited resistance to the third-generation EGFR TKIs, with the major mutation site being C797S on the EGFR gene, as identified by genome sequencing. The mechanisms of drug resistance include cellular-mesenchymal epithelial transition factor (C-MET) amplification, small cell lung cancer transformation, and activation of downstream genes such as Kirsten rat sarcoma viral oncogene (KRAS) or v-Raf murine sarcoma viral oncogene homolog B (BRAF).

5.1.4 Fourth-Generation EGFR TKIs

The fourth-generation EGFR TKIs currently under development primarily target the C797S mutation. Numerous drugs are in the pipeline; however, most are in the early stages of research. To date, only BLU-945 and BBT-176 have reported preliminary clinical trial data.

Using Blueprint Medicines' proprietary compound library, researchers identified a compound with moderate EGFR mutant potency but excellent selectivity over WT-EGFR. The initial phase of optimization focused on improving potency, and a scaffold-hop to a 2,7-naphthyridine enhanced EGFR+/T790M and EGFR+/T790M/C797S enzymatic and cellular potency without compromising WT-EGFR selectivity. Subsequent optimization of kinome selectivity, metabolic stability, and cellular potency resulted in the lead compound. Further analysis revealed a glucuronidation liability leading to high in vivo clearance in cynomolgus monkeys. A strategy of mitigating glucuronidation by sterically encumbering the site, paired with analysis for improved clearance, enabled the identification of compounds with reduced glucuronidation liability. Evaluation of BLU-945 in osimertinib-resistant mouse xenograft models demonstrated robust tumor growth inhibition. BLU-945 is currently being evaluated in a phase I/II clinical trial (NCT04862780) [43]. At the 2022 American Association for Cancer Research (AACR) meeting, the SYMPHONY study showcased the efficacy of BLU-945 in patients with osimertinib-resistant NSCLC. The 2023 AACR presentation of the latest results indicated that treatment with BLU-945 plus osimertinib could improve inhibition of the L858R mutation and provide more durable anticancer efficacy compared to osimertinib alone.

5.2 Targeted PD-1/PD-L1 Signaling Pathway

PD-1/PD-L1 has been recognized as a target for anticancer drugs for many years. To date, several monoclonal antibodies that target the PD-1/PD-L1 signaling pathway have yielded encouraging results in cancer treatment. Immunotherapy has emerged as a new cornerstone of cancer treatment due to the success of immune checkpoint blockade (ICB) drugs, complementing surgery, radiation, chemotherapy, and targeted therapies. However, due to the inherent limitations of antibodies, the development of small-molecule inhibitors targeting the PD-1/PD-L1 signaling pathway has seen a resurgence over the past decades. We now summarize several small-molecule inhibitors based on three distinct therapeutic approaches that interfere with the PD-1/PD-L1 signaling pathway: (1) blocking the direct interaction between programmed cell death protein 1 (PD-1) and programmed cell death 1 ligand 1 (PD-L1), (2) inhibiting the transcription and translation of PD-L1, and (3) promoting the degradation of the PD-L1 protein.

Under normal conditions, the body's immune system performs surveillance for malignancy. It can specifically recognize and eliminate malignant "non-self" cells to prevent tumor growth. However, malignant cells can sometimes inhibit immune responses against tumors by upregulating immunosuppressive molecules or downregulating immune-activating molecules, leading to immune escape and immortalization [44]. The PD-1/PD-L1 axis is the most studied immune checkpoint with a significant role in tumor immune escape. PD-1, a type I transmembrane protein with 288 amino acid residues, is also known as programmed cell death 1 receptor (PDCD1) or CD279 and belongs to the B7/CD28 receptor superfamily [45, 46]. Its two ligands, PD-L1 (CD274) and programmed cell death 1 ligand 2 (PD-L2) (CD273), are type I transmembrane proteins of the same family, consisting of 290 and 270 amino acid residues, respectively. They share 37% sequence homology. PD-L1 is more broadly expressed than PD-L2, which leads to its predominant role in the immune escape of tumor cells [47, 48].

PD-1's structure comprises four parts: an immunoglobulin variable region (IgV), a transmembrane region, immunoreceptor tyrosine-based inhibitory motifs (ITIMs), and immunoreceptor tyrosine-based switch motifs (ITSMs) [49]. Upon interaction with PD-L1, PD-1's ITIMs and ITSMs in the intracellular domain become phosphorylated, leading to the recruitment of tyrosine phosphatases Src homology phosphatase 1 (SHP-1) and Src homology phosphatase 2 (SHP-2) [50]. These phosphatases dephosphorylate key proteins within the T cell antigen receptor (TCR) signaling pathway, repressing downstream signaling pathways, including phosphoinositide 3-kinase (PI3K), protein kinase B (PKB/AKT), mammalian target of rapamycin (mTOR), rat sarcoma (RAS), mitogen-activated protein kinase (MAPK/MEK), and extracellular regulated protein kinase (ERK). This repression inhibits gene transcription, hinders T cell cycle progression and protein expression, and ultimately reduces cytokine production, along with the proliferation and differentiation of T cells, leading to a loss of immune function [51].

Anti-PD-1/PD-L1 monoclonal antibodies have significantly advanced the clinical treatment of various tumors. However, it has been suggested that these macromolecular antibody drugs face challenges in effectively penetrating tumor tissues to reach all tumor regions and accumulate in sufficient concentrations [52]. Additionally, the immunogenicity of antibody drugs may provoke the body to produce anti-drug antibodies, leading to reduced efficacy. Alterations in immune system function by these drugs can lead to an imbalance in immune tolerance, potentially causing unchecked immune responses. This can manifest as autoimmune side effects, damaging normal organs and tissues such as the liver, gastrointestinal tract, lung, skin, and endocrine system [53]. Moreover, clinical data indicate that not all patients respond to monoclonal antibody therapy. While PD-1 antibodies have shown a 50% response rate in melanoma treatment, the response rate for other solid tumors generally remains low at 15–20% [54]. The production difficulties, high costs, and storage and transport inconveniences of monoclonal antibodies could limit the broader clinical application of PD-1/PD-L1 antibody drugs.

Compared to monoclonal antibodies, small-molecule inhibitors offer significant advantages in addressing issues such as tumor penetration and immunogenicity. These inhibitors are more amenable to oral administration and can be engineered to have shorter half-lives, thus reducing target occupancy time and minimizing severe immune-related adverse events. Additionally, their ease of transportation and storage, stability, superior membrane permeability, and potentially better safety profiles make them promising candidates for future clinical treatments [55]. Preclinical studies suggest that small-molecule compounds may be more effective than antibodies in inhibiting tumor growth and migration. They also appear to have favorable biosafety profiles [56]. Despite their current developmental lag behind antibody drugs, small-molecule inhibitors have the potential to resolve the limitations associated with antibody treatments, possibly replacing them or serving as adjunct therapies. Consequently, the discovery of small-molecule inhibitors targeting the PD-1/PD-L1 signaling pathway is crucial to advance tumor immunotherapy.

5.2.1 Direct Interaction Blocking Between PD-1 and PD-L1

Liu Lei's research team employed phage display technology to identify the D-form peptide DPPA-1, composed of 12 amino acids with the sequence NYSKPTDRQYHF, which shows specific affinity for PD-L1. In binding assays, the dissociation constant (Kd) for DPPA-1's interaction with PD-L1 was 0.51 μmol/L. Subsequently, DPPA-1 demonstrated a significant inhibition of tumor growth in a CT26 xenograft mouse model [57]. In 2017, the polypeptide triphenylphosphine compound (TPP-1) was also identified to target PD-L1; it is a 22-amino acid polypeptide with the sequence SGQYASYHCWCWRDPGRSGGSK, which binds to PD-L1 with a Kd of 74 nmol/L. In xenograft mouse models, treatment with TPP-1 led to a notable increase in interferon-γ (IFN-γ) secretion and granzyme B expression, resulting in a reduction of tumor volume [58].

Feng's research group published a series of patents revealing bromobenzyl ether derivatives that significantly block the PD-1/PD-L1 interaction. Structurally similar to BMS's compounds, these derivatives uniquely feature a bromine atom instead of a methyl group in the biphenyl structure. In studies using isolated human monocytes, the derivatives were tested for their ability to inhibit PD-L1, which was added to suppress activated T lymphocytes via anti-CD3/CD28 antibodies. The results indicated that at a concentration of 10 nmol/L, the compounds could partially reverse PD-L1's suppression of IFN-γ secretion. Moreover, in a mouse melanoma cell (B16F10) subcutaneous xenograft mouse model, the sodium salt of compound 7, administered at 15 mg/kg, significantly reduced tumor growth by both volume and weight, achieving a 64.11% inhibition rate of tumor weight.

5.2.2 Inhibiting the Transcription and Translation of PD-L1

Bromodomain-containing protein 4 (BRD4), part of the bromodomain and extraterminal domain (BET) protein family, has two bromodomains that bind to acetylated lysine residues crucial for chromatin remodeling and transcriptional activation [59]. Researchers have shown that BRD4 can upregulate PD-L1 expression [60]. Data from the Cancer Genome Atlas (TCGA) database reveal that many tumors exhibit BRD4 gene amplification, which significantly correlates with PD-L1 expression [61]. Both BRD4 knockdown and the BET bromodomain inhibitor JQ1 have been shown to markedly reduce PD-L1 mRNA and protein levels in lymphoma and epithelial ovarian cancer cells, with the reduction being both time and dose-dependent when treated with JQ1 [59, 60]. Channel intrinsic protein chromatin immunoprecipitation (ChIP) assays demonstrate that BRD4 binds to the PD-L1 promoter, and JQ1 can inhibit this interaction. Additionally, IFN-γ has been found to enhance the binding of BRD4 to the PD-L1 promoter, an effect that can be effectively blocked by JQ1 [60]. Signal transducer and activator of transcription 3 (STAT3) is known to increase PD-L1 transcription by directly binding to its promoter. PD-L1 levels rise following mutations in the oncogene anaplastic lymphoma kinase (ALK), but this increase can be mitigated by knocking down STAT3 [62]. Furthermore, the latent membrane protein 1 (LMP1) elevates PD-L1 by enhancing STAT3 phosphorylation, a process that can be reversed with the Janus kinase 3 (JAK3) inhibitor CP-690550, which inhibits STAT3 phosphorylation [61].

5.2.3 Promoting Degradation of PD-L1 Protein

Current antibody drugs bind to and block surface PD-L1 on tumor cells. However, recent studies have shown that PD-L1 is also present intracellularly within circulating endosomes, the Golgi apparatus, and cellular vesicles. This intracellular PD-L1 contributes to cancer progression and replenishes the surface PD-L1, potentially leading to the failure of antibody drugs. Thus, completely eliminating PD-L1 both inside the cell and on its surface might be a more effective therapeutic approach. Intracellular proteins can be degraded via three main pathways: lysosomal, ubiquitination, and caspase. Scientists are exploring the design of inducers that target PD-L1 for degradation, aiming to reduce its levels in tumor cells and inhibit the cells' ability to evade the immune system, thereby enhancing antitumor responses.

Dr. Xu identified a notable link between Huntingtin-interacting protein 1-related (HIP1R) and PD-L1, revealing that tumor cells with PD-L1 gene amplification frequently exhibit a loss of HIP1R gene copy number, as predicted by the OncoBinder model [63]. Further research demonstrated that HIP1R interacts with PD-L1, targeting it for lysosomal degradation. When HIP1R is depleted, PD-L1 accumulates, dampening T cell cytotoxicity and aiding tumor immune evasion [64, 65]. Subsequent studies identified a lysosomal sorting sequence at HIP1R's carboxy terminus, crucial for PD-L1's transport to the lysosome, facilitated by the adaptor protein complex and the endosomal sorting complexes required for transport [66, 67]. Inspired by this mechanism, the researchers engineered PD-LYLSO, a novel molecule derived from two HIP1R peptides, capable of directing PD-L1 to lysosomal degradation. Functional tests confirmed that PD-LYLSO enhances the lysosomal degradation of PD-L1, thereby boosting T cell-mediated destruction of tumor cells. The research team has patented PD-LYLSO and is advancing preclinical studies to further explore its therapeutic potential [68].

5.2.4 Conclusion and Outlook

From 2011 to 2022, China has seen the development of thousands of antitumor drugs, many of which have received approval. The pace of research and development in this field is commendable. Nonetheless, when compared to European and American countries, China faces a significant gap, especially in the variety of innovative antitumor drugs, which remains limited. To close this gap and achieve clinical breakthroughs, there is a critical need for independent innovation. This will require a thorough understanding of the latest global scientific advancements and the application of new technologies.

References

1. Yoshida T, Zhang G, Haura EB. Targeting epidermal growth factor receptor: central signaling kinase in lung cancer. Biochem Pharmacol. 2010;80:613–23.
2. Jänne PA, Engelman JA, Johnson BE. Epidermal growth factor receptor mutations in non-small-cell lung cancer: implications for treatment and tumor biology. J Clin Oncol. 2005;23:3227–34.
3. Yun CH, Boggon TJ, Li Y, et al. Structures of lung cancer-derived EGFR mutants and inhibitor complexes: mechanism of activation and insights into differential inhibitor sensitivity. Cancer Cell. 2007;11:217–27.
4. Bartholomew C, Eastlake L, Dunn P, et al. EGFR targeted therapy in lung cancer; an evolving story. Respir Med Case Rep. 2017;20:137–40.
5. Kazandjian D, Blumenthal GM, Yuan W, et al. FDA approval of gefitinib for the treatment of patients with metastatic EGFR mutation-positive non-small cell lung cancer. Clin Cancer Res. 2016;22:1307–12.

6. Thatcher N, Chang A, Parikh P, et al. Gefitinib plus best supportive care in previously treated patients with refractory advanced non-small-cell lung cancer: results from a randomised, placebo-controlled, multicentre study (Iressa survival evaluation in lung cancer). Lancet. 2005;366:1527–37.
7. Kim ES, Hirsh V, Mok T, et al. Gefitinib versus docetaxel in previously treated non-small-cell lung cancer (INTEREST): a randomised phase III trial. Lancet. 2008;372:1809–18.
8. Fukuoka M, Wu YL, Thongprasert S, et al. Biomarker analyses and final overall survival results from a phase III, randomized, open-label, first-line study of gefitinib versus carboplatin/paclitaxel in clinically selected patients with advanced non-small-cell lung cancer in Asia (IPASS). J Clin Oncol. 2011;29:2866–74.
9. Inoue A, Kobayashi K, Maemondo M, et al. Updated overall survival results from a randomized phase III trial comparing gefitinib with carboplatin-paclitaxel for chemo-naïve non-small cell lung cancer with sensitive EGFR gene mutations (NEJ002). Ann Oncol. 2013;24:54–9.
10. Mitsudomi T, Morita S, Yatabe Y, et al. Gefitinib versus cisplatin plus docetaxel in patients with non-small-cell lung cancer harbouring mutations of the epidermal growth factor receptor (WJTOG3405): an open label, randomised phase 3 trial. Lancet Oncol. 2010;11:121–8.
11. Zhou C, Wu YL, Chen G, et al. Erlotinib versus chemotherapy as first-line treatment for patients with advanced EGFR mutation-positive non-small-cell lung cancer (OPTIMAL, CTONG-0802): a multicentre, open-label, randomised, phase 3 study. Lancet Oncol. 2011;12:735–42.
12. Zhou C, Wu YL, Chen G, et al. Final overall survival results from a randomised, phase III study of erlotinib versus chemotherapy as first-line treatment of EGFR mutation-positive advanced non-small-cell lung cancer (OPTIMAL, CTONG-0802). Ann Oncol. 2015;26:1877–83.
13. Wu YL, Zhou C, Liam CK, et al. First-line erlotinib versus gemcitabine/cisplatin in patients with advanced EGFR mutation-positive non-small-cell lung cancer: analyses from the phase III, randomized, open-label. ENSURE study. Ann Oncol. 2015;26:1883–9.
14. Zhao Y, Liu J, Cai X, et al. Efficacy and safety of first line treatments for patients with advanced epidermal growth factor receptor mutated, non-small cell lung cancer: systematic review and network meta-analysis. BMJ. 2019;367:l5460.
15. Rosell R, Carcereny E, Gervais R, et al. Erlotinib versus standard chemotherapy as first-line treatment for European patients with advanced EGFR mutation-positive non-small-cell lung cancer (EURTAC): a multicentre, open-label, randomised phase 3 trial. Lancet Oncol. 2012;13:239–46.
16. Chen Y, Wang M, Zhong W, et al. Pharmacokinetic and pharmacodynamic study of gefitinib in a mouse model of non-small-cell lung carcinoma with brain metastasis. Lung Cancer. 2013;82:313–8.
17. Weber B, Winterdahl M, Memon A, et al. Erlotinib accumulation in brain metastases from non-small cell lung cancer: visualization by positron emission tomography in a patient harboring a mutation in the epidermal growth factor receptor. J Thorac Oncol. 2011;6:1287–9.
18. Kim JE, Lee DH, Choi Y, et al. Epidermal growth factor receptor tyrosine kinase inhibitors as a first-line therapy for never-smokers with adenocarcinoma of the lung having asymptomatic synchronous brain metastasis. Lung Cancer. 2009;65:351–4.
19. Park SJ, Kim HT, Lee DH, et al. Efficacy of epidermal growth factor receptor tyrosine kinase inhibitors for brain metastasis in non-small cell lung cancer patients harboring either exon 19 or 21 mutation. Lung Cancer. 2012;77:556–60.
20. Shi Y, Zhang L, Liu X, et al. Icotinib versus gefitinib in previously treated advanced non-small-cell lung cancer (ICOGEN): a randomised, double-blind phase 3 non-inferiority trial. Lancet Oncol. 2013;14:953–61.
21. Shi YK, Wang L, Han BH, et al. First-line icotinib versus cisplatin/pemetrexed plus pemetrexed maintenance therapy for patients with advanced EGFR mutation-positive lung adenocarcinoma (CONVINCE): a phase 3, open-label, randomized study. Ann Oncol. 2017;28:2443–50.

22. Gazdar AF. Activating and resistance mutations of EGFR in non-small-cell lung cancer: role in clinical response to EGFR tyrosine kinase inhibitors. Oncogene. 2009;28(Suppl 1):S24–31.
23. Engelman JA, Zejnullahu K, Mitsudomi T, et al. MET amplification leads to gefitinib resistance in lung cancer by activating ERBB3 signaling. Science. 2007;316:1039–43.
24. Popat S, Wotherspoon A, Nutting CM, et al. Transformation to "high grade" neuroendocrine carcinoma as an acquired drug resistance mechanism in EGFR-mutant lung adenocarcinoma. Lung Cancer. 2013;80:1–4.
25. Suda K, Tomizawa K, Fujii M, et al. Epithelial to mesenchymal transition in an epidermal growth factor receptor-mutant lung cancer cell line with acquired resistance to erlotinib. J Thorac Oncol. 2011;6:1152–61.
26. Metro G, Cappuzzo F. Emerging drugs for small-cell lung cancer. Expert Opin Emerg Drugs. 2009;14:591–606.
27. Solca F, Dahl G, Zoephel A, et al. Target binding properties and cellular activity of afatinib (BIBW 2992), an irreversible ErbB family blocker. J Pharmacol Exp Ther. 2012;343:342–50.
28. Karachaliou N, Molina-Vila MA, Rosell R. The impact of rare EGFR mutations on the treatment response of patients with non-small cell lung cancer. Expert Rev Respir Med. 2015;9:241–4.
29. Blakely CM, Watkins TBK, Wu W, et al. Evolution and clinical impact of co-occurring genetic alterations in advanced-stage EGFR-mutant lung cancers. Nat Genet. 2017;49:1693–704.
30. Engelman JA, Zejnullahu K, Gale CM, et al. PF00299804, an irreversible pan-ERBB inhibitor, is effective in lung cancer models with EGFR and ERBB2 mutations that are resistant to gefitinib. Cancer Res. 2007;67:11924–32.
31. Wu YL, Cheng Y, Zhou X, et al. Dacomitinib versus gefitinib as first-line treatment for patients with EGFR-mutation-positive non-small-cell lung cancer (ARCHER 1050): a randomised, open-label, phase 3 trial. Lancet Oncol. 2017;18:1454–66.
32. Mok TS, Cheng Y, Zhou X, et al. Improvement in overall survival in a randomized study that compared dacomitinib with gefitinib in patients with advanced non-small-cell lung cancer and EGFR-activating mutations. J Clin Oncol. 2018;36:2244–50.
33. Camidge DR, Pao W, Sequist LV. Acquired resistance to TKIs in solid tumours: learning from lung cancer. Nat Rev Clin Oncol. 2014;11:473–81.
34. Tripathi SK, Pandey K, Rengasamy KRR, et al. Recent updates on the resistance mechanisms to epidermal growth factor receptor tyrosine kinase inhibitors and resistance reversion strategies in lung cancer. Med Res Rev. 2020;40:2132–76.
35. Cross DA, Ashton SE, Ghiorghiu S, et al. AZD9291, an irreversible EGFR TKI, overcomes T790M-mediated resistance to EGFR inhibitors in lung cancer. Cancer Discov. 2014;4:1046–61.
36. Soria JC, Ohe Y, Vansteenkiste J, et al. Osimertinib in untreated EGFR-mutated advanced non-small-cell lung cancer. N Engl J Med. 2018;378:113–25.
37. Ramalingam SS, Vansteenkiste J, Planchard D, et al. Overall survival with osimertinib in untreated, EGFR-mutated advanced NSCLC. N Engl J Med. 2020;382:41–50.
38. Yang JC, Camidge DR, Yang CT, et al. Safety, efficacy, and pharmacokinetics of almonertinib (HS-10296) in pretreated patients with EGFR-mutated advanced NSCLC: a multicenter, open-label, phase 1 trial. J Thorac Oncol. 2020;15:1907–18.
39. Lu S, Dong X, Jian H, et al. AENEAS: a randomized phase III trial of aumolertinib versus gefitinib as first-line therapy for locally advanced or metastaticnon-small-cell lung cancer with EGFR exon 19 deletion or L858R mutations. J Clin Oncol. 2022;40:3162–71.
40. Shi Y, Zhang S, Hu X, et al. Safety, clinical activity, and pharmacokinetics of alflutinib (AST2818) in patients with advanced NSCLC with EGFR T790M mutation. J Thorac Oncol. 2020;15:1015–26.
41. Liu XY, Guo ZT, Chen ZD, et al. Alflutinib (AST2818), primarily metabolized by CYP3A4, is a potent CYP3A4 inducer. Acta Pharmacol Sin. 2020;41:1366–76.
42. Shi Y, Chen G, Wang X, et al. Furmonertinib (AST2818) versus gefitinib as first-line therapy for Chinese patients with locally advanced or metastatic EGFR mutation-positive non-small-

cell lung cancer (FURLONG): a multicentre, double-blind, randomised phase 3 study. Lancet Respir Med. 2022;10:1019–28.
43. Eno MS, Brubaker JD, Campbell JE, et al. Discovery of BLU-945, a reversible, potent, and wild-type-sparing next-generation EGFR mutant inhibitor for treatment-resistant non-small-cell lung cancer. J Med Chem. 2022;65:9662–77.
44. Topalian SL, Drake CG, Pardoll DM. Immune checkpoint blockade: a common denominator approach to cancer therapy. Cancer Cell. 2015;27:450–61.
45. Boussiotis VA. Molecular and biochemical aspects of the PD-1 checkpoint pathway. N Engl J Med. 2016;375:1767–78.
46. Tan S, Zhang H, Chai Y, et al. An unexpected N-terminal loop in PD-1 dominates binding by nivolumab. Nat Commun. 2017;8:14369.
47. Chen L. Co-inhibitory molecules of the B7-CD28 family in the control of T-cell immunity. Nat Rev Immunol. 2004;4:336–47.
48. Intlekofer AM, Thompson CB. At the bench: preclinical rationale for CTLA-4 and PD-1 blockade as cancer immunotherapy. J Leukoc Biol. 2013;94:25–39.
49. Lin DY, Tanaka Y, Iwasaki M, et al. The PD-1/PD-L1 complex resembles the antigen-binding Fv domains of antibodies and T cell receptors. Proc Natl Acad Sci USA. 2008;105:3011–6.
50. Lázár-Molnár E, Yan Q, Cao E, et al. Crystal structure of the complex between programmed death-1 (PD-1) and its ligand PD-L2. Proc Natl Acad Sci USA. 2008;105:10483–8.
51. Hui E, Cheung J, Zhu J, et al. T cell costimulatory receptor CD28 is a primary target for PD-1-mediated inhibition. Science. 2017;355:1428–33.
52. Perez HL, Cardarelli PM, Deshpande S, et al. Antibody-drug conjugates: current status and future directions. Drug Discov Today. 2014;19:869–81.
53. Postow MA. Managing immune checkpoint-blocking antibody side effects. Am Soc Clin Oncol Educ Book. 2015:76–83. https://doi.org/10.14694/EdBook_AM.2015.35.76.
54. Hu W, Wei H, Li K, et al. Downregulation of USP32 inhibits cell proliferation, migration and invasion in human small cell lung cancer. Cell Prolif. 2017;50:e12343.
55. Chen S, Lee LF, Fisher TS, et al. Combination of 4-1BB agonist and PD-1 antagonist promotes antitumor effector/memory CD8 T cells in a poorly immunogenic tumor model. Cancer Immunol Res. 2015;3:149–60.
56. Zhan MM, Hu XQ, Liu XX, et al. From monoclonal antibodies to small molecules: the development of inhibitors targeting the PD-1/PD-L1 pathway. Drug Discov Today. 2016;21:1027–36.
57. Chang HN, Liu BY, Qi YK, et al. Blocking of the PD-1/PD-L1 interaction by a D-peptide antagonist for cancer immunotherapy. Angew Chem Int Ed Engl. 2015;54:11760–4.
58. Li C, Zhang N, Zhou J, et al. Peptide blocking of PD-1/PD-L1 interaction for cancer immunotherapy. Cancer Immunol Res. 2018;6:178–88.
59. Hogg SJ, Vervoort SJ, Deswal S, et al. BET-bromodomain inhibitors engage the host immune system and regulate expression of the immune checkpoint ligand PD-L1. Cell Rep. 2017;18:2162–74.
60. Zhu H, Bengsch F, Svoronos N, et al. BET bromodomain inhibition promotes anti-tumor immunity by suppressing PD-L1 expression. Cell Rep. 2016;16:2829–37.
61. Fang W, Zhang J, Hong S, et al. EBV-driven LMP1 and IFN-γ up-regulate PD-L1 in nasopharyngeal carcinoma: implications for oncotargeted therapy. Oncotarget. 2014;5:12189–202.
62. Marzec M, Zhang Q, Goradia A, et al. Oncogenic kinase NPM/ALK induces through STAT3 expression of immunosuppressive protein CD274 (PD-L1, B7-H1). Proc Natl Acad Sci USA. 2008;105:20852–7.
63. Van Coillie S, Liang L, Zhang Y, et al. OncoBinder facilitates interpretation of proteomic interaction data by capturing coactivation pairs in cancer. Oncotarget. 2016;7:17608–15.
64. Juneja VR, McGuire KA, Manguso RT, et al. PD-L1 on tumor cells is sufficient for immune evasion in immunogenic tumors and inhibits CD8 T cell cytotoxicity. J Exp Med. 2017;214:895–904.
65. Li CW, Lim SO, Chung EM, et al. Eradication of triple-negative breast cancer cells by targeting glycosylated PD-L1. Cancer Cell. 2018;33:187–201.e10.

66. Amorim NA, da Silva EM, de Castro RO, et al. Interaction of HIV-1 Nef protein with the host protein Alix promotes lysosomal targeting of CD4 receptor. J Biol Chem. 2014;289:27744–56.
67. Zhai Q, Landesman MB, Robinson H, et al. Identification and structural characterization of the ALIX-binding late domains of simian immunodeficiency virus SIVmac239 and SIVagmTan-1. J Virol. 2011;85:632–7.
68. Wang H, Yao H, Li C, et al. HIP1R targets PD-L1 to lysosomal degradation to alter T cell-mediated cytotoxicity. Nat Chem Biol. 2019;15:42–50.

Chapter 6
Antibodies

Zhe Huang, Jingyi Li, and Miaomiao Zhang

Abstract Antibodies in cancer treatment have revolutionized therapy strategies, offering targeted, immune system-based strategies with a focus on precision. Monoclonal antibodies (mAbs), the most prevalent form, are lab-engineered molecules that mimic the immune system's ability to target cancer cells. These mAbs either directly bind to specific proteins on cancer cells or are conjugated with chemotherapy drugs or radioactive particles, selectively attacking cancer cells while sparing healthy tissue. Additionally, bispecific antibodies, capable of binding to two different targets, such as a cancer cell and a T cell, have emerged, enhancing the immune response against cancer. This shift toward antibody-based therapies signifies a move toward more personalized, effective cancer treatment, demonstrating significant progress in managing previously challenging cancer types and underscoring the growing importance of immunotherapy in cancer treatment.

Keywords Immunity · mAbs · Bispecific antibodies · Combination treatment

6.1 Immune System and Its Role in Cancer

The immune system is an intricate network comprising cells, tissues, and organs that collaborate to defend the body against infections and diseases. A pivotal function of this system is to detect and eradicate abnormal or compromised cells, including those that are cancerous. Nonetheless, cancer cells have developed a multitude of strategies to escape immune surveillance, thereby circumventing detection and destruction by the immune system. They can modify their surface antigens to avoid

Z. Huang (✉) · J. Li · M. Zhang
Department of Medical Oncology, Lung Cancer and Gastrointestinal Unit, Hunan Cancer Hospital/The Affiliated Cancer Hospital of Xiangya School of Medicine, Central South University, Changsha, China
e-mail: huangzhe@hnca.org.cn; e-mail: zhangmiaomiao@hnca.org.cn

© The Author(s), under exclusive license to Springer Nature Singapore Pte Ltd. 2024

Y. Zhang, N. Yang (eds.), *New Anti-cancer Drug Development and Evaluation*,
https://doi.org/10.1007/978-981-97-7274-2_6

recognition, create an immunosuppressive environment, or upregulate immune checkpoint proteins to inhibit an effective immune response [1].

Cancer cells can deploy several strategies to evade immune detection and destruction. One such strategy is to reduce the expression of major histocompatibility complex (MHC) molecules, which are essential for T cell recognition of cancer cells. Diminished MHC expression makes it more challenging for T cells to identify and attack cancer cells. Additionally, cancer cells can secrete immune checkpoint proteins like PD-L1, which bind to inhibitory receptors on T cells, leading to their inactivation. This deactivation of T cells allows cancer cells to avoid immune surveillance and proliferate unchecked. Furthermore, cancer cells may cultivate an immunosuppressive microenvironment by attracting and converting immune cells such as regulatory T cells (Tregs) and myeloid-derived suppressor cells (MDSCs), which suppress the activity of effector T cells and other immune components. This suppression prevents the immune system from recognizing and halting cancer growth and metastasis, further compromising its capacity to eradicate cancer cells.

The tumor microenvironment (TME) is a complex and dynamic entity that epitomizes the interplay between a tumor and the immune system [2]. It consists of cells, the extracellular matrix (ECM), signaling molecules, and physical factors that not only surround but also support tumor growth. This includes cancer cells, stromal cells, immune cells, blood vessels, and lymphatic vessels. The TME is instrumental in tumor initiation, progression, metastasis, and the response to therapy. Interactions between tumor cells and their surrounding microenvironment are bidirectional: cancer cells modify the composition and function of the TME, which in turn influences cancer cell behavior. Tumor-associated stromal cells, such as cancer-associated fibroblasts (CAFs), form a critical component of the TME by producing ECM, cytokines, and growth factors that facilitate tumor growth and angiogenesis. The immune cells within the TME—including T cells, B cells, natural killer (NK) cells, macrophages, and dendritic cells—are pivotal in curbing tumor growth and metastasis by identifying and destroying cancer cells. Nonetheless, tumors can subvert immune surveillance by fostering an immunosuppressive TME, thereby enhancing tumor growth and metastasis. Consequently, a thorough understanding of the intricate interactions between cancer cells and their microenvironment is vital for developing effective cancer treatments that target both the tumor cells and the TME.

The immune system plays a critical role in tumor development and progression. Consequently, there has been a concerted effort to devise therapies that target immune responses to fight cancer. Immunotherapy, a type of cancer treatment, leverages the immune system's capacity to recognize and eliminate cancer cells. It functions by either stimulating the immune system to directly attack cancer cells or by enhancing the immune response to them, thereby exerting antitumor effects. Immunotherapy includes various treatments such as monoclonal antibodies (mAbs), adoptive cell transfer therapy, cancer vaccines, and oncolytic viruses, each designed to strengthen the immune attack on cancer cells. Adoptive cell transfer therapy is a form of immunotherapy that involves extracting T cells from a patient's blood, engineering them to better identify and attack cancer cells, and then reinfusing them into the patient. This strategy has shown effectiveness in treating certain leukemias and lymphomas. Cancer vaccines, another immunotherapy approach, activate the immune system to target cancer cells. These vaccines can be composed of whole cancer cells, parts of cells, or specific cancer antigens, and are delivered via injections, oral administration, or nasal sprays. Oncolytic viruses also show promise in the realm of cancer immunotherapy. These specially designed viruses selectively replicate within and destroy cancer cells while sparing normal cells. Additionally, they can provoke immune responses against cancer, leading to enhanced tumor eradication and better patient outcomes.

Tumor cells can express ligands that bind to immune checkpoints on immune cells, triggering an inhibitory signal that can cause immune cells to undergo apoptosis or become dysfunctional, thus aiding in immune evasion [3]. mAbs are a form of immunotherapy designed to target specific molecules on the surface of cancer cells, including these immune checkpoints. By blocking these checkpoints, mAbs remove inhibitory signals, thereby enhancing the antitumor activity of immune cells and strengthening the immune response against cancer cells. Certain mAbs, such as cetuximab and bevacizumab, target intratumoral vessels instead of tumor or immune cells. Their action reduces intratumoral angiogenesis and normalizes neovascularization, contributing to antitumor effects [4].

6.2 Antibody and Its Biological Function

Antibodies are specialized proteins produced by B lymphocytes in response to antigens. When B lymphocytes differentiate and mature into plasma cells, they produce antigen-specific antibodies with diverse biological functions. Composed of two heavy chains and two light chains linked by disulfide bonds, antibodies have a Y-shaped structure. The variable regions at the tips of the Y bind specific antigens, while the constant region dictates the antibody's class and function [5]. There are five principal classes of antibodies: immunoglobulin A (IgA), immunoglobulin D (IgD), immunoglobulin E (IgE), immunoglobulin G (IgG), and immunoglobulin M (IgM), each with distinct biological roles. IgA antibodies are predominantly found in the mucosal linings of the respiratory, gastrointestinal, and genital tracts, serving as the first line of defense against pathogens. IgD antibodies, which exist on the surface of B lymphocytes, are instrumental in initiating immune responses. IgE antibodies play a key role in allergic reactions by causing the release of histamine and other inflammatory molecules. IgG antibodies are the most abundant in the bloodstream, providing long-term immunity against pathogens. Lastly, IgM antibodies are produced initially by the immune system during the early stages of an infection.

The functions of antibodies in organisms are multifaceted and vital, including:

1. Neutralization and prevention of pathogen invasion: Antibodies can participate in various antigen-antibody binding reactions both in vitro, facilitating antigen or antibody detection and functional assessment, and in vivo, where they neutralize toxins, block pathogen entry, and clear pathogenic microorganisms.

2. Complement activation: Upon binding to antigens, antibodies can activate the complement system via the classical pathway, leading to the formation of membrane attack complexes that lyse and destroy cells.
3. Facilitation of opsonophagocytosis and antibody-dependent cell-mediated cytotoxicity (ADCC): Opsonization involves the Fc segment of IgG antibodies attaching to Fc receptors on neutrophils and macrophages, thereby enhancing phagocytosis. ADCC involves cytotoxic cells, such as NK cells, recognizing the Fc segments of antibodies on target cell surfaces and mediating direct killing.
4. Mediation of Type I hypersensitivity: Antibodies are central to immediate allergic responses, binding to allergens and triggering the release of histamines and other inflammatory substances.
5. Transplacental transport: IgG is the sole antibody class capable of crossing the placental barrier, playing a crucial role in providing neonatal infection protection.
6. Secretory function of IgA: This antibody is important in the local immune defense of mucosal surfaces in the respiratory and digestive tracts.

Antibodies are essential for protecting the body against infections and diseases. Dysfunctions in antibody production or action can lead to significant health issues. For example, individuals with primary immunodeficiency disorders, such as agammaglobulinemia or common variable immunodeficiency, produce fewer antibodies, increasing their susceptibility to infections. Conversely, autoimmune diseases, such as lupus and rheumatoid arthritis, are characterized by an excessive immune response, resulting in antibodies mistakenly targeting the body's own tissues. Antibodies, as critical components of the immune system, offer protection against infectious diseases through their precise binding abilities. They can neutralize pathogens by preventing their entry into cells or by flagging them for elimination by other immune components. Each antibody class has distinct structural features and roles. Disruptions in antibody production or functioning can precipitate a range of health conditions. Therefore, understanding the function of antibodies is crucial for devising effective interventions for both infectious and autoimmune diseases.

6.3 Antibodies in Cancer Treatment

Antibodies serve as formidable agents in cancer treatment, offering distinct benefits over conventional chemotherapy and radiotherapy. They are designed to precisely target cancer cells, thereby minimizing collateral damage to healthy cells and tissues. Moreover, antibodies often exhibit an extended half-life within the body, facilitating sustained and focused assaults on cancerous cells. When used in conjunction with other therapies, such as chemotherapy or radiation, antibodies can significantly boost treatment efficacy [6]. Breast cancer treatment frequently employs antibody-based therapies, notably Herceptin (trastuzumab) for HER2-positive cases. Similarly, lung cancer therapies have incorporated antibodies such as nivolumab and pembrolizumab, which inhibit the PD-1 protein, thus bolstering the immune

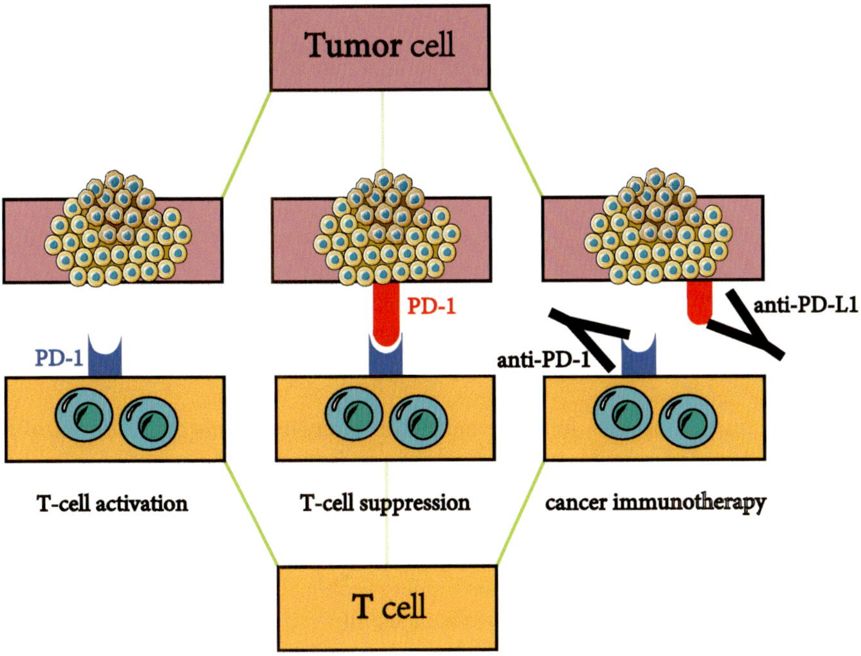

Fig. 6.1 Anti-PD1/L1 for cancer treatment

system's ability to detect and destroy cancer cells (Fig. 6.1). In hematologic malignancies, antibodies like rituximab target the CD20 protein on lymphoma cells. Additionally, blinatumomab uniquely binds to CD19 on B-cell leukemia and lymphomas as well as CD3 on T cells, orchestrating a concerted immune response against cancer cells. Bevacizumab, a monoclonal antibody used in colon cancer therapy, impedes the vascular endothelial growth factor (VEGF) protein, curtailing the tumor's blood supply and decelerating its growth. Continued research is unlocking new avenues and enhancing the application of antibodies in oncology. This progressive approach harbors the promise of advancing patient prognoses with treatments that are both more targeted and potentially less detrimental.

6.3.1 mAbs in Cancer Treatment

6.3.1.1 Introduction to mAbs

In 1975, Köhler and Milstein successfully fused myeloma cells with antibody-producing B lymphocytes to create hybridoma cells. These engineered cells are both stable and tumorigenic, with the remarkable ability to produce uniform antibodies directed against specific antigenic determinants. This pioneering technique, which enables the production of mAbs, has since become a cornerstone in the exploration of immunization and antibody-mediated technologies [7].

mAbs represent a significant leap forward in biotechnological applications, with widespread utilization in both scientific research and clinical practice. Their principal benefit lies in their high specificity, which allows for the precise targeting of select molecules or cells within the body. Such precision renders them indispensable in medical research, diagnostics, and therapeutic interventions.

In the realm of research, mAbs are instrumental in pinpointing and examining particular proteins or cellular components. Diagnostic applications include the detection of specific disease-associated biomarkers. Therapeutically, mAbs have shown considerable promise in immunotherapy, as they are capable of either activating or inhibiting the immune response to combat cancers and autoimmune disorders.

The production process for these antibodies typically entails the selection of a suitable antigen for immunization, administration into animals, harvesting of resultant antibodies, and meticulous screening to ensure specificity. Subsequent steps involve the isolation of B cells to establish hybridomas, which can then generate copious amounts of the target antibody. These antibodies undergo rigorous testing to validate their efficacy, specificity, and safety profile. The medical applications of mAbs are vast and diverse. They have the capability to directly engage cancer cells, marshal immune responses against malignancies, mitigate autoimmune conditions by obstructing particular immune components, and counteract specific pathogens.

Therefore, mAbs are a pivotal innovation in biotechnology and medicine. Their specificity, adaptability, and capacity for targeted treatment underpin their value in research and herald new possibilities for the development of advanced therapies for an array of diseases.

6.3.1.2 Mechanisms of Action for mAbs

Therapeutic antibodies aimed at tumor-associated antigens (TAAs) have the potential to eradicate tumor cells via multiple mechanisms. These include ADCC, complement-dependent cytotoxicity (CDC), antibody-dependent cellular phagocytosis (ADCP), and the direct induction of apoptosis by the antibodies themselves. Furthermore, mAbs can amplify antitumor responses by targeting immune checkpoints such as PD-L1 and cytotoxic T lymphocyte-associated antigen-4 (CTLA-4). This targeting can lead to a reduction in tumor proliferation or the mitigation of lymphocyte suppression, thus contributing to the overall antitumor effect [8].

6.3.1.3 mAbs in China

mAbs have revolutionized cancer treatment and are increasingly adopted as therapeutic options in China. These laboratory-produced proteins emulate the immune system's ability to specifically target cancer cells. The Chinese government's initiatives to enhance cancer therapies, coupled with the country's burgeoning biotechnology sector, have accelerated the development of mAbs. The first mAb approved for cancer treatment in China was bevacizumab, sanctioned by the China Food and Drug Administration (CFDA) in 2010. As a VEGF inhibitor, bevacizumab impedes angiogenesis, which is crucial for tumor growth, and is employed in treating colorectal cancer, non-small cell lung cancer (NSCLC), and renal cell carcinoma. Subsequent approvals include rituximab, trastuzumab, and cetuximab, which have demonstrated efficacy against non-Hodgkin's lymphoma, breast cancer, and head and neck cancer, respectively. A particularly promising area in the Chinese mAb sector is immune checkpoint inhibitors (ICIs). These target regulatory proteins like PD-1 and CTLA-4, which, while protecting normal cells, can also shield cancer cells from the immune response. PD-1 inhibitors, such as nivolumab and pembrolizumab, have yielded impressive results in clinical trials across various cancers.

In 2018, the CFDA approved camrelizumab, a PD-1 inhibitor for classical Hodgkin's lymphoma, marking the first cancer treatment mAb developed domestically. Additionally, bispecific antibodies, capable of targeting two antigens simultaneously, represent another exciting frontier in China's mAb research. Despite these advancements, challenges persist, notably the high costs of these therapies and a still-maturing regulatory landscape, which raise concerns about the quality and safety of some local mAbs. Nonetheless, the Chinese government is actively refining regulatory policies and fostering biotechnological innovation, paving the way for future progress in mAb therapy [9].

In conclusion, mAbs are set to play an increasingly vital role in cancer treatment both within China and globally. The continued evolution of domestically produced mAbs and the growth of the biotech industry in China are poised to spur further innovation and enhance patient access to these treatments. As research advances, mAbs are expected to become a cornerstone of cancer therapy (Fig. 6.2).

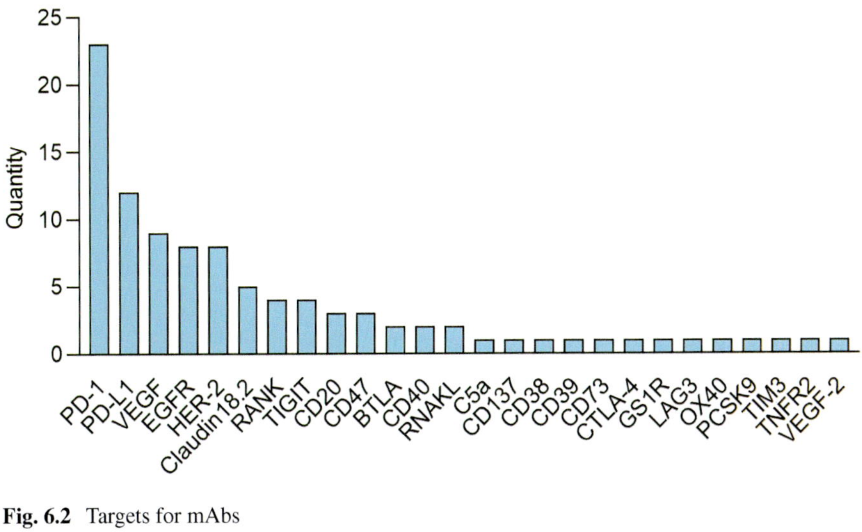

Fig. 6.2 Targets for mAbs

6.3.1.3.1 Sintilimab

On December 24, 2018, the CFDA granted marketing approval to sintilimab (trade name: Tyvyt) for the treatment of relapsed or refractory classical Hodgkin lymphoma in patients who had received at least two prior systemic chemotherapy regimens. This milestone marked the advent of an "era of innovation" in China's antitumor immunotherapy sector. By November 2019, sintilimab had become the sole PD-1 monoclonal antibody listed in the National Health Insurance Catalogue.

Sintilimab was officially launched in mainland China on February 22, 2019. It gained CFDA endorsement in February 2021 for use as a first-line treatment of non-squamous NSCLC, to be administered in conjunction with pemetrexed and platinum-based chemotherapy. Further expanding its therapeutic reach, in June 2021, sintilimab received approval from the State Drug Administration for the first-line treatment of advanced squamous NSCLC in combination with chemotherapy. Additionally, it was approved in combination with bevacizumab injection as a first-line treatment for unresectable or metastatic hepatocellular carcinoma (HCC) in patients who had not previously undergone systemic therapy [10].

In May 2021, the US Food and Drug Administration (FDA) officially accepted the first marketing application for a PD-1 anticancer drug from China. By August 2021, sintilimab, in combination with chemotherapy (oxaliplatin and capecitabine), reached the primary endpoint in an interim analysis of a randomized, double-blind, multicenter phase III clinical trial. This study evaluated its efficacy as a first-line treatment for patients with unresectable locally advanced, recurrent, or metastatic gastric or gastroesophageal junction adenocarcinoma.

Sintilimab, a novel PD-1 inhibitor, boasts global intellectual property rights and meets international quality standards, underscoring China's strides in the innovative drug sector, specifically in cancer immunotherapy. In China, sintilimab has garnered approval for six indications, encompassing lymphoma, liver cancer, gastric cancer, lung cancer, and esophageal cancer, distinguishing it as the sole PD-1 inhibitor sanctioned for first-line therapy across five prevalent tumor types. Furthermore, all approved indications of sintilimab have been integrated into the China National Health Insurance Catalogue, making it the only PD-1 immunotherapy drug approved for gastric cancer that is covered by health insurance.

6.3.2 Bispecific Antibodies for Cancer Treatment

6.3.2.1 Introduction to Bispecific Antibodies

Bispecific antibodies are synthetic molecules that amalgamate antigen recognition sites from two distinct antibodies, thus enabling simultaneous binding to diverse antigens or epitopes. Produced through chemical heteroconjugation, hybridoma technology, or recombinant DNA technology, these methods enhance the stability and reduce the immunogenicity of bispecific antibodies, bolstering their promise for clinical application [11].

In antitumor therapy, bispecific antibodies employ various mechanisms, such as recruiting T cells or NK cells to eliminate tumor cells, inhibiting multiple signal transduction pathways to curtail tumor growth, proliferation, and survival, and concurrently targeting multiple tumor antigens or epitopes to augment specificity and cytotoxic efficacy. Effective treatment with bispecific antibodies requires optimal pharmacokinetic (PK) properties, achievable through precise molecular modifications [12]. Overall, bispecific antibodies have great potential for improving cancer therapy and warrant further research and development.

6.3.2.2 Preparation and Classification

Natural antibodies are typically specific to a single antigen. While mAbs have been extensively used in cancer immunotherapy, their clinical efficacy often falls short of expectations due to drawbacks such as severe adverse reactions in many patients and the potential for developing resistance, leading to disease recurrence. Consequently, in recent years, the focus has shifted toward bispecific antibodies to address these challenges.

Bispecific antibodies, which do not occur naturally, must be intricately designed and synthesized using advanced techniques from biochemical, synthetic biology, and genetic engineering fields. Common production methods include chemically linking two different antibodies or antibody fragments, fusing two hybridoma cells that produce different antibodies to create dual hybridoma lines, and utilizing genetic engineering to restructure conventional antibodies into various formats.

Structurally, bispecific antibodies are categorized as either IgG-like or non-IgG-like. IgG-like bispecific antibodies comprise two antigen-binding Fab fragments and one Fc fragment, allowing them to target different antigens while maintaining Fc-mediated effector functions. Non-IgG-like bispecific antibodies, lacking the Fc segment, consist solely of Fab fragments, which results in a lower molecular weight, faster in vivo clearance, and improved tissue penetration.

The production process for IgG-like bispecific antibodies is well-established, with the Fc fragment enhancing solubility and stability during purification. Notable examples include Triomab, the "knobs-into-holes" technology, dual-variable domain Ig (DVD-Ig), and single-chain Fv (scFv) formats. On the other hand, non-IgG-like bispecific antibodies, such as dual-affinity re-targeting molecules (DARTs), nanobodies, and bivalent and bispecific T cell engagers (BiTEs), are prominent in this class.

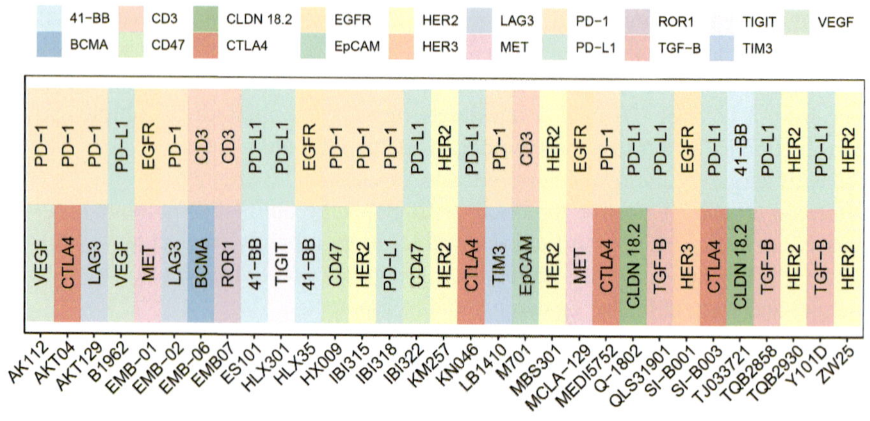

Fig. 6.3 Targets for bispecific antibodies

6.3.2.3 Bispecific Antibodies in China

We reviewed the clinical studies registered for bispecific antibodies on the clinical study website, focusing on those conducted in China and involving drugs developed and produced by Chinese enterprises. Our screening identified 30 bispecific antibody drugs (Fig. 6.3). In line with previous findings on mAbs, 19 of these drugs were bispecific, targeting PD-1 or PD-L1 along with another target. Additionally, eight drugs were found to target either EGFR or HER2, comprising about 30% of the total screened. Reflecting current trends in drug development, immune checkpoints continue to be a major focus of research, though the exploration of other targets is also progressing [13].

6.3.2.3.1 Candonilimab (AK104)

The 2022 American Society on Contemporary Ophthalmology (ASCO) conference abstracts, published on the official website, highlight the significant advancements in cervical cancer treatment with AK104. This innovative PD-1/CTLA-4 dual anti-AK104, used in conjunction with standard therapy, has shown remarkable efficacy in first-line cervical cancer treatment. In a study of 45 subjects across three subgroups, the objective response rate (ORR) ranged from 68.8% to 92.3%. The updated clinical data from ASCO 2022 underscored AK104's superior efficacy and reduced adverse effects compared to existing treatments. This drug is poised to be a groundbreaking addition to cancer immunotherapy, with a unique mechanism that preferentially targets tumor-infiltrating lymphocytes, thereby offering precise treatment with fewer side effects [14]. AK104 is notable for being the first PD-1-based bispecific antibody drug submitted for global marketing application and the first such drug independently developed in China. It received orphan drug designation from the US FDA for cervical cancer treatment. On September 24, 2021, China's National Medical Products Administration (NMPA) granted it priority review.

6.3.3 Antibody-Drug Conjugates (ADCs) for Cancer Treatment

6.3.3.1 Introduction to ADCs

In recent years, ADCs have rapidly grown to become a leading class of cancer therapeutics. Initially developed for hematologic cancers, ADCs have since expanded to target a variety of tumor types. Notably, innovative ADCs targeting HER2, such as Kadcyla and Enhertu, have delivered breakthrough results in the treatment of solid tumors, marking a significant advancement in the field. Furthermore, ADCs aimed at other molecular targets are showing promising outcomes in preclinical studies, indicating a broad potential for this therapeutic approach in diverse cancer types [15].

Since the US FDA approved the first ADC drug, gemtuzumab ozogamicin (Mylotarg), in 2000, a milestone in cancer therapy, the field has seen significant growth, with 14 ADCs now approved worldwide. Among these, vetuximab stands out as the first ADC independently developed and marketed by Chinese pharmaceutical companies, highlighting China's advancing capabilities in this area. Additionally, four internationally marketed ADCs—Adcetris, Kadcyla, Bessponsorsa, and Trodelvy—have also received approval for marketing in China, further expanding the range of treatments available to Chinese patients.

In regulatory advancements, the US FDA released a draft guideline titled "Considerations for Antibody-Conjugated Drug Development" in February 2022. This guideline aims to streamline the development process for ADCs. Similarly, the Center for Drug Evaluation (CDE) of the China NMPA has issued a draft of "Technical Guidelines for Non-clinical Studies of Antibody-conjugated Drugs." This move is indicative of a global effort to refine and enhance the research and development processes for ADCs, promising more efficient and effective therapies for cancer patients.

The safety and efficacy of ADCs, which are designed to deliver potent cytotoxic agents directly to cancer cells, are foundational principles in their development. However, there is potential toxicity associated with ADCs, primarily due to their binding to unintended or nonspecific sites in the blood, leading to off-target effects. Therefore, a key focus in the development of ADCs is conducting thorough metabolic studies. These studies are essential to understand the mechanisms of payload release and the metabolic pathways involved. Furthermore, exploring the construction core of ADCs is critical in enhancing their antitumor mechanisms and ensuring targeted delivery of the cytotoxic payload. Given the complex nature of these drugs, ongoing research and development are vital to optimize their safety and efficacy, ensuring they achieve their therapeutic potential with minimal adverse effects.

6.3.3.2 Construction of ADCs

The construction of ADCs involves three crucial components: an mAb, a linker, and a cytotoxic payload. The mAb, typically a humanized or fully human antibody, is designed to specifically target antigens on cancer cells. It is engineered for high affinity to the antigen, a long serum half-life, and low potential to trigger an immune response. Most ADCs use the IgG1 subtype of IgG antibodies due to its favorable properties for cancer targeting [16].

Linkers, which attach the cytotoxic payload to the mAb, are categorized as either cleavable or non-cleavable. This classification is based on how they release the payload within the cell, a crucial aspect for the drug's efficacy. The payloads are typically potent agents like tubulin inhibitors, DNA-damaging agents, or immunomodulators, chosen for their ability to effectively kill cancer cells.

The method of conjugation significantly influences an ADC's drug-to-antibody ratio (DAR), PK, pharmacodynamics (PD), and overall therapeutic index. Current conjugation methods include random conjugation, involving lysine or cysteine residue coupling, and site-directed conjugation. While random conjugation can result in heterogeneity and variable DAR in each batch, site-specific methods such as THIOMAB technology, enzyme-catalyzed coupling, and glycosylation coupling offer more uniformity in DAR, higher efficiency, better stability, and increased safety. These more consistent and predictable characteristics of site-directed conjugation can enhance the clinical effectiveness of ADCs.

6.3.3.3 Antitumor Mechanism of ADCs

ADCs are a targeted cancer treatment system that utilizes mAbs as carriers. These mAbs guide the ADCs to tumor sites, where they bind specifically to target antigens expressed on tumor cells or within the TME. The primary role of these mAbs is to deliver the cytotoxic small molecule drugs—the "warheads"—directly to the tumor cells [17].

The cytotoxic drugs are a pivotal component of ADCs, as the antitumor effect primarily depends on their ability to kill cancer cells. Linkers, another crucial element, attach these cytotoxic drugs to the mAbs. They provide stability, water solubility, and ensure the controlled release of the cytotoxic drugs at the tumor site. Once administered intravenously, ADCs circulate in the bloodstream and bind to antigens on tumor cells. They are typically internalized by the cells through a process known as clathrin-mediated endocytosis. Inside the tumor cells, ADCs are transported to lysosomes, where the cytotoxic drugs are released. These drugs then bind to key cellular components like DNA, RNA, and tubulin, disrupting vital processes such as replication or mitosis, leading to the destruction of the tumor cells. In addition to the cytotoxic action, ADCs can exploit the mAb's ability to block tumor cell receptor signaling pathways and leverage immune responses mediated by the antibody's Fc domain and the payload. This multifaceted approach enhances the overall efficacy of the treatment.

The success of an ADC hinges on the careful selection of its components: antibodies, target antigens, cytotoxins, linkers, and conjugation methods. Each element plays a vital role in ensuring that ADCs effectively target and destroy cancer cells while minimizing effects on healthy tissue.

6.3.3.4 ADCs in China

Numerous ADCs are currently under investigation in China, encompassing both preclinical and clinical studies. To compile data on ADC clinical trials conducted in China, we specifically selected ADCs that have been independently developed within the country. Among the 24 ADCs chosen for clinical study, the majority target HER-2, representing about 37.5% of the total (Fig. 6.4). Additionally, ADCs developed to target a range of other antigens have also been explored.

6.3.3.4.1 Disitamab

Disitamab vedotin, also known as RC48 and marketed as vetuximab (trade name: Edisec), is a pioneering ADC therapy targeting HER2-overexpressing cancer cells. It represents a significant advancement in targeted cancer treatment, combining an antibody with a cytotoxic drug to precisely attack cancer cells, such as those found in breast and gastric cancers [18]. The drug has shown promising efficacy in initial clinical trials for HER2-positive solid tumors and is currently undergoing further advanced-stage clinical trials.

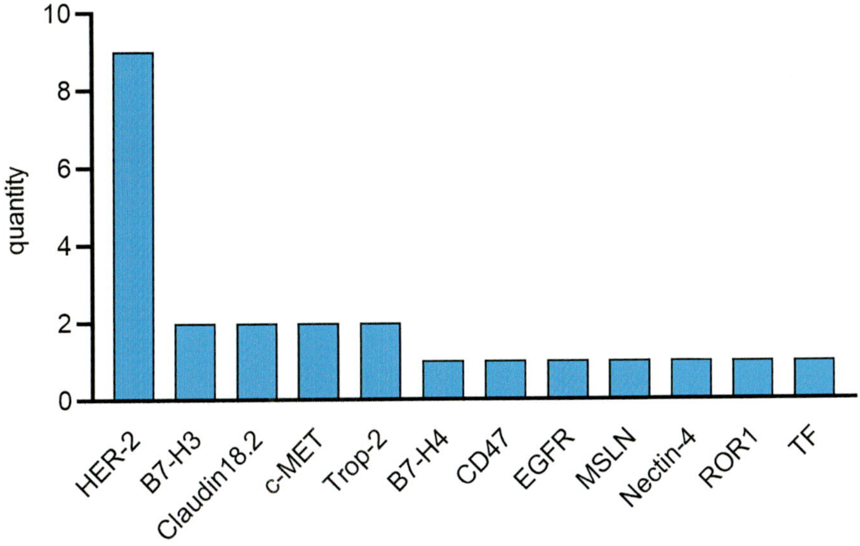

Fig. 6.4 Targets for ADCs

On June 9, 2021, the CFDA conditionally approved vetuximab for patients with locally advanced or metastatic gastric cancer, including gastroesophageal junction adenocarcinoma, who have undergone at least two systemic chemotherapies. This marked a milestone as RC48 was the first ADC drug to enter clinical studies in China. Its development involved advanced humanized antibodies with high affinity and efficient endocytosis, coupled with potent small molecule toxin drugs.

Vetuximab was officially launched in China on July 2, 2021. Professor Shi Yuankai highlighted its efficacy not only in gastric and breast cancer but also in tumors with low HER-2 expression. Expanding its therapeutic reach, on January 5, 2022, the NMPA approved vedetuximab for treating patients with urothelial cancer, marking another step forward in cancer treatment. Furthermore, Rongchang Biopharmaceutical (Yantai) Co., Ltd. announced the acceptance of a new drug clinical study application for vedetuximab combined with terriplumab for muscle-invasive bladder cancer (MIBC) by the NMPA, indicating ongoing research and potential new therapeutic applications. In summary, vedetuximab is a breakthrough in biopharmaceuticals targeting HER2-overexpressing tumors, showing significant efficacy in gastric, breast, and urothelial cancers. Its development and successive approvals underscore China's progress in the field of targeted cancer therapy, with promising implications for future patient treatment.

6.3.4 ICIs for Cancer Treatment

6.3.4.1 Introduction to ICIs

In recent years, there has been remarkable progress in cancer treatment, particularly with the advancement of ICIs. These medications work by blocking the signals cancer cells use to evade the immune system, allowing the body's natural defense mechanisms to target and destroy cancer cells. The first immune checkpoint inhibitor, ipilimumab, was approved by the US FDA in 2011 for treating metastatic melanoma. Since then, several other checkpoint inhibitors, such as pembrolizumab and nivolumab, have been approved for various cancers, including lung, kidney, and bladder cancer.

The development of ICIs in China began in the early 2000s. Researchers first identified the PD-1 checkpoint as a promising cancer treatment target. PD-1 is a protein that helps regulate the immune system, but cancer cells can hijack this process by producing ligands that bind to PD-1 and turn off immune responses. Researchers at Peking University were among the first to discover this mechanism and to develop drugs that block the interaction between PD-1 and its ligands, reactivating the immune system against cancer cells.

In 2018, China became the first country to approve a PD-1 inhibitor for cancer treatment. The drug, sintilimab [19], developed by Innovent Biologics, has been effective in treating several cancer types, including lung, liver, and esophageal cancer. Since then, other PD-1 inhibitors, such as toripalimab, camrelizumab, and tislelizumab, have been approved in China.

Besides PD-1 inhibitors, Chinese scientists are developing drugs targeting other immune checkpoints, such as CTLA-4 and lymphocyte activation gene-3 (LAG-3). CTLA-4 is another protein that cancer cells use to evade the immune system, and blocking it has been effective in treating melanoma and other cancers. LAG-3, a protein that can suppress T cell function, has shown promise in early clinical trials for various cancers.

Cadonilimab (AK104) [14], the first domestically approved bispecific antibody, is also the world's first PD-1/CTLA-4 bispecific antibody. It's a symmetric, tetravalent bispecific antibody with an Fc-null design. Cadonilimab works by concurrently blocking the PD-1 and CTLA-4 immune checkpoint pathways, indirectly freeing and activating immune cells, thus enhancing antitumor effects.

The large patient population in China provides ample opportunities for clinical trials of these drugs. Chinese researchers have conducted trials in various cancers, including lung, liver, and gastric cancer, showing significant improvements in patients' survival rates. Another advantage is China's relatively low cost of drug development. Compared to the US and Europe, China has lower labor costs and a less burdensome regulatory environment, fostering a boom in biotech companies like BeiGene, Innovent, and Junshi Biosciences, which develop and produce ICIs.

However, challenges remain. Gaining acceptance from the global medical community, particularly in the United States and Europe, is crucial. Chinese companies must demonstrate their drugs' safety and effectiveness in rigorous clinical trials and gain approval from the US FDA and the European Medicines Agency to enter these markets. Another challenge is protecting intellectual property. Many ICIs developed in China are based on technologies first discovered in the West. Navigating the complex landscape of patent law and intellectual property rights is essential to avoid legal disputes and ensure profitability.

6.3.4.2 Mechanisms of Action for ICIs

ICIs have become increasingly important in treating various cancers, working through several key mechanisms involving T cells, antigen-presenting cells (APCs), and cytokines. These drugs target complex signaling pathways and interactions within the immune system to enhance the body's antitumor response.

One primary mechanism of ICIs is the blockade of the PD-1 pathway. PD-1, a receptor on T cells, interacts with PD-L1 and PD-L2 on cancer and immune cells. This interaction typically reduces T cell activity, suppressing the immune response against cancer. ICIs like pembrolizumab and nivolumab block this interaction, reactivating T cells to attack cancer cells. Another key mechanism involves inhibiting the CTLA-4 pathway. CTLA-4, expressed on T cells, interacts with CD80 and CD86 on APCs, similarly dampening the immune response. ICIs targeting CTLA-4, such as ipilimumab [20], prevent this interaction, boosting T cell activity against cancer.

ICIs also affect other immune cells in the TME. For instance, they can reduce the number of Tregs, which are known for suppressing other immune cells. By decreasing Tregs, drugs like ipilimumab allow for more robust T cell activation. Additionally, ICIs modulate cytokines, which are immune signaling molecules. Some ICIs increase pro-inflammatory cytokines like IL-2, enhancing T cell efficacy, while others target immune-suppressive cells like MDSCs and tumor-associated macrophages (TAMs) to amplify the immune response. Moreover, ICIs can enhance the effects of traditional cancer treatments like chemotherapy and radiation therapy. These treatments release tumor antigens, triggering an immune response, but they can also harm immune cells. ICIs can amplify the immune system's response to these released antigens, improving overall treatment efficacy.

ICIs work through various mechanisms, including blocking immune checkpoints like PD-1 and CTLA-4, modulating immune cells and cytokines in the tumor environment, and enhancing traditional cancer therapies. These complex interactions underscore the significance of ICIs in cancer treatment.

6.3.4.3 The Rationale for Combining Different Antibodies for Cancer Treatment

One promising approach to improving cancer treatment involves combining different antibodies that target various aspects of the TME. Antibodies, as immune proteins, can recognize and bind to specific targets on cancer or immune cells, thereby influencing cell growth, survival, and immune responses. Some can also recruit immune cells, such as T cells and NK cells, to directly or indirectly attack cancer cells.

The rationale for using different antibody combinations is multifaceted. Firstly, cancer cells often evade immune surveillance through immunosuppressive cells and molecules in their microenvironment. Different antibodies targeting various immune checkpoints or pathways can enhance the immune response against cancer. For instance, combining anti-PD-1 and anti-CTLA-4 antibodies has been effective in treating melanoma and other solid tumors [21].

Secondly, cancer cells can develop resistance to targeted therapies, such as tyrosine kinase inhibitors (TKIs), through mutations, activation of alternative pathways, or increased drug efflux. Combining antibodies that target different pathways can overcome these resistances. A notable example is the combination of trastuzumab (anti-HER2) and pertuzumab (anti-HER3) in HER2-positive breast cancer, which improves response rates in patients resistant to trastuzumab alone.

Thirdly, combining antibodies can result in synergistic effects, enhancing efficacy and reducing toxicity. For example, bevacizumab [22] (anti-VEGF) combined with cetuximab [23] (anti-EGFR) has shown increased antitumor activity and reduced toxicity in metastatic colorectal cancer. This synergy may arise from their complementary effects on tumor angiogenesis and immune evasion. However, this approach presents challenges, such as increased toxicity, complex dosing and administration, and high costs of development and production. PK and PD interactions in combined therapies can also affect efficacy and safety.

Finally, combination therapy with different antibodies can address tumor heterogeneity and complexity. Tumors exhibit a range of genetic and epigenetic alterations, express various antigens, and activate different signaling pathways. A cocktail of antibodies targeting multiple targets increases the likelihood of addressing all relevant cancer cells, potentially reducing the risk of relapse or progression.

6.3.4.4 Examples of ICIs in Cancer Treatment

In recent years, the clinical application of drugs in cancer treatment has been significantly influenced by factors such as indications, safety, efficacy, and, notably, accessibility. This is particularly evident in the context of ICIs in China. For instance, toripalimab, the first domestic PD-1 monoclonal antibody, has been approved for six indications, including melanoma, urothelial cancer, and recurrent/metastatic nasopharyngeal carcinoma (R/M NPC) [24], with three covered by health insurance. Similarly, camrelizumab, targeting PD-1, treats eight cancer types, including NSCLC [25] and esophageal squamous cell carcinoma (ESCC), all under health insurance coverage.

Sugemalimab, which targets PD-L1, is notable for its effect on NSCLC. The GEMSTONE-301 study showed that sugemalimab significantly improves progression-free survival (PFS) in unresectable stage III NSCLC patients post-chemoradiotherapy, with a 35% reduction in disease progression or death risk [26].

Adebrelimab, a domestically developed PD-L1 inhibitor, is used for extensive-stage small cell lung cancer (ES-SCLC) as a first-line therapy in combination with carboplatin and etoposide. The CAPSTONE-1 study demonstrated its efficacy, with a 15.3-month overall survival (OS) improvement and a 31.3% 2-year survival rate [27].

Cadonilimab, the world's first PD-1/CTLA-4 bispecific antibody and the first in China, shows four advantages: blocking both PD-1 and CTLA-4 pathways; an optimized Fc segment to avoid adverse immune reactions; enhanced stability and reduced protein residue; and strong antitumor activity, particularly in advanced cervical cancer.

CTLA-4 inhibitors, still under research, face challenges like limited response rates and resistance in monotherapy for solid tumors. Future research may focus on combining CTLA-4 mAbs with PD-1/PD-L1 drugs and chemotherapy or developing dual-target CTLA-4/PD-(L)1 antibodies to provide more effective and safer treatment options. These developments in ICIs highlight the progress in cancer treatment in China, with a focus on improving accessibility for patients who previously could not afford such advanced therapies.

6.4 Examples of Combination Therapies for Cancer Treatment

Combination therapy, involving the use of multiple drugs or treatment modalities, has become increasingly prevalent in cancer treatment. This approach is particularly effective because it targets cancer cells through various mechanisms, thereby enhancing the chances of successful treatment. Among the successful strategies is the combination of chemotherapy with immunotherapy.

Chemotherapy, which utilizes drugs to destroy rapidly dividing cancer cells, has been a cornerstone of cancer treatment. On the other hand, immunotherapy aims to harness and activate the body's immune system to recognize and attack cancer cells. Recent research has shown that when used together, chemotherapy and immunotherapy can work synergistically to improve outcomes in cancer patients. Chemotherapy can also induce immunogenic cell death, a process in which dying cancer cells release signals that alert and activate the immune system. Drugs such as anthracyclines, oxaliplatin, and mitoxantrone are known to trigger this effect, enhancing the immune response facilitated by immunotherapy.

Moreover, chemotherapy can modulate the TME [28], a complex network around cancer cells that influences cancer progression and treatment response. By reducing immune-suppressive elements within the TME, such as Tregs and MDSCs, chemotherapy creates a more conducive environment for immunotherapy. Additionally, chemotherapy can increase the expression of tumor-associated antigens on cancer cells, making them more recognizable to the immune system. This increased visibility aids immunotherapy in targeting and eliminating cancer cells.

Finally, chemotherapy contributes to the development of memory T cells, a type of immune cell that retains the "memory" of cancer antigens. These cells provide long-term surveillance and protection against cancer recurrence, thereby enhancing the sustained effectiveness of immunotherapy. The combination of chemotherapy and immunotherapy represents a powerful approach to cancer treatment. By employing multiple mechanisms, this combination offers a more comprehensive and effective strategy against cancer, potentially improving patient outcomes significantly.

Nasopharyngeal carcinoma, with the highest incidence in Southern China, poses significant challenges in cancer treatment. Patients in the early and middle stages often achieve favorable outcomes with radiotherapy alone or concurrent chemoradiotherapy, boasting a 5-year OS rate of up to 90%. However, in cases of recurrence and metastasis, the 5-year survival rate drops dramatically to 20–40%, necessitating a more comprehensive treatment approach. One successful strategy in cancer treatment is combining chemotherapy and immunotherapy. In particular, for nasopharyngeal carcinoma, recent studies such as JUPITER-02, CAPTAIN-1st [29], and RATIONALE-309 [30] have demonstrated the efficacy of combining immunotherapy with chemotherapy, marking a significant shift in treatment paradigms. However, immunotherapy has its limitations, with only 10–30% of patients responding to ICIs. This limited response is intricately linked to the complex nature of cancer cells, the immune system, and the TME.

The PACIFIC trial, a phase III clinical study, illustrates the effectiveness of combining the PD-L1 monoclonal antibody durvalumab with chemoradiotherapy in treating inoperable stage III NSCLC. This combination therapy has now become the first-line standard regimen for such patients, as recommended by the National Comprehensive Cancer Network (NCCN) guidelines in the United States and endorsed by the European Society for Medical Oncology (ESMO) and the Chinese Society of Clinical Oncology (CSCO) guidelines.

Another successful approach is the combination of radiotherapy with immunotherapy. Radiotherapy, which uses high-energy radiation to target cancer cells, has the added benefit of exposing tumor antigens, thereby facilitating in situ vaccine production that can enhance tumor antigen presentation. This process not only helps reverse immunosuppressive factors in the TME but also synergizes with immunotherapy. For example, radiotherapy can counteract resistance to immunotherapy by reshaping the TME and reactivating the suppressed immune microenvironment, thereby boosting the effectiveness of immunotherapy. However, the use of radiotherapy is not without its challenges. It can cause long-term and irreversible side effects, including damage to healthy tissues near the tumor. Therefore, it is crucial to carefully consider the potential benefits and risks of radiotherapy, tailored to each patient's unique circumstances. In short, the treatment of nasopharyngeal carcinoma in China involves a multifaceted approach, leveraging the strengths of both radiotherapy and immunotherapy, while also addressing their respective challenges and limitations.

In 1953, the discovery of the "abscopal effect" [31] from radiotherapy highlighted a phenomenon where localized radiation could trigger regression in distant, nonirradiated lesions, illustrating the immunomodulatory impact of radiotherapy. While clinically observed cases of the abscopal effect are rare, radiotherapy invariably induces molecular and genetic changes, such as the release of cancer cell antigens and damage-associated molecular patterns (DAMPs). These changes, occurring in the irradiated area, are crucial for activating a systemic immune response, with cytokines and chemokines playing a significant role.

It's notable that low-dose radiotherapy, which does not primarily aim to kill cancer cells, may be more effective in modulating the immune microenvironment and reducing the immunosuppression often associated with high-dose radiotherapy, thereby complementing immunotherapy.

The effectiveness and safety of immune checkpoint radiotherapy (iRT) depend on several factors:

1. Dose and fractionation of radiotherapy: The immune response modulation by radiotherapy is dose-dependent within a certain range.
2. Irradiation site: Studies indicate that radiation exposure to metastases at different sites can variably affect the systemic immune response.
3. Timing of radiotherapy: A major debate in the field is whether to administer immunotherapy and radiotherapy sequentially or concurrently. The PACIFIC study's immune consolidation model, involving chemoradiotherapy followed by immunotherapy, was successful but showed a relatively high incidence of pneu-

monia in sequentially treated patients. Some patients also struggled with tolerating subsequent immuno-maintenance therapy. Conversely, studies like KEYNOTE-799 [32] suggest that concurrent administration of immunotherapy and radiotherapy may enhance efficacy with a safety profile comparable to sequential therapy. This approach has garnered significant interest in recent clinical research.

One notable study led by Professor You Lu's team introduces a novel triple therapy mode for treating tumors. This approach combines in-situ hypofractionated radiotherapy, low-dose radiotherapy for distant tumors, and ICIs. In their study using a mouse model, this triple therapy resulted in significant control of distant tumor growth, with five out of nine mice achieving complete remission. The mechanism involves hypofractionated radiotherapy inducing tumor cell apoptosis, exposing tumor-specific antigens for "in situ vaccination," and sensitizing tumor-specific T cells. Low-dose radiotherapy facilitates the migration of these T cells into distant tumors and modulates the immune microenvironment. PD-1 inhibitors then enhance T cell activity by releasing inhibitory controls, amplifying the systemic antitumor effect [33].

Another successful strategy is the combination of targeted therapy and immunotherapy. Unlike immunotherapy, which primarily stimulates the immune system to fight cancer, targeted therapy focuses on specific molecules and pathways essential for cancer cell growth and spread. In the context of HCC, drugs like sorafenib, lenvatinib, and the antiangiogenic monoclonal antibody bevacizumab have been approved for use. They are often combined with ICIs such as atezolizumab and pembrolizumab.

The ORIENT-32 study [34], a phase III clinical trial for HCC treatment, exemplifies this approach. It compared the efficacy of sintilimab plus a bevacizumab biosimilar against sorafenib monotherapy in unresectable HCC patients. The study demonstrated significantly better OS and PFS in the combination group, leading to its approval as a first-line treatment for unresectable or metastatic HCC in China on June 25, 2021.

In conclusion, these combination therapies, leveraging different treatment modalities, have shown improved response rates, PFS, and OS compared to monotherapy. They represent a promising direction in cancer treatment, with the potential to significantly enhance patient outcomes through continued research and development.

6.5 Challenges and Outlook

Antibody therapy has shown significant promise in cancer treatment, yet several challenges and limitations require attention. A primary issue is the development of resistance to antibody therapy. The complexity of the TME can suppress immune responses, limiting the efficacy of checkpoint inhibitors. Tumors may activate alternative immune evasion pathways or undergo genetic changes, diminishing their susceptibility to immune attack. Combining checkpoint inhibitors with other cancer therapies, such as targeted therapies or chemotherapy, has emerged as a potential solution. These combinations can enhance antitumor effects and overcome resistance by inducing immunogenic cell death and facilitating tumor antigen release. The effectiveness and safety of these therapies also hinge on identifying reliable biomarkers. Current markers like tumor mutational burden and PD-L1 expression offer limited predictive value. Given the high cost of these drugs and their potential for severe immune-related adverse events, better biomarkers are urgently needed. Cost is another significant barrier. Antibodies are complex to develop and manufacture, resulting in high costs transferred to patients. In China, only a limited number of PD-1, PD-L1, and bispecific antibodies are included in the National Health Insurance Directory, impacting accessibility.

Side effects present additional challenges. Camrelizumab, a checkpoint inhibitor in China, can cause adverse reactions, including autoimmune responses, fatigue, nausea, diarrhea, and serious skin reactions [35]. These side effects necessitate close monitoring and can complicate treatment decisions. Furthermore, antibodies may not be universally effective across all cancer types. Some cancers lack the target antigen or develop resistance to antibody therapy, reducing therapeutic efficacy. The development of new antibodies is a lengthy and expensive process, often requiring years and substantial financial investment, with no guaranteed success.

While antibody therapy offers promising avenues in cancer treatment, addressing these challenges is crucial for improving effectiveness and patient accessibility. Future developments, including new generations of checkpoint inhibitors with improved properties and the discovery of novel immune targets, may enhance the antitumor activity of these drugs. Another challenge in using antibodies for cancer treatment is the potential for side effects. Antibodies can cause a range of adverse reactions, including infusion-related reactions, hypersensitivity reactions, and autoimmune reactions.

Recent advancements in antibody-based cancer therapies have underscored their potential as a powerful form of immunotherapy. However, challenges such as tumor resistance and variable efficacy among patients necessitate further research to enhance their effectiveness.

One promising direction is the development of more specific and potent antibodies. By targeting tumor-specific antigens, these therapies can minimize damage to healthy tissues while effectively combating cancer cells. Additionally, more potent antibodies could significantly improve clinical responses by efficiently destroying cancer cells.

Combination treatments also hold great promise. By simultaneously targeting various pathways or mechanisms, these combinations could overcome tumor resistance and boost therapeutic responses. For instance, integrating antibody-based therapy with chemotherapy or radiation might sensitize tumors to treatment. Similarly, combining checkpoint inhibitors with antibodies targeting specific cancer cell markers could yield improved outcomes. The development of bispecific antibodies, capable of binding to both cancer and immune cells, is another exciting area of exploration.

Personalized treatment strategies, based on specific biomarkers or genetic profiles, represent another important avenue. Identifying patients likely to respond to certain therapies can optimize treatment effectiveness and reduce unnecessary exposure to potentially ineffective drugs.

Enhancing the delivery of antibody-based therapies to tumor sites is also crucial. Innovations like nanoparticles and targeted delivery systems promise to direct therapies more precisely to cancer cells, sparing healthy tissue. Techniques such as the use of microbubbles or light-activated therapies could further improve targeted delivery.

Understanding and overcoming tumor resistance remains a critical challenge. Research into combination therapies and adaptive strategies is key to addressing resistance. By targeting multiple resistance pathways or adjusting treatments based on changes in the TME, the efficacy of antibody-based therapies can be significantly improved. While antibody-based cancer therapies have shown considerable promise, overcoming their current limitations through more targeted, potent, and personalized strategies is essential for maximizing their therapeutic potential.

6.6 Conclusion

China has emerged as a significant player in the global market for antibody-based cancer therapies, driven by its aging population and a surge in cancer diagnoses. This has spurred extensive research and development, particularly by Chinese companies focusing on novel antibody-based therapies for a range of cancers. Contributing factors include rising disposable incomes and improvements in healthcare infrastructure, which have boosted demand for innovative cancer treatments.

Among the most notable advancements is the development of bispecific antibodies. These innovative therapies, such as cadonilimab and Keynote-046, target two different cancer cell proteins simultaneously, potentially enhancing efficacy and reducing drug resistance. Cadonilimab, developed by Akeso, is a novel PD-1/CTLA-4 bispecific tumor immunotherapy drug, while Keynote-046 [36], developed by Corning Jereh, is a PD-L1/CTLA-4 bispecific antibody undergoing clinical trials for various tumor types.

However, the rapid expansion of clinical trials in China has raised concerns about their quality, particularly in terms of patient safety and data integrity. To address these challenges, there is a pressing need to improve the quality of these trials.

The Chinese government has provided support for the development of these therapies, as evidenced by the NMPA's approval of the first antibody-based cancer therapy developed by a Chinese company in 2018. This marked a major milestone for the industry. Another significant challenge is the high cost of these treatments. Many patients in China cannot afford these therapies, prompting government actions such as the 2018 launch of a national medical insurance program covering some high-cost cancer treatments, including antibody-based therapies.

The Chinese pharmaceutical industry also faces the challenge of market homogenization. The lack of differentiation in drug development poses difficulties for companies trying to stand out. Addressing this requires a shift in research and development strategies, focusing on patient-oriented designs and a willingness to pursue unconventional approaches.

Despite these challenges, the prospects for antibody-based cancer therapies in China remain positive. With a large market for cancer treatments and increasing investment in innovative therapies, coupled with the NMPA's growing list of approved treatments, the cost of these therapies is expected to decrease, making them more accessible to patients. The future of antibody-based cancer therapies in China looks promising, with potential for significant advancements in the treatment of various cancers.

References

1. Parkin J, Cohen B. An overview of the immune system. Lancet. 2001;357:1777–89.
2. Hinshaw DC, Shevde LA. The tumor microenvironment innately modulates cancer progression. Cancer Res. 2019;79:4557–66.
3. Jiang X, Wang J, Deng X, et al. Role of the tumor microenvironment in PD-L1/PD-1-mediated tumor immune escape. Mol Cancer. 2019;18:10.
4. Fu Z, Li S, Han S, et al. Antibody drug conjugate: the "biological missile" for targeted cancer therapy. Signal Transduct Target Ther. 2022;7:93.
5. Schroeder HW Jr, Cavacini L. Structure and function of immunoglobulins. J Allergy Clin Immunol. 2010;125:S41–52.
6. Chen W, Yuan Y, Jiang X. Antibody and antibody fragments for cancer immunotherapy. J Control Release. 2020;328:395–406.
7. Alejandra WP, Miriam Irene JP, Fabio Antonio GS, et al. Production of monoclonal antibodies for therapeutic purposes: a review. Int Immunopharmacol. 2023;120:110376.
8. Tsao LC, Force J, Hartman ZC. Mechanisms of therapeutic antitumor monoclonal antibodies. Cancer Res. 2021;81:4641–51.
9. Liu JW, Yang YH, Wu N, et al. Biosimilar monoclonal antibodies in China: a patent review. Bioengineered. 2022;13:14503–18.
10. Lu Z, Wang J, Shu Y, et al. Sintilimab versus placebo in combination with chemotherapy as first line treatment for locally advanced or metastatic oesophageal squamous cell carcinoma (ORIENT-15): multicentre, randomised, double blind, phase 3 trial. BMJ. 2022;377:e068714.
11. Shim H. Bispecific antibodies and antibody-drug conjugates for cancer therapy: technological considerations. Biomol Ther. 2020;10:4764.
12. Wei J, Yang Y, Wang G, et al. Current landscape and future directions of bispecific antibodies in cancer immunotherapy. Front Immunol. 2022;13:1035276.
13. Zhang J, Yi J, Zhou P. Development of bispecific antibodies in China: overview and prospects. Antib Ther. 2020;3:126–45.
14. Pang X, Huang Z, Zhong T, et al. Cadonilimab, a tetravalent PD-1/CTLA-4 bispecific antibody with trans-binding and enhanced target binding avidity. MAbs. 2023;15:2180794.
15. Hafeez U, Parakh S, Gan HK, et al. Antibody-drug conjugates for cancer therapy. Molecules. 2020;25:4764.

16. Baah S, Laws M, Rahman KM. Antibody-drug conjugates-a tutorial review. Molecules. 2021;26:2943.
17. Chau CH, Steeg PS, Figg WD. Antibody-drug conjugates for cancer. Lancet. 2019;394:793–804.
18. Shi F, Liu Y, Zhou X, et al. Disitamab vedotin: a novel antibody-drug conjugates for cancer therapy. Drug Deliv. 2022;29:1335–44.
19. Shi Y, Wu L, Yu X, et al. RETRACTED: ORIENT-3: a randomized, open-label, phase III study of sintilimab versus docetaxel in previously treated advanced/metastatic squamous non-small cell lung cancer (sqNSCLC). Ann Oncol. 2020;31(Suppl 7):S1428.
20. Rohaan MW, Borch TH, van den Berg JH, et al. Tumor-infiltrating lymphocyte therapy or ipilimumab in advanced melanoma. N Engl J Med. 2022;387:2113–25.
21. Gide TN, Quek C, Menzies AM, et al. Distinct immune cell populations define response to anti-PD-1 monotherapy and anti-PD-1/anti-CTLA-4 combined therapy. Cancer Cell. 2019;35:238–255 e6.
22. Prager GW, Taieb J, Fakih M, et al. Trifluridine-tipiracil and bevacizumab in refractory metastatic colorectal cancer. N Engl J Med. 2023;388:1657–67.
23. Tabernero J, Grothey A, Van Cutsem E, et al. Encorafenib plus cetuximab as a new standard of care for previously treated BRAF V600E-mutant metastatic colorectal cancer: updated survival results and subgroup analyses from the BEACON study. J Clin Oncol. 2021;39:273–84.
24. Wang FH, Wei XL, Feng J, et al. Efficacy, safety, and correlative biomarkers of toripalimab in previously treated recurrent or metastatic nasopharyngeal carcinoma: a phase II clinical trial (POLARIS-02). J Clin Oncol. 2021;39:704–12.
25. Zhou C, Chen G, Huang Y, et al. Camrelizumab plus carboplatin and pemetrexed versus chemotherapy alone in chemotherapy-naive patients with advanced non-squamous non-small-cell lung cancer (CameL): a randomised, open-label, multicentre, phase 3 trial. Lancet Respir Med. 2021;9:305–14.
26. Zhou Q, Chen M, Jiang O, et al. Sugemalimab versus placebo after concurrent or sequential chemoradiotherapy in patients with locally advanced, unresectable, stage III non-small-cell lung cancer in China (GEMSTONE-301): interim results of a randomised, double-blind, multicentre, phase 3 trial. Lancet Oncol. 2022;23:209–19.
27. Wang J, Zhou C, Yao W, et al. Adebrelimab or placebo plus carboplatin and etoposide as first-line treatment for extensive-stage small-cell lung cancer (CAPSTONE-1): a multicentre, randomised, double-blind, placebo-controlled, phase 3 trial. Lancet Oncol. 2022;23:739–47.
28. Barkley D, Moncada R, Pour M, et al. Cancer cell states recur across tumor types and form specific interactions with the tumor microenvironment. Nat Genet. 2022;54:1192–201.
29. Yang Y, Qu S, Li J, et al. Camrelizumab versus placebo in combination with gemcitabine and cisplatin as first-line treatment for recurrent or metastatic nasopharyngeal carcinoma (CAPTAIN-1st): a multicentre, randomised, double-blind, phase 3 trial. Lancet Oncol. 2021;22:1162–74.
30. Yang Y, Pan J, Wang H, et al. Tislelizumab plus chemotherapy as first-line treatment for recurrent or metastatic nasopharyngeal cancer: a multicenter phase 3 trial (RATIONALE-309). Cancer Cell. 2023;41:1061–1072 e4.
31. Ngwa W, Irabor OC, Schoenfeld JD, et al. Using immunotherapy to boost the abscopal effect. Nat Rev Cancer. 2018;18:313–22.
32. Jabbour SK, Lee KH, Frost N, et al. Pembrolizumab plus concurrent chemoradiation therapy in patients with unresectable, locally advanced, stage III non-small cell lung cancer: the phase 2 KEYNOTE-799 nonrandomized trial. JAMA Oncol. 2021;7:1–9.
33. Yin L, Xue J, Li R, et al. Effect of low-dose radiation therapy on abscopal responses to hypofractionated radiation therapy and anti-PD1 in mice and patients with non-small cell lung cancer. Int J Radiat Oncol Biol Phys. 2020;108:212–24.
34. Ren Z, Xu J, Bai Y, et al. Sintilimab plus a bevacizumab biosimilar (IBI305) versus sorafenib in unresectable hepatocellular carcinoma (ORIENT-32): a randomised, open-label, phase 2-3 study. Lancet Oncol. 2021;22:977–90.

35. Luo H, Lu J, Bai Y, et al. Effect of camrelizumab vs placebo added to chemotherapy on survival and progression-free survival in patients with advanced or metastatic esophageal squamous cell carcinoma: the ESCORT-1st randomized clinical trial. JAMA. 2021;326:916–25.
36. Stein MN, Fong L, Tutrone R, et al. ADXS31142 immunotherapy +/− pembrolizumab treatment for metastatic castration-resistant prostate cancer: open-label phase I/II KEYNOTE-046 study. Oncologist. 2022;27:453–61.

Chapter 7
Cell-Guided Drugs

Haoyue Qin and Guowei Zhou

Abstract This chapter delves into the innovative domain of cell-guided drugs in tumor therapy, showcasing groundbreaking developments in this area. The focus of cell-guided therapy is primarily on two cell types: stem cells and immune cells. While stem cell transplants are a mainstay in treating hematological malignancies, their broader use as drug agents in cancer therapy remains limited. Therefore, this chapter places a special emphasis on adoptive cell therapy (ACT), a more promising approach that leverages immune cells to target and destroy cancer cells. We offer a thorough introduction to ACT, discussing its principal methods, such as Lymphokine-Activated Killer (LAK) cells, Cytokine-Induced Killer (CIK) cells, Tumor-Infiltrating Lymphocytes (TILs), T Cell Receptor (TCR) therapy, Chimeric Antigen Receptor (CAR) T cell therapy, and Natural Killer (NK) cell therapy. Beyond outlining these advanced techniques, the chapter traces their historical development and evolution. It provides a critical analysis of clinical trials, sheds light on the drugs that have gained approval, and explores the future prospects and potential of ACT in the ongoing fight against cancer.

Keywords ACT · ALK · CIK · TILs · CAR-T · NK cell

H. Qin (✉)
Department of Medical Oncology, Lung Cancer and Gastrointestinal Unit, Hunan Cancer Hospital/The Affiliated Cancer Hospital of Xiangya School of Medicine, Central South University, Changsha, China
e-mail: qinhaoyue@hnca.org.cn

G. Zhou
Xiangya Hospital, Central South University, Changsha, China
e-mail: guowei_zhou@csu.edu.cn

© The Author(s), under exclusive license to Springer Nature Singapore Pte Ltd. 2024

Y. Zhang, N. Yang (eds.), *New Anti-cancer Drug Development and Evaluation*,
https://doi.org/10.1007/978-981-97-7274-2_7

7.1 Adoptive Cell Therapy (ACT)

Adoptive cell therapy (ACT) represents a pioneering approach in cancer treatment. The first step of ACT involves the in vitro expansion and activation of autologous immune cells. Then, these enhanced cells are reintroduced into patients, where they aggressively target and destroy tumor cells in vivo. Currently, ACT primarily employs lymphocytes, particularly T lymphocytes, which are genetically engineered for enhanced tumor recognition and eradication capabilities [1]. Back in 1986, Rosenberg et al. first isolated lymphocytes from mouse tumors and transplanted them into other tumor-bearing mice after amplification. The transplanted lymphocytes demonstrated effective inhibition of tumor growth [2], which led to the first clinical trials in metastatic melanoma [3], marking a milestone in the development of ACT. Following the initial development of ACT, tumor-infiltrating lymphocytes (TILs) have gained regulatory approval for clinical trials. With the development of genetic engineering technology, the focus has shifted to lymphocytes expressing specialized T cell receptors (TCRs) and chimeric antigen receptors (CARs), which are adept at identifying and attacking tumor-specific antigens [4, 5], further enriching the therapeutic means of ACT. Besides T lymphocytes, natural killer (NK) cells, macrophages, and dendritic cells (DC) have also been adopted in ACT and have shown promising clinical prospects [6–8].

The nature of immune cells endows ACT with unique advantages over other cancer treatments, particularly in long-lasting efficacy. After entering the tumor microenvironment (TME), the immune cells can be stimulated by specific antigens to produce long-lasting therapeutic effects [9]. Moreover, immune cells can easily traverse anatomical barriers, possess a longer half-life, and distribute more widely within tissues compared to traditional drugs [10]. Despite these advantages, ACT's successful application has been predominantly in hematological malignancies, with its efficacy in solid tumors still in nascent stages [11]. Critical challenges for future research include enhancing the precision of immune cell targeting to tumor sites, prolonging cell survival, and overcoming the immunosuppressive signals within the TME. Addressing these issues will be crucial in realizing the full potential of ACT in cancer therapy [12–14].

7.2 LAK Therapy

Lymphokine-Activated Killer (LAK) cells are derived from lymphocytes found in peripheral blood (PB) or lymph nodes from nonmetastatic regions. These lymphocytes are transformed into potent LAK cells through activation and proliferation induced by the lymphokine interleukin (IL)-2 in vitro [15]. It is important to note that LAK cells are not a distinct subpopulation but rather a composite of various immune cells, including NK cells, T cells, and NKT cells. When exposed to high doses of IL-2 in vitro, these immune cells evolve into a specific group of cells capable of targeting and destroying tumor cells that are typically resistant to NK and cytotoxic T lymphocytes (CTL) [15, 16].

The first development of LAK therapy can be traced back to 1982, when Grimm et al. discovered that treating peripheral blood mononuclear cells (PBMCs) with IL-2 for 4–6 days in vitro could lead to the formation of these nonspecific but effective killer cells [17]. Later, Dr. Rosenberg's research team first used IL-2 in combination with LAK to treat 25 patients with renal cell carcinoma, melanoma, lung cancer, and colon cancer and reported the results of the clinical trial in 1985 [18]. This study demonstrated remarkable results: out of 25 patients, 11 experienced over 50% tumor regression, and one melanoma patient achieved complete tumor remission. Remarkably, adverse events, such as fluid retention, subsided once IL-2 administration was terminated [18]. In a subsequent study conducted in 1988, Rosenberg's team presented their findings from treating 222 patients with the IL-2 and LAK cell combination. This extensive study revealed that 16 patients had complete tumor metastasis regression, while 26 experienced more than 50% tumor reduction. The therapy showed particular promise in patients with metastatic renal cell carcinoma, melanoma, colon cancer, and non-Hodgkin's lymphoma, marking a significant advancement in the field of ACT and opening new avenues for cancer treatment [19].

While LAK therapy combined with IL-2 has demonstrated remarkable efficacy in treating certain tumors, it has also encountered numerous challenges that have hindered its broader clinical application. Initial promising results reported by Dr. Rosenberg were not consistently replicated by other researchers, indicating variability in treatment outcomes. Furthermore, the logistical and biological limitations of LAK therapy have become increasingly apparent. The production of LAK cells involves extracting substantial quantities of peripheral blood from patients, followed by a prolonged co-culture with IL-2 to activate the cells. This process is time-consuming and costly, as it requires multiple infusions of LAK cells each week.

Additionally, the lack of tumor specificity in LAK cells presents a significant drawback. Originating from a diverse array of progenitor cells, such as those found in the thymus, spleen, and lymph nodes, LAK cells differentiate into a broad spectrum of killer cells. They adopt a generalized, rather than a targeted, approach to tumor eradication. Upon infusion into the body, LAK cells predominantly accumulate in the lungs and liver. There is evidence suggesting their cytotoxic effects extend to vital cells, including myocardial cells, hepatocytes, and renal tubular epithelial cells.

Moreover, the high doses of IL-2 used in LAK therapy are associated with serious toxic and side effects, most notably capillary leak syndrome (CLS), which can lead to severe complications like pleural effusion, pulmonary interstitial edema, and congestive heart failure. The pathogenesis of CLS may be related to IL-2-induced endothelial cell damage and the release of vasoactive substances [15, 16]. These considerable limitations and adverse effects of LAK therapy have prompted researchers to pursue a deeper understanding of the immune system and the role of inflammatory mediators like cytokines. As a result, the focus in the field has gradually shifted toward alternative ACT strategies that offer greater efficacy and reduced risk, continuing the evolution of cancer treatment modalities.

7.3 CIK Therapy

Cytokine-Induced Killer (CIK) cells are derived from human PBMCs, which are cultured in vitro with a cocktail of cytokines, including anti-CD3 monoclonal antibody (mAb), IL-2, interferon-γ (IFN-γ), and IL-1α. In this diverse cell population, the CD3+ CD56+ cells are identified as the primary effector cells. Specifically, these cells uniquely combine the potent antitumor capabilities of T lymphocytes with the non-major histocompatibility complex-restricted tumor-targeting ability inherent to NK cells [15]. CIK cells are adept at recognizing and destroying tumor cells while sparing normal cells, making them highly effective, particularly in post-surgical, radiotherapy, or chemotherapy settings for eradicating residual metastatic lesions. Consequently, CIK cells are instrumental in hindering cancer cell spread and recurrence, as well as bolstering the body's immune response during maintenance therapy.

CIK cells exert their tumor-killing effects through multiple mechanisms. Firstly, CIK cells recognize tumor cells through various pathways and release cytotoxic molecules such as granzyme and perforin, causing tumor cell lysis. Secondly, CIK cells can secrete a variety of cytokines, including IFN-γ, tumor necrosis factor-alpha (TNF-α), and IL-2, which directly inhibit tumor cells and also indirectly attack them by modulating the body's immune response. Finally, CIK cells can express Fas Ligand (FasL) on their membranes, which binds to Fas proteins on tumor cells and triggers apoptosis [20, 21].

The in vitro expansion of CIK cells is a simple process that starts with the addition of 1000 IU/ml IFN-γ, which increases the activation of IL-2 responder cells and activates monocytes to regulate the immunomodulator IL-12 [22]. Subsequently, 50 ng/ml anti-CD3 mAb, 100 IU/ml IL-1β, and 600 IU/ml IL-2 are introduced into the medium [23, 24]. Note that IL-2 and fresh medium need to be supplemented regularly until after 2–3 weeks. While IL-2 remains the original part of the activation/expansion mixture, IL-2 support is no longer required after CIK cell infusion [15].

First reported by Schmidt Wolf et al. from Stanford University in 1991 [24], CIK cells have since been the subject of numerous clinical trials. An International Registry on CIK Cells (IRCC) was established to monitor progress in the field, ensuring quality standards in clinical trials and publishing reports every 5 years [22]. Between 1999 and 2019, CIK therapy was tested in over 30 different cancers, with the majority of cases involving lung cancer (26.4%), hepatocellular carcinoma (18.9%), gastric cancer (16.0%), renal cell carcinoma (15.1%), and lymphoma (15.1%) [22]. Most trials used autologous CIK cells, though there were experiments with allogeneic CIK and cord blood-derived CIK cells, showing significant improvements in progression-free and overall survival rates [25]. Side effects were generally mild (e.g., fever, chills, fatigue, headache, and rash), with low fever being the most common, while severe toxicities like leukopenia, neutropenia, and thrombocytopenia were rare [22].

Combining CIK with DC therapy has shown promising results in enhancing CIK's proliferation and antitumor activity. This synergy significantly prolongs overall survival and disease-free survival rates, bolstering the T lymphocyte response [26]. As of early 2023, over 70 CIK therapy-related clinical trials have been registered in China, with CIK therapy being recommended as adjuvant therapy post-hepatectomy by the Chinese Society of Clinical Oncology (CSCO) in 2022. Looking forward, CIK therapy stands as a pivotal component of ACT, with ongoing challenges to enhance its clinical efficacy and prolong its therapeutic effects.

7.4 Tumor-Infiltrating Lymphocyte Therapy

7.4.1 Introduction

TIL therapy is a targeted method for treating primary or secondary tumors. It involves isolating TILs directly from the tumor tissue, amplifying them in vitro, and then reintroducing them into patients to enhance the immune response against cancer [27]. Distinct from LAK and CIK therapies, which utilize cells from PBMCs or other normal tissues, TIL therapy specifically employs heterogeneous lymphocytes harvested from the tumor itself. Specifically, TILs are a diverse group of lymphocytes in the tumor interstitium, including T cells, B cells, and NK cells, mainly CD4+ and CD8+ T cells [28, 29]. The role of activated CD8+ T cells in TIL therapy is critical, as they produce pro-inflammatory cytokines that lead to tumor cell death. CD4+ T cells, on the other hand, support plasma cells in producing antibodies and are instrumental in activating CD8+ T cell responses. Hence, TILs are capable of recognizing, combating, and eradicating tumors. Numerous studies have indicated that the presence and quantity of TILs within tumor tissues can significantly influence patient prognosis [29].

TILs that naturally exist in tumors often fail to effectively eliminate tumor cells. This failure is primarily attributed to two factors: firstly, tumor cells can evade recognition and destruction by TILs through immune escape mechanisms, such as expressing immunosuppressive molecules like PD-1 and CTLA-4 [30, 31]. Secondly, the quantity and activity level of TILs may be insufficient to combat the volume of tumor cells present [32, 33]. TIL therapy addresses these issues by enhancing the in vitro amplification and activation of these immune cells, thereby increasing their efficacy in targeting and killing tumor cells. This approach provides a more direct and potentially powerful means of leveraging the body's natural immune response against cancer.

7.4.2 Implementation Procedure of TIL Therapy

TIL therapy can be divided into three distinct stages. In the initial stage, tumor tissue is surgically removed from the patient and then either enzymatically broken down into a single-cell solution or mechanically sectioned into smaller pieces. These fragments serve as the foundation for the next phase of TIL amplification [27].

The second stage involves culturing the single-cell solution or tissue fragments in a medium rich in IL-2, leading to the growth of what are termed young TILs (yTILs). Over a period of 10–40 days, these yTILs undergo rapid expansion through the addition of high-dose IL-2, irradiated PBMCs, and anti-CD3, typically over a 2-week period [34]. However, it's important to note that this amplification process begins with the initial identification and isolation of tumor-specific TILs, which can be time-consuming, taking approximately 6–8 weeks. Additionally, prolonged in vitro culture can lead to TIL exhaustion [35]. This can significantly impact the efficacy of the treatment and limit its clinical application [36]. To address this, the "Young TIL" approach was developed, which bypasses the need for in vitro screening of TILs, enabling faster administration and demonstrating comparable efficacy to traditional TILs in melanoma patients [37, 38].

The third and final stage involves preparing the patients for lymphocyte infusion through a lymphodepletion regimen, which usually includes administering cyclophosphamide (60 mg/kg) for 2 days and fludarabine (25 mg/m^2) for 5 days [39]. This regimen is followed by the intravenous administration of the expanded TILs, complemented by high doses of IL-2 (720,000 IU/kg IV) every 8 h up to 15 times or to a toxic dose [27]. Though the mechanism of lymphodepletion is not entirely understood, studies suggest that it enhances ACT's effectiveness [40, 41] by diminishing immunosuppressive cell populations like Tregs and myeloid-derived suppressor cells (MDSCs), and by removing cellular cytokine sinks [27]. Initially demonstrated in mouse models, the effectiveness of TILs post-lymphodepletion was also validated in human studies [42]. In 1994, Rosenberg et al. reported higher overall response rates (ORR) in patients with metastatic melanoma who underwent lymphodepletion (34%) compared to those who did not (31%) [43]. Dudley et al. also proved that the adoptive transfer of TILs resulted in better ORR after using a lymphodepletion regimen in 2002 [40]. However, it's crucial to recognize that most patients experience side effects from the lymphodepletion regimen, such as lymphopenia, coagulation dysfunction, and gastrointestinal symptoms [44, 45]. To mitigate these side effects, Santos et al. designed a lymphodepletion regimen using oncolytic adenovirus instead of chemotherapy, which obtained better efficacy and survival rates, and significantly reduced toxicity [46].

7.4.3 Development Progression of TIL Therapy

The pioneering work in TIL therapy was conducted by Dr. Steven Rosenberg and his team at the National Institutes of Health (NIH). Initially, they established that TILs, once isolated and amplified in vitro, could induce tumor regression, successfully treating advanced tumor-bearing mice with liver and lung metastases. They also identified the critical role of IL-2 in stimulating the growth and survival of effector T cells. When combined with TIL infusion, IL-2 significantly enhances the therapeutic effect [2, 47].

Building on these fundamental discoveries, Rosenberg's team initiated the first human study of TILs in 1988. They isolated lymphocytes from excised melanoma specimens, amplified them in vitro, and administered them to patients along with IL-2 following chemotherapy with cyclophosphamide. Their groundbreaking findings revealed an ORR of 55% in patients treated with TILs. Despite some adverse events related to IL-2, these were found to be reversible [3], underscoring the relative safety and efficacy of TIL therapy [11].

Subsequent research has continued to explore the efficacy of TIL therapy in melanoma. A comprehensive meta-analysis by Dafni et al. examined patients with advanced cutaneous melanoma treated with TILs and IL-2 from 1988 to 2016, noting an ORR of 41% and a complete response rate of 12%. This analysis highlighted that the combination of TILs with high-dose IL-2 could provide more durable clinical benefits [48]. However, this study did not include uveal melanoma, a rarer and more refractory form of the disease. In 2017, Chandran et al. reported the effective application of TIL therapy in treating uveal melanoma, achieving an ORR of 35%. The common adverse events in these patients were primarily associated with the lymphodepletion regimen, indicating TIL therapy's potential in this challenging area [49].

Beyond melanoma, TIL therapy has demonstrated considerable clinical benefits in various solid tumors, including non-small cell lung cancer (NSCLC) [50], ovarian cancer [51], colorectal cancer [52], breast cancer [53], and cervical cancer [54]. These successes suggest a broad clinical application potential for TIL therapy in solid tumors. However, the effectiveness of TIL therapy in other solid tumors can vary significantly. This variability is likely due to the heterogeneity in mutation load, neoantigen load, and the infiltration of lymphocytes and myeloid cells in different tumors [55]. As such, while TIL therapy represents a promising avenue in cancer treatment, its application and efficacy must be considered in the context of each unique tumor type.

7.4.4 Optimization of TIL Therapy

As research into TIL therapy progresses, it has become increasingly clear that combining TILs with other cancer treatments can yield enhanced clinical outcomes. A notable development in this context is the emergence of immune checkpoint inhibitors (ICIs) in cancer therapy. ICIs work by blocking the co-inhibitory signaling pathways between tumor cells and the immune system, thereby activating an antitumor immune response and promoting the immune-mediated destruction of tumor cells [56]. Many studies have established a close correlation between the efficacy of ICIs and the presence of TILs within tumors [33, 57]. The synergy between TIL therapy and ICIs is particularly promising. While ICIs counteract the immune evasion tactics of tumor cells, TIL therapy boosts the number of activated immune cells. Theoretically, their combined application can provide a more potent therapeutic effect. Early clinical trials combining TIL therapy with ICIs have shown encouraging results [50, 58]. However, it has been observed that prolonged exposure to immune checkpoint inhibition signals can lead to apoptosis or abnormal differentiation of CD8+ T cells, reducing the number of TILs in tumor tissues [59]. Therefore, to maximize the effectiveness of TILs, ICIs should ideally be administered both prior to the resection and initial amplification of tumor tissue for TIL extraction, as well as after TIL infusion [60–62]. A Phase II clinical trial in 2021 by Sarnaik et al. using the TIL product Lifileucel (LN-144) showed promising results for advanced melanoma patients who had progressed following ICI and targeted therapy [63]. The trial reported an ORR of 36%, with complete and partial responses at 3% and 33%, respectively, and an impressive disease control rate of 80%. This suggests that TIL therapy could be a viable new treatment approach for advanced melanoma patients who have not responded to ICIs and targeted therapies.

Furthermore, TIL therapy has been effectively combined with targeted inhibitors like vrafmurine sarcoma viral oncogene homolog B (BRAF) inhibitors, which can decrease immunosuppressive signals, enhance lymphocyte infiltration, and improve tumor antigen presentation [64]. Clinical studies have reported a 64% ORR in patients with metastatic melanoma treated with a combination of TILs and BRAF inhibitors, indicating this combination's tolerability and safety [65]. Additionally, the potential of combining TIL therapy with DC vaccines and oncolytic viruses is being explored. These treatments can activate and increase the number of TILs, further enhancing their antitumor efficacy. Such combination therapies represent a growing area of interest and hold the promise of further improving outcomes in cancer treatment [47].

7.4.5 TIL-Related Clinical Trials and Drugs

Currently, TIL therapy predominantly serves as a second-line treatment option, with melanoma being the primary focus in most clinical trials [47]. Over the decade from 2011 to 2020, a significant number of TIL therapy trials were conducted: 79 in total, involving 22 different TIL products. Geographically, the distribution of these trials has been notably concentrated, with over half (51%) taking place in the United States and 15% in China [66]. By February 2023, the scope of TIL therapy research had expanded substantially, with more than 600 clinical trials registered globally, as per data from ClinicalTrials.gov. Of these, China accounts for a significant portion, with over 60 trials, roughly 10% of the global total. The commitment to TIL therapy research within China is further underscored by progress in product development and regulatory acceptance. To date, four TIL therapy products have received approval from the National Medical Products Administration (NMPA) in China, indicating a growing interest and investment in this therapeutic approach within the country (Table 7.1).

Table 7.1 Four TIL therapy products accepted by NMPA

Acceptance number	Enterprise	TILs product	Date
CXSL2200061	Suzhou GRIT Biotechnology Co., Ltd.	GT101	2022-01-30
CXSL2200070	Shanghai Junsai Biotechnology Co., Ltd.	GC101	2022-02-09
CXSL2200552	Guangzhou Zhiling Biomedical Co., Ltd.	ZLT-001	2022-11-02
CXSL2200574	Hangzhou Houwu Biomedical Technology Co., Ltd. and Guangdong Tiankeya Biomedical Technology Co., Ltd.	HV-101	2022-11-16

7.4.6 Future Prospects of TIL Therapy

TIL therapy presents distinct advantages over other forms of ACT. A key feature of TILs is their composition: they are made up of multiple TCR clones derived directly from the patient's own immune system. This unique origin not only endows TILs with a lower toxicity profile but also enables them to effectively recognize tumor-specific antigens [67]. Meanwhile, memory T cells within the TILs, upon stimulation by tumor antigens, express chemokine receptors that facilitate their infiltration into tumor tissues, enhancing their effectiveness in targeting cancer cells [47].

However, TIL therapy is not without its limitations. One primary challenge is its dependence on autologous, or self-derived, effector T cells with antitumor activity within the tumor. Not all patients possess a sufficient number of these necessary cells within their tumors, which limits the applicability of TIL therapy. Another significant challenge is isolating a sufficient quantity of these effector immune cells that can not only recognize and eliminate tumor cells, but also maintain their viability and functionality over extended periods in vitro. Although the use of IL-2 in TIL therapy is crucial for promoting lymphocyte proliferation and activation, it also raises the issue of associated adverse events. Moreover, the immunosuppressive nature of the TME, which can lead to the exhaustion of infiltrating cytotoxic T cells, remains a significant challenge. Identifying and targeting effective molecular markers to improve this environment is an area that requires further research and exploration [47, 66].

7.5 TCR-Gene Engineered T Cells Therapy

7.5.1 Introduction

TCR-T therapy is a form of ACT that involves a process in which T cells are isolated from tumor patients, genetically modified to enhance their ability to specifically recognize tumor antigens, and then reintroduced into the patients to combat tumors. The crux of this therapy lies in the TCR, a specific receptor on T cells. The TCR pairs with CD3 to form the TCR-CD3 complex through non-covalent bonds. This complex plays a crucial role in recognizing tumor antigens presented by the major histocompatibility complex (MHC), leading to the activation of T cells [68].

In cancer patients, T cells that can specifically target tumor antigens naturally exist. However, their activity and numbers are typically insufficient to substantially impact tumor growth. To address this limitation, researchers isolate and amplify T cells responsive to the same antigen, or they identify and extract the TCR-encoding gene. This gene is then introduced into regular T cells, effectively endowing them with the ability to specifically target tumors. The resulting T cells, which express specific TCR sequences, are known as TCR-T cells [69]. When these engineered TCR-T cells are transfused back into patients, they can specifically target tumor cells and induce their apoptosis.

A notable difference between TCR-T therapy and TIL therapy lies in the nature of the T cells used. While TIL therapy utilizes a diverse array of T cells with multiple TCR clones, TCR-T therapy predominantly uses monoclonal cells that recognize a single epitope. As a result, TCR-T therapy offers stronger tumor specificity compared to TIL therapy, providing a more focused attack on cancer cells [70, 71]. This specificity is one of the critical strengths of TCR-T therapy, allowing for a tailored approach to cancer treatment that targets specific tumor antigens with enhanced precision.

7.5.2 Implementation of TCR-T Therapy

The procedure for TCR-T therapy shares some similarities with TIL therapy, particularly in the initial steps of extracting T cells from tumor tissue, amplifying these cells in vitro, and then reinfusing them into patients. However, TCR-T therapy distinguishes itself with an additional critical step: the selection and modification of T cells to specifically recognize tumor antigens through their TCR [71].

TCR-T cells rely on TCR to bind to the antigenic peptide-MHC molecular complex (pMHC) for their activation and tumor-targeting ability. Therefore, patients undergoing TCR-T therapy must first undergo human leukocyte antigen (HLA) typing [72] to ensure the compatibility and efficacy of the TCR-T cells against the tumor. After determining the HLA type, patients need to undergo tumor biopsies to screen for tumor-specific antigens. Subsequently, white blood cells are extracted from the patient's blood. The use of anti-CD3 and CD28 antibodies facilitates the isolation and pre-activation of PBMCs.

Given the variable and often uncertain number of specific TCR-T cells obtainable from tumor patients, target-specific TCRs are typically isolated from healthy donors. These TCRs are then extensively characterized and modified. Lentiviral vectors are employed to introduce these target-specific TCRs into T cells. The modified T cells are then rapidly expanded over 3–5 days, after which they are cryopreserved until needed. After release testing is complete, the TCR-T cells are transfused into the patients.

It is important to note that, similar to TIL therapy, TCR-T cell therapy requires a lymphodepletion regimen prior to cell infusion. Additionally, it may be combined with IL-2 injections to support the expansion of the infused T cells. Post-infusion, patients undergo long-term monitoring, sometimes extending up to 15 years, to observe any delayed adverse events [71].

7.5.3 Evolution of TCR-T Therapy

TCR-T therapy has gone through a series of evolutions since its first discovery. Back in 1980, Dembic et al. first discovered that the α and β chains of the TCR are crucial for T cells' specific antigen recognition [73]. In 2006, Dr. Steven Rosenberg along with his colleagues reported the first clinical application of TCR-T cells targeting the melanoma antigen recognized by T cells (MART-1) in melanoma patients [74]. Remarkably, two patients with rapidly progressing metastatic melanoma showed complete clinical responses, highlighting the potential of TCR-T cell therapy in clinical settings. The same team further demonstrated the efficacy of TCR-T cells targeting the cancer/testis antigen NY-ESO-1 in patients with melanoma and synovial sarcoma [75]. Clinical responses were observed in patients with both cancer types, with no significant toxicity or adverse effects noted. Beyond NY-ESO-1, the melanoma antigen genes (MAGE) antigen, present in various cancer types, has also been targeted. A study in 2013 involving anti-MAGE-A3 TCR-T cells showed clinical regression in five out of nine patients, reinforcing the broad applicability of TCR-T cell therapy in cancer treatment [76].

The advancement of high-throughput sequencing technology enabled the identification of specific cancer-related mutations between tumors and healthy tissue. Dr. Steven Rosenberg and his team reported that exome sequencing can be used to explore human tumor neoantigens recognized by tumor-reactive T cells in 2013 [77]. By employing this approach, Dr. Steven Rosenberg's team later identified a group of patients with advanced refractory cholangiocarcinoma harboring ERBB2IP point mutations. The patients then received reactive human epidermal growth factor receptor 2 (ERBB2IP)-specific T cell infusion and experienced significant tumor remission and prolonged survival time [78]. This case emphasizes the potential of TCR-T therapy in precision medicine: the TCR-T cells can be specifically modified to target patients with certain genetic features, which may enhance the specificity of the therapy and reduce side effects.

Recently, TCR-T therapy has witnessed more breakthroughs. In 2016, researchers reported that T cells isolated from healthy individuals could respond to neoplastic antigens expressed in melanoma, suggesting that naive T cells from healthy donors could serve as a viable source for TCR-T cells. This finding also supported the use of TCR-T cells derived from allogeneic sources [79]. TCR-T cell therapy has since shown promising clinical outcomes in treating a range of solid tumors, including melanoma, colorectal cancer, sarcoma, metastatic human papilloma virus

(HPV)16-associated cervical cancer, and multiple myeloma [80]. Concurrently, the development of more tumor-specific antigens, including those mediated by viruses like HPV and EB virus, as well as tumor neoantigens, has further expanded the range of target antigens for TCR-T cell therapy.

7.5.4 *Optimization of TCR-T Therapy*

The efficacy of TCR-T cell therapy is significantly influenced by the ability of TCR-T cells to recognize the peptide-MHC complex (pMHC), making the expression and affinity of the TCR important factors in TCR-T cell therapy [69]. The cytotoxic activity of T cells is closely linked to the affinity of the TCR for its target [81]. To enhance this affinity, several methods have been developed, including the random mutation of pMHC recognition sites, phage display techniques, and the identification of high-affinity TCRs through humanized immune system mouse models [69]. However, excessively high TCR affinity can paradoxically diminish the effectiveness of TCR-T cells by leading to premature exhaustion upon encountering their target antigen, which can limit their sustained cytotoxic effect on tumor cells [82]. Therefore, balancing the affinity of TCRs is critical for the success of TCR-T cell therapy.

In addition to affinity, high expression of the TCR and its correct assembly on T cell surfaces are essential. Research has indicated that specific residues in the TCR variable domain framework can enhance TCR expression on T cells [83]. Modifying these variable domains could lead to increased expression and improved functionality of TCRs.

Recent advancements have also shown promise in using CRISPR-Cas9 technology to replace endogenous TCRs with transgenic TCRs. One major challenge with using transgenic TCRs is that the endogenous TCR may compete with the transgenic TCR for cell surface expression, forming mixed dimers that could potentially lead to autoreactive specificities. The use of CRISPR-Cas9 to knock out endogenous TCRs addresses this issue by preventing competitive binding with CD3 and the endogenous TCR [84, 85]. Although no serious adverse events have been reported in clinical trials involving genome editing with CRISPR-Cas9, the genome integrity needs to be carefully evaluated for such therapy [86].

7.5.5 *TCR-T-Related Clinical Trials and Drugs*

The first TCR-T clinical trial was initiated by Dr. Steven Rosenberg in 2004, targeting the melanoma differentiation antigen gp100 (NCT00085462). This pioneering trial set the stage for subsequent developments in the field. Since then, there has been a notable increase in the number of new TCR-T therapy trials, particularly

Table 7.2 Six TCR-T therapy products accepted by NMPA

Acceptance number	Enterprise	TCR-T product	Date
CXSL1800128	Guangdong Xiangxue Life Science and Technology Co., Ltd.	TAEST16001	2018-12-29
CXSL2101306	Guangdong Tiankeya Biomedical Technology Co., Ltd.	TC-E202	2021-09-02
CXSL2101494	Dalian Xinghande Biopharmaceutical Co., Ltd.	SCG101	2021-12-22
CXSL2200481	Shenzhen Pregene Biopharma Co., Ltd.	Targeting HLA-A*02:01/NY-ESO-1	2021-12-31
CXSL2200058	Guangdong Xiangxue Life Science and Technology Co., Ltd.	TAEST1901	2022-01-29
CXSL2300144	Hengruiyuanzheng Biotechnology Co., Ltd.	HRYZ-T101	2023-02-21

between 2017 and 2019, a period that saw the initiation of 51 new TCR-T clinical trials [87]. As of February 2023, over 60 clinical trials related to TCR-T therapy have been registered, the majority of which are phase I trials. Notably, there have been no phase III clinical trials registered for TCR-T therapy to date.

China has been a significant contributor to this research, with over 20 clinical trials registered in the country, according to data from ClinicalTrials.gov. There have been six TCR-T cell therapy drugs newly accepted by the National Medical Products Administration (NMPA) in China (Table 7.2). A landmark development in the international acceptance of TCR-T cell therapy occurred with the approval of the TCR-T cell therapy drug KSH01, developed by Biotech Valley Park. This drug received official approval from the US FDA, marking the first time a TCR-T cell therapy drug developed in China has been recognized by the FDA (NCT05539833).

7.5.6 *Future Prospects of TIL Therapy*

TCR-T therapy, with its enhanced ability to precisely target tumor-specific antigens, offers a more individualized treatment approach compared to TIL therapy. However, it confronts several significant challenges. A primary concern is the therapy's cytotoxicity, which is often linked to the expression of tumor-associated antigens (TAA) by normal cells [88–90]. This issue is exacerbated when the affinity of TCR-T cells is increased through genetic modifications, potentially elevating the therapy's toxicity. Hence, there is an urgent need for the development of preclinical strategies to evaluate TCR-related cross-reactivity and mitigate potential adverse effects.

Another significant challenge for TCR-T therapy is drug resistance. The primary resistance mechanism is often attributed to low or heterogeneous expression of the target antigen by tumor cells or an inherent resistance of tumor cells to T cell-mediated cytotoxicity [91]. Secondary resistance mechanisms involve the upregulation of immune checkpoint ligands on tumor cells and the activation of immune checkpoint receptors, or the loss and diminishment of MHC Class I molecules on tumor cells [69]. Understanding and overcoming these resistance mechanisms are crucial for enhancing the efficacy of TCR-T therapy.

Moving forward, the future of TCR-T cell therapy will likely focus on better selection of tumor-associated antigens and the optimization of T cell engineering. These efforts aim to minimize toxicity risks and improve therapeutic outcomes. Such advancements are vital for fully realizing the potential of TCR-T therapy as a powerful and precise tool in the fight against cancer, offering a more tailored and effective treatment option for patients.

7.6 CARs-Mediated Cell Immunotherapy

7.6.1 Introduction

CAR therapy represents a significant advancement in cancer treatment, featuring CARs as synthetic modular proteins that function as specific receptors. CARs enable immune cells to recognize and eliminate cells expressing a relevant target ligand [92]. CARs have undergone iterative optimization and now comprise three primary functional domains: the extracellular domain, the transmembrane domain, and the intracellular domain.

The extracellular domain is characterized by a single-chain variable fragment (scFv), which plays a pivotal role in antigen recognition and binding of the mAb to the antigen. This domain is akin to an mAb and is connected to the transmembrane domain by a linking hinge region. The scFv is crucial for the specific binding of tumor-associated antigens (TAA), consisting of the variable regions of the light (VL) and heavy (VH) chains of an antibody, linked together by a peptide [93]. This configuration maintains the antibody's specificity and affinity for its antigen. Notably, the scFv enables CAR-T cells to specifically recognize and bind target antigens independently of MHC. This feature is vital as it prevents tumor cells from evading immune responses by modulating MHC molecules and allows CAR-T cells to target non-peptide antigens [94].

The hinge region, which varies in length, connects the scFv to the transmembrane structural domain. Derived typically from the hinge of IgG or the CD8α/CD28 extracellular region, the length of the hinge region is crucial as it can influence CAR-T cell activation. The appropriate length ensures an optimal distance between CAR-T cells and target cells, mitigating the effects of large phosphatases that can weaken the CAR signal during antigen-antibody interaction. In cases where antigen epitopes are less accessible, a longer hinge region might be necessary to enable efficient antigen binding [95].

The transmembrane structural domain serves as the link between the extracellular and intracellular domains of CARs, anchoring the receptor to the cell's membrane. Common sources for this domain include CD4, CD8α, and CD28, with CD8α and CD28 transmembrane domains being particularly effective in enhancing CAR expression on the cell surface. These domains are widely used in most clinical trials due to their ability to promote cell surface expression of CARs, further optimizing the efficacy of CAR-T cell therapy [96].

The intracellular domain of CAR plays a crucial role in the functionality of CAR-T cell therapy, serving as the nexus for signal transduction and T cell activation. This domain typically comprises two key components: the costimulatory domain and the signal transduction domain. The costimulatory domain is essential for enhancing the proliferation, durability, and overall efficacy of CAR-T cells. Commonly used costimulatory molecules include CD28, 4-1BB (CD137), and OX40 (CD134). Each of these molecules contributes uniquely to the therapy; for instance, CD28 provides robust initial activation and proliferation of CAR-T cells, while 4-1BB enhances the persistence and endurance of these cells. Meanwhile, the signal transduction domain, usually derived from the CD3ζ chain, is integral to initiating the T cell activation cascade. It contains Immunoreceptor Tyrosine-based Activation Motifs (ITAMs), which, upon antigen recognition by the CAR's extracellular domain, become phosphorylated. This phosphorylation triggers a series of intracellular signaling events leading to T cell activation, proliferation, cytokine production, and the development of cytotoxic activity against tumor cells.

7.6.2 Implementation of CARs Therapy

In the development of CAR-T cell therapy, a specific antigen receptor gene that recognizes TAA is first engineered in vitro. This recombinant gene is then incorporated into T cells extracted from a patient's blood. The integration enables these T cells to express TAAs on their surface, effectively programming them to target cancer cells. After genetic modification, these T cells undergo purification and large-scale amplification to prepare them for infusion back into the patient.

Typically, the patient's own T cells are employed in this process, primarily to circumvent the risks associated with immune rejection and graft-versus-host disease (GVHD). The use of autologous T cells, being genetically identical to the patient's immune system, ensures better compatibility and reduces potential complications. However, there are instances where a patient's own T cells may not be viable for harvesting or might fail during the engineering process. In such situations, donor-derived T cells can be considered as an alternative. Using donor-derived T cells introduces more complexity, as it necessitates additional steps to mitigate the risks of GVHD. These steps may include careful donor-patient matching and the implementation of immunosuppressive measures.

7.6.3 Development Progression of CARs Therapy

7.6.3.1 CARs and T Cells

The evolution of CAR-T cell therapy, a critical component of ACT, has seen remarkable developments since its inception. The journey began in 1986 with Dr. Steven A. Rosenberg's pioneering use of TILs extracted from patients with advanced melanoma [2]. However, the efficacy of TIL therapy was largely limited to highly immunogenic tumors like malignant melanoma, where various lymphocytes, particularly T cells, could recognize and combat tumor cells. For less immunogenic tumors with suppressed MHC molecule expression, the effectiveness of this approach was significantly reduced. Addressing this limitation, in 1989, Israeli scientist Zelig Eshhar conceptualized a non-MHC-restricted method to direct T cell specificity. Specifically, Zelig developed CAR by fusing scFv receptors (γ chains) or CD3 complexes (ζ chains), enabling T cells to recognize TAAs independently of MHC. These genetically engineered T cells, termed T-bodies, marked the creation of the first-generation CAR-T cells.

Although first-generation CAR-T cells could activate T cells effectively [97], their clinical efficacy was limited due to their inability to sustain T cell proliferation and cytokine secretion [98, 99]. In fact, the full activation of T cells requires stimulation by a dual signal. The first signal comes from TCR recognition of antigen peptide-MHC complexes (p-MHC) on the surface of antigen-presenting cells (APCs), ensuring the specificity of the immune response; meanwhile, the second signal comes from the interaction of co-stimulatory molecules (e.g., B7 and CD28, from the surface of APCs and T cells, respectively) between T cells and APCs, which is critical for the induction of antigen-specific T cell responses, ensuring that the immune response occurs under the required conditions.

Recognizing the importance of dual stimulation, Carl H. June and his team at the University of Pennsylvania innovated second-generation CAR-T cells. Incorporating a co-stimulatory domain like CD137 (4-1BB) alongside the CAR structure, these cells exhibited enhanced and prolonged antitumor activity, proliferation, and cytokine secretion, resulting in significant clinical efficacy [100–102]. A testament to this success was Emily Whitehead, the first person "cured" of acute lymphoblastic leukemia using second-generation CAR-T cells, marking a milestone in medical history.

The advent of third-generation CAR-T cells incorporated two co-stimulatory domains (e.g., CD28 and CD137) into the intracellular structural domain, facilitated by retroviruses carrying larger gene fragments. However, studies have indicated that the safety and efficacy of third-generation CAR-T cells may not surpass those of the second generation [103–105]. Despite enhanced efficacy, second- and third-generation CAR-T cells have been associated with severe toxic side effects like cytokine release syndrome and neurotoxicity.

To address the toxicity challenge, fourth-generation CAR-T cells, or armored T cells, introduce additional cytokines (e.g., IL-12, IL-15, IL-18, etc.) and co-stimulatory ligands to counteract the tumor immune microenvironment and incorporate suicide genes for better control and reduced toxicity. Still, CAR-T cell therapy is highly personalized and involves modifying and transfusing a patient's own T cells, making it a costly and complex treatment. The ongoing development of fifth-generation CAR-T cell therapy aims to overcome these limitations, seeking to create universal CARs applicable at scale, though this endeavor faces high technical barriers and stringent safety requirements.

7.6.3.2 CARs and Other Immune Cells

The advancement of CAR therapies has broadened beyond T cells to encompass a diverse range of immune cells, each offering unique mechanisms and potential in cancer treatment.

CAR-NK: NK cells, as innate lymphocytes, play a crucial role in the first-line immune response and possess the innate ability to kill tumor cells without prior sensitization. The development of CAR-NK cells mirrors that of CAR-T cells, evolving from the first generation with a CD3ζ domain to subsequent generations incorporating additional co-stimulatory domains. More advanced iterations, such as the fourth and fifth generations, have introduced new functionalities, including the ability to target multiple tumor antigens. The sixth-generation CAR-NK cells uniquely feature both activating and inhibiting CARs (aCAR and iCAR), allowing for precise targeting of tumor cells while sparing healthy tissue. The seventh generation, or dual-specific CARs, combines FcRγIII (CD16A) and tumor-specific epitope-binding sites, enhancing the diversity and potential of CAR-NK cells.

CAR-Macrophage: Macrophages, key players in the immune system, have recently gained attention in CAR therapy research. Targeting the immune checkpoint CD47 on macrophages holds promise for activating their antitumor activity. However, challenges such as severe anemic responses caused by CD47 antibodies targeting normal red blood cells and platelets pose significant hurdles in clinical development.

CAR-NKT: Natural Killer T cells (NKT) represent a unique subset of T cells that express both TCR and NK cell markers. They are notable for their cytokine production, such as IL-4 and INF-γ, and can mediate antitumor effects either directly through cell lysis or indirectly through cytokine secretion and immune cell activation.

CAR-γδT: γδT cells account for 1% to 5% of peripheral blood T lymphocytes and are predominantly found in mucosal and epithelial tissues. The γδT cells straddle the line between adaptive and innate immunity. Transforming these cells into CAR-γδT cells allows for the precise recognition and efficient eradication of tumor cells, presenting new possibilities for treating solid tumors.

CAR-Treg: Regulatory T cells (Treg) play a critical role in maintaining immune homeostasis and self-tolerance and are implicated in tumor immune evasion. Initially focused on autoimmune diseases, CAR-Treg therapies are now venturing into oncology. By harnessing the regulatory functions of Treg cells, these therapies aim to balance effective tumor targeting while mitigating excessive immune responses.

7.6.4 CARs-Related Clinical Trials and Drugs

7.6.4.1 CARs and T Cells

There are currently six CAR-T products approved for marketing by the FDA and two CAR-T products approved for marketing by the NMPA, as shown in Table 7.3.

Based on the pivotal ZUMA-1 study [106], Fosun Kite's CAR-T product, axi-cabtagene ciloleucel (axi-cel), was approved for marketing in China in June 2021. Specifically, axi-cel is an autologous CAR-T cell product targeting human CD19. This approval marked it as the first CAR-T therapy in China for the treatment of adult patients with relapsed/refractory large B cell lymphoma (r/r LBCL) who have undergone two or more lines of systemic therapy. In August 2021, axi-cel received clinical trial approval from the NMPA for an additional indication: the treatment of relapsed or refractory indolent non-Hodgkin's lymphoma (r/r iNHL) after two or more lines of systemic therapy. This expanded indication was also included in China's Breakthrough Therapy Drug Program. Subsequently, in April and October 2022, the US FDA and the European Medicines Agency (EMA) approved axi-cel for treating adult patients with LBCL refractory to first-line chemoimmunotherapy or those who relapsed within 12 months after first-line chemoimmunotherapy [107]. Furthermore, in October 2022, the China Center for Drug Evaluation (CDE) accepted a drug registration application for axi-cel for a second-line indication, prioritizing its review.

Table 7.3 Eight approved CAR-T products worldwide

CAR-T product	Target	Enterprise	Key registration clinical studies	Institution for permission	Listing date
Kymriah	CD19	Novartis	ELIANA	FDA	February 2017
Yescarta	CD19	Gilead Sciences	ZUMA-1	FDA	October 2017
Teacart's	CD19	Gilead Sciences	ZUMA-3	FDA	July 2020
Breyanzi	CD19	Bristol-Myers Squibb	TRANSCEND	FDA	February 2021
Abecma	BCMA	Bluebird Bio	KarMMa	FDA	March 2021
Carvykti	BCMA	Nanjing Legend Biotech	CARTITUDE-1	FDA	February 2022
Axi-cel	CD19	FosunKite	ZUMA-1	NMPA	June 2021
Relma-cel	CD19	Juno Therapeutics	RELIANCE	NMPA	September 2021

In a parallel development, in September 2021, the NMPA approved another CAR-T product, relmacabtagene autoleucel (relma-cel), for treating adult patients with r/r LBCL after second-line or higher systemic therapy. Distinct from axi-cel, relma-cel was supported by the National Major New Drug Creation Program in China and received its first clinical study approval in 2018, targeting CD19. Developed by Yaoming Juno based on JCAR017 from Juno Therapeutics, relma-cel is the first CAR-T product approved as a Class 1 biologic in China, reflecting a significant leap in the indigenous development of CAR-T therapies. The development process adhered to stringent Class 1 new drug standards, involving extensive review and expert evaluation in China.

A pivotal clinical study, RELIANCE, led by Professors Zhu Jun and Song Yuqin from Peking University Cancer Hospital and Research Institute, demonstrated the high efficacy and safety profile of relma-cel in treating patients with relapsed or refractory follicular lymphoma [108]. This led to the NMPA's approval in October 2022 of relma-cel for a new indication: the treatment of adult patients with refractory or relapsed follicular lymphoma within 24 months (r/r FL) after second-line or higher systemic therapy.

To date, more than 900 clinical studies on CAR-T cells have been registered in the ClinicalTrials.gov registry worldwide, with approximately 500 registered in China. Additionally, over 200 CAR-T cell therapy clinical studies are registered in the Chinese Clinical Trial Registry. These figures underscore the rapid and comprehensive advancement of CAR-T cell therapy research and development in China, signaling a new era of accelerated progress in this transformative medical technology.

7.6.4.2 CARs and Other Immune Cells

Despite the advances in fundamental research, no product utilizing CAR technology in immune cells other than T cells has been approved for marketing. However, significant progress is being made in early stage development and clinical trials.

CAR-NK cells: Pioneering work by the University of California, San Diego, and the University of Minnesota in 2018 led to the development of NK-CAR-iPSC-NK cells from the NK-92 cell line, which showed promising antitumor effects in xenograft mouse models of ovarian cancer [109]. In the same year, Tang et al. constructed CD33-CAR NK-92 cells, demonstrating enhanced cytotoxicity against the HL-60 leukemia cell line in vitro, leading to the first clinical study of CAR-NK cells (NCT02944162) [110]. In 2020, the MD Anderson Cancer Center reported promising results from a Phase I/II clinical trial of CAR-NK cells. Specifically, 8 of 11 patients (73%) responded to treatment. Notably, seven patients achieved complete remission, and no significant toxic reactions, such as cytokine release syndrome or neurotoxicity, were observed during the course of treatment [111]. Also in 2020, a Chinese team led by Professors Wuling Zhu and Ping Lu published the effectiveness of CCCR-NK92, a modified CAR-NK cell, in advanced NSCLC in animal models [112], initiating a clinical study (NCT 03656705). In November 2021, the CDE approved the first Chinese clinical trial for CAR-NK cells targeting ovarian cancer. Later, Fate Therapeutics presented promising interim data from the Phase 1 study of FT596, a CAR-NK cell targeting CD19, in patients with relapsed/refractory B cell lymphoma (BCL).

CAR-Macrophage: Researchers from the University of Pennsylvania in 2017 demonstrated that CAR-modified macrophages significantly inhibited solid tumor growth with favorable safety profiles [113]. Further research in 2020 showed that these CAR-M cells, targeting HER2 antigens, can also differentiate into a pro-inflammatory M1 macrophage type. In this way, these CAR-M cells not only target and phagocytose tumor cells but also alter the microenvironment around the tumor by secreting pro-inflammatory cytokines, while presenting tumor antigens to T cells to activate the T cell immune response against the tumor [114]. In 2021, Carisma Therapeutics announced the first patient dosing of CAR-M therapy (CT-0508) targeting HER2 (NCT04660929), marking a significant step in CAR-M therapy for solid tumors.

CAR-NKT: A Phase I clinical trial at Baylor College of Medicine and Texas Children's Hospital is evaluating the effectiveness and safety of CAR-NKT cell therapy in children with recurrent neuroblastoma (NCT03294954).

CAR-γδT: There are currently five clinical research projects on CAR-γδT cells, all initiated in China, as per ClinicalTrials.gov records. This indicates a growing interest in leveraging the unique properties of γδT cells in cancer therapy.

CAR-Treg: Initially focused on autoimmune diseases, CAR-Treg cell therapies are now being explored in oncology. Though still in the early stages of research, they hold potential for oncology therapy, particularly in modulating immune responses to prevent excessive damage.

7.6.5 Prospects of CARs Therapy

The emergence of CAR technology has significantly transformed tumor immunotherapy, particularly with the rapid advancements in CAR-T cell therapy. CAR-T cell therapy has revolutionized the treatment of hematological cancers, but it also brings serious adverse events like cytokine release syndrome and neurotoxicity, necessitating ongoing attention and improvement. Strategies such as drug blockade or genetic knockout of IFN-γ in CAR-T cells have shown promise in reducing toxicity while enhancing persistence and antitumor efficacy [115]. In addition, innovative approaches like gated switch CARs are being explored to mitigate adverse reactions by controlling excessive activation through antibodies or small molecules. Additionally, the incorporation of safety mechanisms, such as the inducible caspase 9 (iCas9) system, into CAR structures provides a means to trigger apoptosis in cases of severe toxic events, serving as a crucial safety net [111]. However, the efficacy and safety of these new approaches still require validation through larger clinical trials.

A significant challenge for patients undergoing CAR-T cell therapy is tumor antigen escape, which can lead to clonal proliferation and recurrence. Developing multi-targeted CAR-T cells or combining different CAR-T cell targets may help overcome this issue. In particular, the treatment of solid tumors with CAR-T cells remains suboptimal due to the high heterogeneity of tumor cells, the inhibitory effect of the TME on CAR-T cell infiltration, and suppression of the host's antitumor immunity. To address these challenges, optimizing the CAR structure to enhance CAR-T cell expansion and efficacy is crucial [116]. Genetically engineering CAR-T cells to produce specific cytokines, such as IL-7 and CCL19, can help recruit and activate other immune cells, counteracting TME-mediated immunosuppression and improving immune cell infiltration at tumor sites [117].

While precision regulation emerges as a key area of focus, identifying new and more representative antigenic targets is another key issue in the advancement of CAR-T therapy. Potential targets like glypican-3 (GPC3), Claudin18.2, B7H3, and EphA2 show promise but are still in the early stages of research and require further clinical validation to ascertain their efficacy. These developments signify the dynamic and ever-evolving nature of CAR-T cell therapy, highlighting both its potential and the challenges that lie ahead in its journey toward becoming a mainstay in cancer treatment.

7.7 NK Cell Therapy

7.7.1 Introduction

NK cells, a distinct type of lymphocyte, play a vital role in the body's immune response. They rapidly respond to threats without the need for prior antigen sensitization and can effectively target cells that either lack or have low expression of MHC class I molecules [118]. Their ability to eliminate malignant and virus-infected cells makes them highly promising candidates for tumor immunotherapy [119, 120]. Notably, their therapeutic potential is enhanced by their inherent cellular toxicity and their ability to function independently of MHC molecular antigen presentation.

The current NK cell therapy can be roughly divided into three categories:

1. Nongenetically engineered (unmodified) NK cells

Utilizing the natural tumor-killing ability of NK cells, this therapy uses either autologous or allogeneic NK cells that are nongenetically modified to enhance their cytotoxic effectiveness against cancer cells:

- **Cytokine therapy:** This involves directly infusing cytokines like IL-2 into the patient's body to activate NK cells. For example, IL-2 can directly stimulate the activation and proliferation of T cells and NK cells but is limited in vivo by toxic effects and activation of immunosuppressive regulatory T cells (Treg).

- **mAb therapy:** NK cells can be activated by IgG antibodies to induce antibody-dependent cellular cytotoxicity (ADCC). Antibodies infused into patients can target NK cell inhibitory receptors or tumor-associated antigens, thereby activating NK cells for tumor cell destruction. Examples include monalizumab, which targets NKG2A and activates NK cells to kill tumor cells, and cetuximab, which targets EGFR on the tumor cells and induces ADCC effects via NK cells.
- **NK cell adapters**: These bispecific or trispecific antibodies target both tumor cell antigens and NK cell activation receptors, recruiting NK cells to tumor sites and stimulating them to attack cancer cells.
- **Adoptive NK cell therapy:** Similar to cytokine therapy but conducted ex vivo, NK cells are activated and enhanced before being transfused back into the patient. Sources of NK cells for this therapy can be diverse, including healthy allogeneic donors.

2. Genetically engineered NK cells

This method involves the infusion of NK cells that have been genetically modified to enhance their ability to specifically target and kill tumor cells. A prime example of this approach is CAR-NK cell therapy, where NK cells are engineered to express CARs. These receptors enable NK cells to recognize and bind to specific antigens on the surface of cancer cells, thereby directing their cytotoxic activity toward the tumor. This genetic modification not only improves the inherent antitumor capabilities of NK cells but also broadens their applicability against a variety of cancer types, making this a promising area of advancement in cancer immunotherapy:

- **Hybrid NK cell therapy (combination therapy):** This method combines surgery, radiotherapy, and targeted agents with immunotherapy to enhance overall clinical outcomes. Specifically, immunotherapy agents such as NK cell activators, ACT, monoclonal antibodies, and NK cell adapters are being explored for their potential to enhance the efficacy of NK cell therapy. By combining these different treatment strategies, researchers aim to create more comprehensive and effective therapeutic regimens that can tackle the complexities of cancer more efficiently and with potentially greater success.

7.7.2 Implementation of NK Cell Therapy

The technical process of NK cell therapy shares several similarities with CAR therapy. Initially, NK cells are isolated from various sources, such as peripheral blood (PB), umbilical cord blood (UCB), human embryonic stem cells (HESC), induced pluripotent stem cells (iPSC), and established NK cell lines. This wide range of sources provides a rich pool of cells for therapy. Notably, unlike CAR-T cells, NK cells can be derived from both autologous and allogeneic sources. This flexibility is due to the less stringent requirement for HLA matching with NK cells and their reduced risk of causing GVHD, a significant concern in CAR-T cell therapy.

After isolation, NK cells can be activated and their cytotoxicity augmented through cytokine therapy and mAb therapy. These treatments involve the direct administration of cytokines or antibodies to stimulate NK cell activity. Following this activation, NK cells are further enhanced either via exogenous substances or through genetic engineering techniques. They are then expanded in vitro and eventually reintroduced into the patient's body through transfusion.

It should also be noted that a key advantage of CAR-NK cell therapy over CAR-T therapy is the lower likelihood of serious adverse events like cytokine release syndrome and neurotoxicity. This enhanced safety profile is attributed to the nature of cytokines released by NK cells upon activation, primarily IFN-γ and granulocyte-macrophage colony-stimulating factor (GM-CSF). The distinct cytokine release profile and the inherent properties of NK cells make CAR-NK cell therapy a promising and potentially safer alternative in cancer immunotherapy.

7.7.3 Development Progression of NK Cell Therapy

The discovery and characterization of NK cells were first performed in the 1970s. Initially described by Rosenberg et al. in Canada and later independently identified by Professors Herberman in the United States and Kiessling in Sweden, NK cells were named for their natural ability to spontaneously kill tumor cells observed in tumor-bearing animals [121–123]. The concept of NK cells was further refined in 1981 when Professors Kärre and Ljunggren proposed the "missing self" hypothesis [124], suggesting that NK cells can recognize and eliminate cells with reduced expression of MHC class I molecules. This hypothesis laid the groundwork for a deeper understanding of NK cell biology and their potential role in combating cancer and other diseases.

Early studies focused on expanding autologous NK cells in vitro and then reintroducing them into the patient's body. These studies demonstrated some antitumor effects in various cancers, including renal cell carcinoma [125], lymphoma, breast cancer [126], lung cancer, and colon cancer [127]. A significant milestone was achieved in 2002 when Ruggeri and colleagues published their findings, showing that five out of nine patients with acute myeloid leukemia treated with healthy donor NK cells achieved complete hematological remission [128]. Their study provided strong clinical trial evidence for the efficacy and safety of the antitumor effects of NK cells and pulled back the curtain on allogeneic NK cell therapy. Subsequent studies by Krause, Miller, Arai, Rubnitz, and others have confirmed the safety and efficacy of allogeneic-derived NK cells in patients with hematological or solid tumors [127, 129–131]. Subsequently, the development of CAR technology has given further impetus to the development of NK cells and CAR-NK cell therapies, which are expected to exhibit enhanced efficacy against solid tumors.

7.7.4 NK Cell Therapy-Related Clinical Trials and Drugs

In the last two decades, the field of NK cell therapy has witnessed a significant boost in clinical trials, reflecting growing interest and investment in this area of research. Currently, over 600 clinical research projects worldwide focus on NK cell therapies, as registered on platforms like ClinicalTrials.gov, with nearly 200 of these trials being conducted in China. Data from Global Data's analytical database further highlight China's prominent role in NK cell therapy development, with the country housing nearly one-third of the world's institutions engaged in this research, making it a global leader in this field.

Although no NK cell therapy products have yet received global approval, numerous autologous and allogeneic NK cell therapies are in Phase I and II clinical studies. Over the next few years, it is anticipated that NK cell therapies will progress into pivotal clinical phases and potentially achieve marketing approval. Importantly, a landmark development in China was the approval for clinical trials of an investigational new drug (IND) for targeted mesothelin (MSLN) chimeric antigen receptor NK cell (CAR-NK) injection, specifically for the treatment of advanced epithelial ovarian cancer (Fig. 7.1).

7.7.5 Prospects of NK Cell Therapy

CAR-NK cell therapy has emerged as a promising area, particularly in the treatment of solid tumors, because it effectively addresses some limitations of CAR-T cell therapy. Compared to CAR-T cells, CAR-NK cells offer several advantages: they are abundant in sources, have a strong safety profile, lower toxicity risk, and can attack cancer cells through multiple pathways. These advantages position CAR-NK cells as strong candidates for "universal" products, potentially overcoming challenges associated with the long production cycles and individualized requirements characteristic of current CAR-T therapies.

However, similar to CAR-T cells, CAR-NK cells face several clinical application challenges. These include extending the survival of NK cells post-infusion, enhancing their migration and infiltration abilities, overcoming the immunosuppressive effects of the TME, and addressing the heterogeneity of target antigens. Identifying new and more representative antigenic targets, along with continuous exploration of molecular substances and innovative cell structure optimization, remains crucial for the advancement of NK cell therapies.

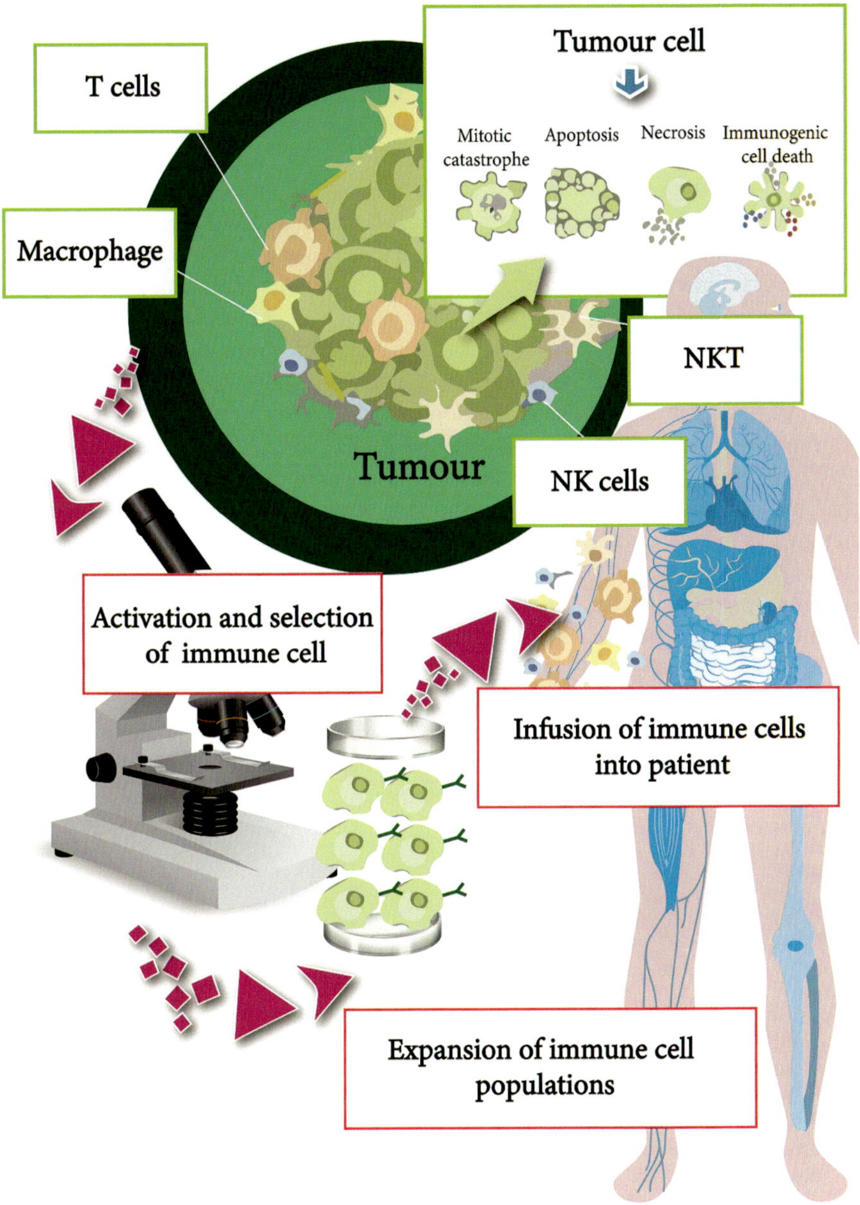

Fig. 7.1 ACT for cancer treatment

7.8 Summary

Immunotherapy stands at the forefront of oncological advancements, particularly with the rise of immune cell therapy in recent years. This innovative approach has revolutionized the treatment of hematological cancers as well as solid tumors. Regarded as a future direction for drug development, immune cell therapy encompasses a range of techniques from nonspecific therapies like LAK, CIK, and NK cells to specific therapies, including TILs, TCR-T, and CAR-T cells. As the field evolves, researchers are broadening their scope to explore other immune cells such as macrophages, DCs, NKT cells, γδT cells, and Treg cells, seeking to employ and amplify their antitumor capabilities. This expansion, however, brings its own set of challenges, including managing adverse events, selecting and targeting antigens, addressing antigen heterogeneity, and optimizing immune cell migration, infiltration, and CAR design within the suppressive TME.

While most current clinical studies in cellular immunotherapy are in the early phases, their results are consistently promising. A significant advantage of immunotherapy lies in its potential to synergize with various therapeutic modalities, enhancing overall treatment efficacy. Immune cell-based therapies are increasingly becoming pivotal in cancer treatment and managing other diseases, with a growing trend toward trials that integrate cellular immune technologies with safer, more effective drugs. In light of these developments, a concerted effort from governments, academic institutions, and the pharmaceutical industry is crucial. Collaborative strategies focused on technological innovation, clinical research, product development, and integration into routine clinical practice are essential to realize the full potential of cellular immunotherapy, paving the way for it to become a cornerstone in modern medical treatment.

References

1. Wang Z, Cao YJ. Adoptive cell therapy targeting neoantigens: a frontier for cancer research. Front Immunol. 2020;11:176.
2. Rosenberg SA, Spiess P, Lafreniere R. A new approach to the adoptive immunotherapy of cancer with tumor-infiltrating lymphocytes. Science. 1986;233:1318–21.
3. Rosenberg SA, Packard BS, Aebersold PM, et al. Use of tumor-infiltrating lymphocytes and interleukin-2 in the immunotherapy of patients with metastatic melanoma. A preliminary report. N Engl J Med. 1988;319:1676–80.
4. Sadelain M, Riviere I, Brentjens R. Targeting tumours with genetically enhanced T lymphocytes. Nat Rev Cancer. 2003;3:35–45.
5. Sadelain M, Riviere I, Riddell S. Therapeutic T cell engineering. Nature. 2017;545:423–31.
6. Myers JA, Miller JS. Exploring the NK cell platform for cancer immunotherapy. Nat Rev Clin Oncol. 2021;18:85–100.
7. Anderson NR, Minutolo NG, Gill S, et al. Macrophage-based approaches for cancer immunotherapy. Cancer Res. 2021;81:1201–8.
8. Wculek SK, Cueto FJ, Mujal AM, et al. Dendritic cells in cancer immunology and immunotherapy. Nat Rev Immunol. 2020;20:7–24.

9. Rosenberg SA, Restifo NP. Adoptive cell transfer as personalized immunotherapy for human cancer. Science. 2015;348:62–8.
10. Xue Y, Che J, Ji X, et al. Recent advances in biomaterial-boosted adoptive cell therapy. Chem Soc Rev. 2022;51:1766–94.
11. Kirtane K, Elmariah H, Chung CH, et al. Adoptive cellular therapy in solid tumor malignancies: review of the literature and challenges ahead. J Immunother Cancer. 2021;9:e002723.
12. Weber EW, Maus MV, Mackall CL. The emerging landscape of immune cell therapies. Cell. 2020;181:46–62.
13. Binnewies M, Roberts EW, Kersten K, et al. Understanding the tumor immune microenvironment (TIME) for effective therapy. Nat Med. 2018;24:541–50.
14. Rafiq S, Hackett CS, Brentjens RJ. Engineering strategies to overcome the current roadblocks in CAR T cell therapy. Nat Rev Clin Oncol. 2020;17:147–67.
15. Lasvergnas J, Naigeon M, Chouahnia K, et al. Adoptive cell therapies in thoracic malignancies. Cancer Immunol Immunother. 2022;71:2077–98.
16. Lindemann A, Herrmann F, Oster W, et al. Lymphokine activated killer cells. Blut. 1989;59:375–84.
17. Grimm EA, Mazumder A, Zhang HZ, et al. Lymphokine-activated killer cell phenomenon. Lysis of natural killer-resistant fresh solid tumor cells by interleukin 2-activated autologous human peripheral blood lymphocytes. J Exp Med. 1982;155:1823–41.
18. Rosenberg SA, Lotze MT, Muul LM, et al. Observations on the systemic administration of autologous lymphokine-activated killer cells and recombinant interleukin-2 to patients with metastatic cancer. N Engl J Med. 1985;313:1485–92.
19. Mertelsmann R. Lymphohaematopoietic growth factors in cancer therapy. Heidelberg: Springer Berlin; 1990.
20. Lee HK, Kim YG, Kim JS, et al. Cytokine-induced killer cells interact with tumor lysate-pulsed dendritic cells via CCR5 signaling. Cancer Lett. 2016;378:142–9.
21. Zhang Q, Liu XY, Zhang T, et al. The dual-functional capability of cytokine-induced killer cells and application in tumor immunology. Hum Immunol. 2015;76:385–91.
22. Zhang Y, Schmidt-Wolf IGH. Ten-year update of the international registry on cytokine-induced killer cells in cancer immunotherapy. J Cell Physiol. 2020;235:9291–303.
23. Gao X, Mi Y, Guo N, et al. Cytokine-induced killer cells as pharmacological tools for cancer immunotherapy. Front Immunol. 2017;8:774.
24. Schmidt-Wolf IG, Negrin RS, Kiem HP, et al. Use of a SCID mouse/human lymphoma model to evaluate cytokine-induced killer cells with potent antitumor cell activity. J Exp Med. 1991;174:139–49.
25. Niu Q, Wang W, Li Y, et al. Cord blood-derived cytokine-induced killer cells biotherapy combined with second-line chemotherapy in the treatment of advanced solid malignancies. Int Immunopharmacol. 2011;11:449–56.
26. Wang X, Tang S, Cui X, et al. Cytokine-induced killer cell/dendritic cell-cytokine-induced killer cell immunotherapy for the postoperative treatment of gastric cancer: a systematic review and meta-analysis. Medicine (Baltimore). 2018;97:e12230.
27. Granhoj JS, Witness Praest Jensen A, Presti M, et al. Tumor-infiltrating lymphocytes for adoptive cell therapy: recent advances, challenges, and future directions. Expert Opin Biol Ther. 2022;22:627–41.
28. Liu D, Heij LR, Czigany Z, et al. The role of tumor-infiltrating lymphocytes in cholangiocarcinoma. J Exp Clin Cancer Res. 2022;41:127.
29. Paijens ST, Vledder A, de Bruyn M, et al. Tumor-infiltrating lymphocytes in the immunotherapy era. Cell Mol Immunol. 2021;18:842–59.
30. Farhood B, Najafi M, Mortezaee K. CD8(+) cytotoxic T lymphocytes in cancer immunotherapy: a review. J Cell Physiol. 2019;234:8509–21.
31. Molgora M, Esaulova E, Vermi W, et al. TREM2 modulation remodels the tumor myeloid landscape enhancing anti-PD-1 immunotherapy. Cell. 2020;182:886–900 e17.

32. Bonaventura P, Shekarian T, Alcazer V, et al. Cold tumors: a therapeutic challenge for immunotherapy. Front Immunol. 2019;10:168.
33. Rosenbaum SR, Wilski NA, Aplin AE. Fueling the fire: inflammatory forms of cell death and implications for cancer immunotherapy. Cancer Discov. 2021;11:266–81.
34. Andersen R, Borch TH, Draghi A, et al. T cells isolated from patients with checkpoint inhibitor-resistant melanoma are functional and can mediate tumor regression. Ann Oncol. 2018;29:1575–81.
35. Powell DJ Jr, Dudley ME, Robbins PF, et al. Transition of late-stage effector T cells to CD27+ CD28+ tumor-reactive effector memory T cells in humans after adoptive cell transfer therapy. Blood. 2005;105:241–50.
36. Wu R, Forget MA, Chacon J, et al. Adoptive T-cell therapy using autologous tumor-infiltrating lymphocytes for metastatic melanoma: current status and future outlook. Cancer J. 2012;18:160–75.
37. Donia M, Junker N, Ellebaek E, et al. Characterization and comparison of 'standard' and 'young' tumour-infiltrating lymphocytes for adoptive cell therapy at a Danish translational research institution. Scand J Immunol. 2012;75:157–67.
38. Tran KQ, Zhou J, Durflinger KH, et al. Minimally cultured tumor-infiltrating lymphocytes display optimal characteristics for adoptive cell therapy. J Immunother. 2008;31:742–51.
39. Rosenberg SA, Yang JC, Sherry RM, et al. Durable complete responses in heavily pretreated patients with metastatic melanoma using T-cell transfer immunotherapy. Clin Cancer Res. 2011;17:4550–7.
40. Dudley ME, Wunderlich JR, Robbins PF, et al. Cancer regression and autoimmunity in patients after clonal repopulation with antitumor lymphocytes. Science. 2002;298:850–4.
41. Nguyen LT, Saibil SD, Sotov V, et al. Phase II clinical trial of adoptive cell therapy for patients with metastatic melanoma with autologous tumor-infiltrating lymphocytes and low-dose interleukin-2. Cancer Immunol Immunother. 2019;68:773–85.
42. Spiess PJ, Yang JC, Rosenberg SA. In vivo antitumor activity of tumor-infiltrating lymphocytes expanded in recombinant interleukin-2. J Natl Cancer Inst. 1987;79:1067–75.
43. Rosenberg SA, Yannelli JR, Yang JC, et al. Treatment of patients with metastatic melanoma with autologous tumor-infiltrating lymphocytes and interleukin 2. J Natl Cancer Inst. 1994;86:1159–66.
44. Nissani A, Lev-Ari S, Meirson T, et al. Comparison of non-myeloablative lymphodepleting preconditioning regimens in patients undergoing adoptive T cell therapy. J Immunother Cancer. 2021;9:e001743.
45. Dudley ME, Yang JC, Sherry R, et al. Adoptive cell therapy for patients with metastatic melanoma: evaluation of intensive myeloablative chemoradiation preparative regimens. J Clin Oncol. 2008;26:5233–9.
46. Santos JM, Cervera-Carrascon V, Havunen R, et al. Adenovirus coding for interleukin-2 and tumor necrosis factor alpha replaces lymphodepleting chemotherapy in adoptive T cell therapy. Mol Ther. 2018;26:2243–54.
47. Zhao Y, Deng J, Rao S, et al. Tumor Infiltrating Lymphocyte (TIL) therapy for solid tumor treatment: progressions and challenges. Cancers (Basel). 2022;14:4160.
48. Dafni U, Michielin O, Lluesma SM, et al. Efficacy of adoptive therapy with tumor-infiltrating lymphocytes and recombinant interleukin-2 in advanced cutaneous melanoma: a systematic review and meta-analysis. Ann Oncol. 2019;30:1902–13.
49. Chandran SS, Somerville RPT, Yang JC, et al. Treatment of metastatic uveal melanoma with adoptive transfer of tumour-infiltrating lymphocytes: a single-centre, two-stage, single-arm, phase 2 study. Lancet Oncol. 2017;18:792–802.
50. Creelan BC, Wang C, Teer JK, et al. Tumor-infiltrating lymphocyte treatment for anti-PD-1-resistant metastatic lung cancer: a phase 1 trial. Nat Med. 2021;27:1410–8.
51. Andersen R, Donia M, Westergaard MC, et al. Tumor infiltrating lymphocyte therapy for ovarian cancer and renal cell carcinoma. Hum Vaccin Immunother. 2015;11:2790–5.

52. Tran E, Robbins PF, Lu YC, et al. T-cell transfer therapy targeting mutant KRAS in cancer. N Engl J Med. 2016;375:2255–62.
53. Zacharakis N, Chinnasamy H, Black M, et al. Immune recognition of somatic mutations leading to complete durable regression in metastatic breast cancer. Nat Med. 2018;24:724–30.
54. Stevanovic S, Helman SR, Wunderlich JR, et al. A phase II study of tumor-infiltrating lymphocyte therapy for human papillomavirus-associated epithelial cancers. Clin Cancer Res. 2019;25:1486–93.
55. Radvanyi LG. Tumor-infiltrating lymphocyte therapy: addressing prevailing questions. Cancer J. 2015;21:450–64.
56. Darvin P, Toor SM, Sasidharan Nair V, et al. Immune checkpoint inhibitors: recent progress and potential biomarkers. Exp Mol Med. 2018;50:1–11.
57. Zhang Y, Zhang Z. The history and advances in cancer immunotherapy: understanding the characteristics of tumor-infiltrating immune cells and their therapeutic implications. Cell Mol Immunol. 2020;17:807–21.
58. Wang C, Li M, Wei R, et al. Adoptive transfer of TILs plus anti-PD1 therapy: an alternative combination therapy for treating metastatic osteosarcoma. J Bone Oncol. 2020;25:100332.
59. McLane LM, Abdel-Hakeem MS, Wherry EJ. CD8 T cell exhaustion during chronic viral infection and cancer. Annu Rev Immunol. 2019;37:457–95.
60. Kverneland AH, Pedersen M, Westergaard MCW, et al. Adoptive cell therapy in combination with checkpoint inhibitors in ovarian cancer. Oncotarget. 2020;11:2092–105.
61. Hall M, Liu H, Malafa M, et al. Expansion of tumor-infiltrating lymphocytes (TIL) from human pancreatic tumors. J Immunother Cancer. 2016;4:61.
62. Besser MJ, Shapira-Frommer R, Itzhaki O, et al. Adoptive transfer of tumor-infiltrating lymphocytes in patients with metastatic melanoma: intent-to-treat analysis and efficacy after failure to prior immunotherapies. Clin Cancer Res. 2013;19:4792–800.
63. Sarnaik AA, Hamid O, Khushalani NI, et al. Lifileucel, a tumor-infiltrating lymphocyte therapy, in metastatic melanoma. J Clin Oncol. 2021;39:2656–66.
64. Cooper ZA, Frederick DT, Juneja VR, et al. BRAF inhibition is associated with increased clonality in tumor-infiltrating lymphocytes. Onco Targets Ther. 2013;2:e26615.
65. Deniger DC, Kwong ML, Pasetto A, et al. A pilot trial of the combination of vemurafenib with adoptive cell therapy in patients with metastatic melanoma. Clin Cancer Res. 2017;23:351–62.
66. Wang S, Sun J, Chen K, et al. Perspectives of tumor-infiltrating lymphocyte treatment in solid tumors. BMC Med. 2021;19:140.
67. Schumacher TN, Schreiber RD. Neoantigens in cancer immunotherapy. Science. 2015;348:69–74.
68. Chen L, Flies DB. Molecular mechanisms of T cell co-stimulation and co-inhibition. Nat Rev Immunol. 2013;13:227–42.
69. Baulu E, Gardet C, Chuvin N, et al. TCR-engineered T cell therapy in solid tumors: state of the art and perspectives. Sci Adv. 2023;9:eadf3700.
70. Zhao Q, Jiang Y, Xiang S, et al. Engineered TCR-T cell immunotherapy in anticancer precision medicine: pros and cons. Front Immunol. 2021;12:658753.
71. Tsimberidou AM, Van Morris K, Vo HH, et al. T-cell receptor-based therapy: an innovative therapeutic approach for solid tumors. J Hematol Oncol. 2021;14:102.
72. Liu Y, Yan X, Zhang F, et al. TCR-T immunotherapy: the challenges and solutions. Front Oncol. 2021;11:794183.
73. Dembic Z, Haas W, Weiss S, et al. Transfer of specificity by murine alpha and beta T-cell receptor genes. Nature. 1986;320:232–8.
74. Morgan RA, Dudley ME, Wunderlich JR, et al. Cancer regression in patients after transfer of genetically engineered lymphocytes. Science. 2006;314:126–9.
75. Robbins PF, Morgan RA, Feldman SA, et al. Tumor regression in patients with metastatic synovial cell sarcoma and melanoma using genetically engineered lymphocytes reactive with NY-ESO-1. J Clin Oncol. 2011;29:917–24.

76. Morgan RA, Chinnasamy N, Abate-Daga D, et al. Cancer regression and neurological toxicity following anti-MAGE-A3 TCR gene therapy. J Immunother. 2013;36:133–51.
77. Robbins PF, Lu YC, El-Gamil M, et al. Mining exomic sequencing data to identify mutated antigens recognized by adoptively transferred tumor-reactive T cells. Nat Med. 2013;19:747–52.
78. Tran E, Turcotte S, Gros A, et al. Cancer immunotherapy based on mutation-specific CD4+ T cells in a patient with epithelial cancer. Science. 2014;344:641–5.
79. Stronen E, Toebes M, Kelderman S, et al. Targeting of cancer neoantigens with donor-derived T cell receptor repertoires. Science. 2016;352:1337–41.
80. Rath JA, Arber C. Engineering strategies to enhance TCR-based adoptive T cell therapy. Cells. 2020;9:1485.
81. Zhong S, Malecek K, Johnson LA, et al. T-cell receptor affinity and avidity defines antitumor response and autoimmunity in T-cell immunotherapy. Proc Natl Acad Sci USA. 2013;110:6973–8.
82. Campillo-Davo D, Flumens D, Lion E. The quest for the best: how TCR affinity, avidity, and functional avidity affect TCR-engineered T-cell antitumor responses. Cells. 2020;9:1720.
83. Thomas S, Mohammed F, Reijmers RM, et al. Framework engineering to produce dominant T cell receptors with enhanced antigen-specific function. Nat Commun. 2019;10:4451.
84. Legut M, Dolton G, Mian AA, et al. CRISPR-mediated TCR replacement generates superior anticancer transgenic T cells. Blood. 2018;131:311–22.
85. Roth TL, Puig-Saus C, Yu R, et al. Reprogramming human T cell function and specificity with non-viral genome targeting. Nature. 2018;559:405–9.
86. Nahmad AD, Reuveni E, Goldschmidt E, et al. Frequent aneuploidy in primary human T cells after CRISPR-Cas9 cleavage. Nat Biotechnol. 2022;40:1807–13.
87. Shafer P, Kelly LM, Hoyos V. Cancer therapy with TCR-engineered T cells: current strategies, challenges, and prospects. Front Immunol. 2022;13:835762.
88. Johnson LA, Morgan RA, Dudley ME, et al. Gene therapy with human and mouse T-cell receptors mediates cancer regression and targets normal tissues expressing cognate antigen. Blood. 2009;114:535–46.
89. Chodon T, Comin-Anduix B, Chmielowski B, et al. Adoptive transfer of MART-1 T-cell receptor transgenic lymphocytes and dendritic cell vaccination in patients with metastatic melanoma. Clin Cancer Res. 2014;20:2457–65.
90. Parkhurst MR, Yang JC, Langan RC, et al. T cells targeting carcinoembryonic antigen can mediate regression of metastatic colorectal cancer but induce severe transient colitis. Mol Ther. 2011;19:620–6.
91. Larson RC, Kann MC, Bailey SR, et al. CAR T cell killing requires the IFNgammaR pathway in solid but not liquid tumours. Nature. 2022;604:563–70.
92. Jackson HJ, Rafiq S, Brentjens RJ. Driving CAR T-cells forward. Nat Rev Clin Oncol. 2016;13:370–83.
93. Bird RE, Hardman KD, Jacobson JW, et al. Single-chain antigen-binding proteins. Science. 1988;242:423–6.
94. Posey AD Jr, Schwab RD, Boesteanu AC, et al. Engineered CAR T cells targeting the cancer-associated Tn-Glycoform of the membrane mucin MUC1 control adenocarcinoma. Immunity. 2016;44:1444–54.
95. James SE, Greenberg PD, Jensen MC, et al. Antigen sensitivity of CD22-specific chimeric TCR is modulated by target epitope distance from the cell membrane. J Immunol. 2008;180:7028–38.
96. Kochenderfer JN, Wilson WH, Janik JE, et al. Eradication of B-lineage cells and regression of lymphoma in a patient treated with autologous T cells genetically engineered to recognize CD19. Blood. 2010;116:4099–102.
97. Gross G, Waks T, Eshhar Z. Expression of immunoglobulin-T-cell receptor chimeric molecules as functional receptors with antibody-type specificity. Proc Natl Acad Sci USA. 1989;86:10024–8.

98. Kershaw MH, Westwood JA, Parker LL, et al. A phase I study on adoptive immunotherapy using gene-modified T cells for ovarian cancer. Clin Cancer Res. 2006;12:6106–15.
99. Park JR, Digiusto DL, Slovak M, et al. Adoptive transfer of chimeric antigen receptor re-directed cytolytic T lymphocyte clones in patients with neuroblastoma. Mol Ther. 2007;15:825–33.
100. Song DG, Ye Q, Carpenito C, et al. In vivo persistence, tumor localization, and antitumor activity of CAR-engineered T cells is enhanced by costimulatory signaling through CD137 (4-1BB). Cancer Res. 2011;71:4617–27.
101. Kandalaft LE, Powell DJ Jr, Coukos G. A phase I clinical trial of adoptive transfer of folate receptor-alpha redirected autologous T cells for recurrent ovarian cancer. J Transl Med. 2012;10:157.
102. Brentjens RJ, Davila ML, Riviere I, et al. CD19-targeted T cells rapidly induce molecular remissions in adults with chemotherapy-refractory acute lymphoblastic leukemia. Sci Transl Med. 2013;5:177ra38.
103. Morgan RA, Yang JC, Kitano M, et al. Case report of a serious adverse event following the administration of T cells transduced with a chimeric antigen receptor recognizing ERBB2. Mol Ther. 2010;18:843–51.
104. Yi Z, Prinzing BL, Cao F, et al. Optimizing EphA2-CAR T cells for the adoptive immunotherapy of glioma. Mol Ther Methods Clin Dev. 2018;9:70–80.
105. Abate-Daga D, Lagisetty KH, Tran E, et al. A novel chimeric antigen receptor against prostate stem cell antigen mediates tumor destruction in a humanized mouse model of pancreatic cancer. Hum Gene Ther. 2014;25:1003–12.
106. Locke FL, Ghobadi A, Jacobson CA, et al. Long-term safety and activity of axicabtagene ciloleucel in refractory large B-cell lymphoma (ZUMA-1): a single-arm, multicentre, phase 1-2 trial. Lancet Oncol. 2019;20:31–42.
107. Elsawy M, Chavez JC, Avivi I, et al. Patient-reported outcomes in ZUMA-7, a phase 3 study of axicabtagene ciloleucel in second-line large B-cell lymphoma. Blood. 2022;140:2248–60.
108. Ying Z, Zou D, Yang H, et al. Preliminary efficacy and safety of Relmacabtagene autoleucel (Carteyva) in adults with relapsed/refractory follicular lymphoma in China: a phase I/II clinical trial. Am J Hematol. 2022;97:E436–8.
109. Li Y, Hermanson DL, Moriarity BS, et al. Human iPSC-derived natural killer cells engineered with chimeric antigen receptors enhance anti-tumor activity. Cell Stem Cell. 2018;23:181–192.e5.
110. Tang X, Yang L, Li Z, et al. Erratum: first-in-man clinical trial of CAR NK-92 cells: safety test of CD33-CAR NK-92 cells in patients with relapsed and refractory acute myeloid leukemia. Am J Cancer Res. 2018;8:1899.
111. Liu E, Marin D, Banerjee P, et al. Use of CAR-transduced natural killer cells in CD19-positive lymphoid tumors. N Engl J Med. 2020;382:545–53.
112. Lu C, Guo C, Chen H, et al. A novel chimeric PD1-NKG2D-41BB receptor enhances antitumor activity of NK92 cells against human lung cancer H1299 cells by triggering pyroptosis. Mol Immunol. 2020;122:200–6.
113. Alvey CM, Spinler KR, Irianto J, et al. SIRPA-Inhibited, Marrow-derived macrophages engorge, accumulate, and differentiate in antibody-targeted regression of solid tumors. Curr Biol. 2017;27:2065–2077.e6.
114. Klichinsky M, Ruella M, Shestova O, et al. Human chimeric antigen receptor macrophages for cancer immunotherapy. Nat Biotechnol. 2020;38:947–53.
115. Bailey SR, Vatsa S, Larson RC, et al. Blockade or deletion of IFNgamma reduces macrophage activation without compromising CAR T-cell function in hematologic malignancies. Blood Cancer Discov. 2022;3:136–53.
116. June CH, Sadelain M. Chimeric antigen receptor therapy. N Engl J Med. 2018;379:64–73.
117. Adachi K, Kano Y, Nagai T, et al. IL-7 and CCL19 expression in CAR-T cells improves immune cell infiltration and CAR-T cell survival in the tumor. Nat Biotechnol. 2018;36:346–51.

118. Del Vecchio F, Martinez-Rodriguez V, Schukking M, et al. Professional killers: the role of extracellular vesicles in the reciprocal interactions between natural killer, CD8+ cytotoxic T-cells and tumour cells. J Extracell Vesicles. 2021;10:e12075.
119. Vivier E, Raulet DH, Moretta A, et al. Innate or adaptive immunity? The example of natural killer cells. Science. 2011;331:44–9.
120. Vivier E, Artis D, Colonna M, et al. Innate lymphoid cells: 10 years on. Cell. 2018;174:1054–66.
121. Rosenberg EB, Herberman RB, Levine PH, et al. Lymphocyte cytotoxicity reactions to leukemia-associated antigens in identical twins. Int J Cancer. 1972;9:648–58.
122. Herberman RB, Nunn ME, Lavrin DH. Natural cytotoxic reactivity of mouse lymphoid cells against syngeneic acid allogeneic tumors. I. Distribution of reactivity and specificity. Int J Cancer. 1975;16:216–29.
123. Kiessling R, Klein E, Wigzell H. "Natural" killer cells in the mouse. I. Cytotoxic cells with specificity for mouse Moloney leukemia cells. Specificity and distribution according to genotype. Eur J Immunol. 1975;5:112–7.
124. Ljunggren HG, Karre K. In search of the 'missing self': MHC molecules and NK cell recognition. Immunol Today. 1990;11:237–44.
125. Hercend T, Farace F, Baume D, et al. Immunotherapy with lymphokine-activated natural killer cells and recombinant interleukin-2: a feasibility trial in metastatic renal cell carcinoma. J Biol Response Mod. 1990;9:546–55.
126. Miller JS, Tessmer-Tuck J, Pierson BA, et al. Low dose subcutaneous interleukin-2 after autologous transplantation generates sustained in vivo natural killer cell activity. Biol Blood Marrow Transplant. 1997;3:34–44.
127. Krause SW, Gastpar R, Andreesen R, et al. Treatment of colon and lung cancer patients with ex vivo heat shock protein 70-peptide-activated, autologous natural killer cells: a clinical phase i trial. Clin Cancer Res. 2004;10:3699–707.
128. Ruggeri L, Capanni M, Urbani E, et al. Effectiveness of donor natural killer cell alloreactivity in mismatched hematopoietic transplants. Science. 2002;295:2097–100.
129. Miller JS, Soignier Y, Panoskaltsis-Mortari A, et al. Successful adoptive transfer and in vivo expansion of human haploidentical NK cells in patients with cancer. Blood. 2005;105:3051–7.
130. Arai S, Meagher R, Swearingen M, et al. Infusion of the allogeneic cell line NK-92 in patients with advanced renal cell cancer or melanoma: a phase I trial. Cytotherapy. 2008;10:625–32.
131. Rubnitz JE, Inaba H, Ribeiro RC, et al. NKAML: a pilot study to determine the safety and feasibility of haploidentical natural killer cell transplantation in childhood acute myeloid leukemia. J Clin Oncol. 2010;28:955–9.

Chapter 8
Gene-Guided Drugs

Yuda Zhang and Tian Xu

Abstract Gene therapy in cancer treatment represents a cutting-edge approach, targeting the genetic alterations that drive cancer growth. By introducing, removing, or modifying genes within a patient's cells, gene therapy seeks to treat or prevent cancer. Techniques include replacing a mutated gene that causes disease with a healthy copy, inactivating a mutated gene that is functioning improperly, or introducing a new or modified gene to help fight the cancer. Gene therapy offers a highly personalized treatment option, potentially overcoming the limitations of traditional therapies like chemotherapy and radiotherapy. Its development signifies a major leap in precision medicine, offering new hope for targeting specific cancer types and improving patient outcomes, while ongoing research continues to refine and enhance its efficacy and safety.

Keywords Gene therapy · AAV · *CRISPR*

8.1 Definition of Gene Therapy

Gene therapy is a biomedical technology that involves the insertion of normal or therapeutic exogenous genes into target cells to repair or replace defective genes, ultimately treating diseases. The concept of gene therapy can be divided into broad and narrow senses [1]. In the narrow sense, it pertains specifically to substituting or

Y. Zhang (✉)
Department of Medical Oncology, Lung Cancer and Gastrointestinal Unit, Hunan Cancer Hospital/The Affiliated Cancer Hospital of Xiangya School of Medicine, Central South University, Changsha, China
e-mail: zhangyuda@hnca.org.cn

T. Xu
Department of Medical Oncology, Lung Cancer and Gastrointestinal Unit, The Second Xiangya Hospital, Changsha, China
e-mail: 208211134@csu.edu.cn

© The Author(s), under exclusive license to Springer Nature Singapore Pte Ltd. 2024

Y. Zhang, N. Yang (eds.), *New Anti-cancer Drug Development and Evaluation*,
https://doi.org/10.1007/978-981-97-7274-2_8

supplementing defective genes in patients with normally functioning genes, in order to achieve therapeutic outcomes. On the other hand, the broad sense refers to the transfer of genetic material into a patient, allowing for its expression and ultimately treating a disease [2]. As the understanding of genetic material and its mechanisms of action continues to evolve, scientists have developed the ability to modify certain target genes at the molecular level through advancements in genetic technology [3].

8.2 Techniques of Gene Therapy

Currently, the most cutting-edge technologies in gene therapy encompass adeno-associated virus (AAV) vector delivery, CRISPR (Clustered Regularly Interspaced Short Palindromic Repeats) gene editing, single/double-base editing, and oncolytic virus gene modification techniques [4] (Fig.8.1).

8.2.1 AAV Vector Delivery Technology

Adeno-associated virus (AAV) was initially discovered in adenovirus preparations in the 1960s and subsequently identified in human tissues. Due to its unique properties, such as nonpathogenicity, efficient gene expression, ease of gene manipulation, and low immune response, AAV has became a leading platform for in vivo gene delivery [5]. AAV stands out as a promising vector for gene therapy due to its low potential for causing genetic damage in humans. In fact, there is limited direct evidence that the use of recombinant AAV (rAAV) results in host genome-mediated genotoxicity in humans. This is due in part to the fact that the rAAV genome mostly persists in the host nucleus as episomes, which are nonintegrated genetic elements [6].

The most recent advancements in the design of the AAV genome allow for the inclusion of self-complementary sequences, which can be carried within the capsid as single-stranded DNA. One key advantage of this design is that it eliminates the need for single-stranded DNA replication into double-stranded DNA, resulting in faster and more efficient gene expression compared to traditional single-stranded AAV genomes. However, it is important to note that this design reduces the carrying capacity of AAV by half, and further studies are required to optimize this approach [6].

8.2.2 CRISPR Gene Editing Technology

CRISPR gene editing technology represents the latest generation of DNA nuclease-based gene editing approaches. The CRISPR/Cas9 system is composed of two main components: a Cas9 protein and a single-stranded guide RNA (sgRNA) [7]. By

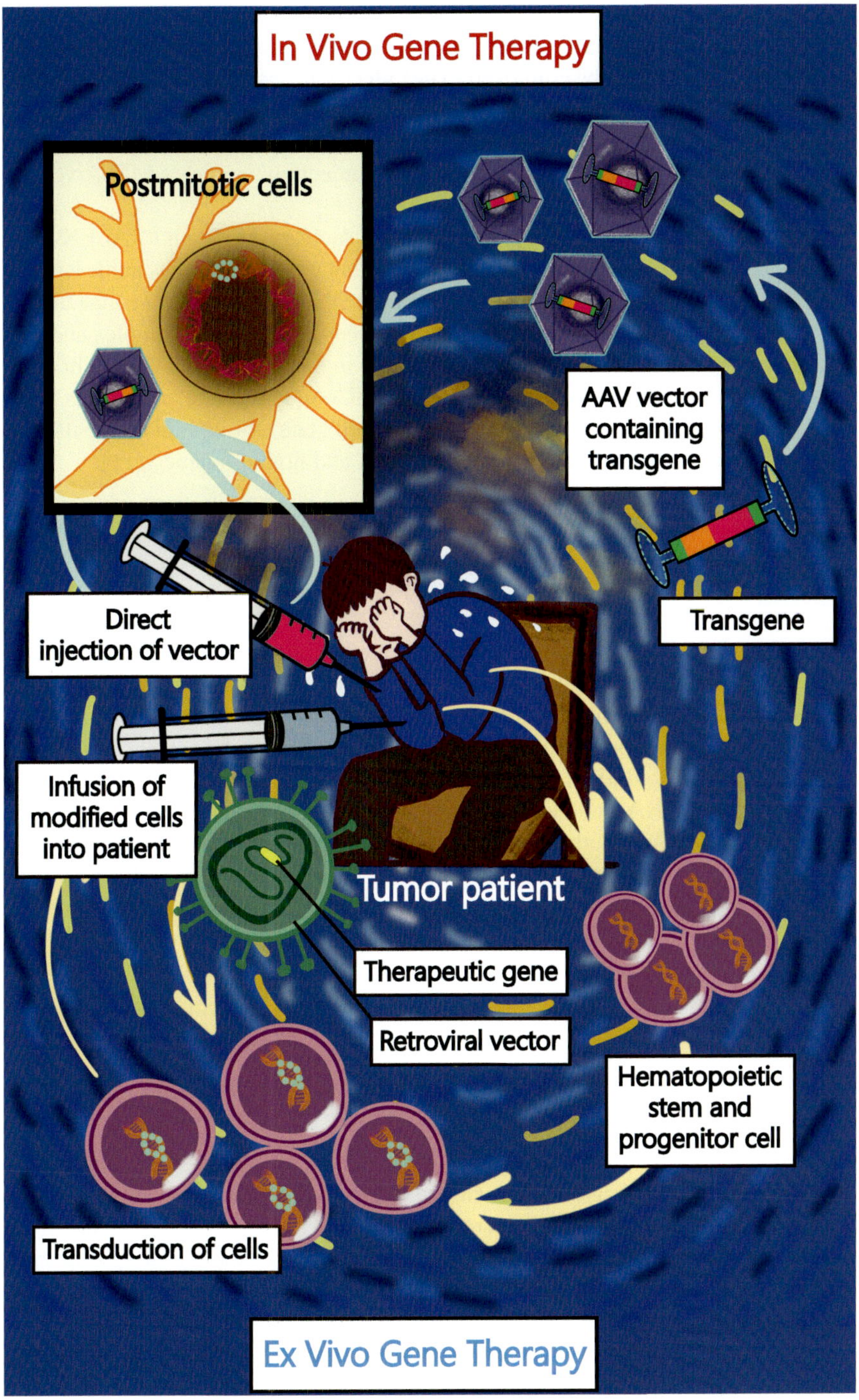

Fig. 8.1 Scheme for gene therapy

utilizing the guiding function of the sgRNA, the Cas9 protein can precisely cleave target sites within the DNA, inducing double-stranded breaks through base pairing [8]. This system can then be employed to introduce various types of mutations at the cleavage sites. These include random mutations through non-homologous end joining (NHEJ) repair or specific mutations or insertions through homologous directed repair (HDR). The latter can be achieved by co-injecting engineered DNA vectors homologous to the target DNA [9].

In contrast to earlier gene editing methods such as ZFNs and TALENs, the CRISPR/Cas9 system boasts several distinct advantages. It employs a guide RNA to precisely guide the Cas9 nuclease to the intended DNA locus, thereby enhancing its specificity. Additionally, unlike previous approaches that required complex and precise protein design or assembly, the Cas9 protein in the CRISPR/Cas9 system functions as a monomer under the guidance of the sgRNA [10]. These advantages make CRISPR/Cas9 the most widely studied and utilized gene editing tool due to its simplicity in synthesis, short cycle time, ease of use, and high efficiency [11].

8.2.3 Single/Double-Base Editing Technique

Although the CRISPR system has demonstrated proficiency in inducing precise double-strand breaks in DNA, its efficacy in facilitating homology-directed repair has encountered certain limitations. Other gene editing technologies, such as ZFN and TALEN, suffer from similar issues, including a lack of control over editing outcomes and the potential for off-target effects [12]. Additionally, these methods rely on inducing DNA double-strand breaks, which can result in unexpected outcomes within the edited cells [13]. To address these concerns, the David Liu laboratory at Harvard University developed a single-base editor in 2016 that uses a Cas9 fusion protein. This innovative approach significantly improves the efficiency of base editing and allows for precise targeting of single-base errors without inducing double-strand breaks in the DNA [14].

8.2.4 Oncolytic Virus Genetic Modification Technology

An oncolytic virus is a type of virus with the unique ability to target and destroy cancer cells while leaving healthy cells unharmed [15]. It achieves this through a two-pronged attack: firstly, the virus replicates within the tumor cells, causing them to burst and die. Secondly, as the infected cells die, they release tumor-specific antigens that trigger the body's immune system to mount an attack against the remaining cancer cells [16]. Furthermore, scientists can modify oncolytic viruses by inserting therapeutic genes into them, which enhances their ability to kill cancer cells. This approach avoids the problem of drug resistance that commonly occurs with traditional cancer treatments that target a single molecule or pathway. Overall, oncolytic viruses hold great promise as a novel and effective approach to fighting cancer [17].

8.3 Process for Gene Therapy Drug Development

When it comes to developing gene therapy drugs, the focus is on achieving two critical goals: efficacy and safety. To enhance efficacy, researchers need to identify suitable targets based on the underlying genetics and genomics of the disease [18]. They then need to carefully choose the appropriate viral vectors that can effectively deliver the therapeutic genes to the target cells. Furthermore, optimizing the delivery process is crucial to ensure that the genes reach the desired cells and produce the intended effects while avoiding serious adverse events. Assessing the efficacy and safety of gene therapy drugs involves conducting a series of complex and time-consuming preclinical trials. The production process for viral vectors is also highly specialized, with each vector requiring a tailored approach that accounts for its unique chemistry, production, and control [19]. These challenges make the large-scale production of gene therapy drugs a complex task that requires a deep understanding of the underlying processes involved. Therefore, it is essential to design each gene therapy drug with a customized and meticulous approach that takes into account its unique features and production requirements [20].

The development process of gene therapy drugs mainly includes the following three stages (Fig. 8.2):

1. The design and optimization of viral vectors
2. The proof of concept of viral vectors in vitro and in vivo
3. The clinical evaluation of drugs

8.3.1 Virus Vector Design and Optimization

Various types of viral vectors have distinct packaging and production systems, especially for large vectors like herpes simplex virus carriers or vaccinia virus vectors. These vectors offer significant advantages in loading exogenous genomes, but their modification can be challenging. To overcome this challenge, researchers have developed two widely used modification methods: bacterial artificial chromosome (BAC) and CRISPR [21].

BAC technology is a powerful method that allows for the preservation and manipulation of viral genomes using artificial chromosomes in bacteria. This technique offers several benefits [21]. Firstly, the viral genome is inserted into the BAC, and because the viral promoter cannot function properly in bacteria, the viral genes are replicated by bacterial polymerase. Hence, no selective pressure is exerted on the viral genome, ensuring that there are no mutations in the viral genes. Secondly,

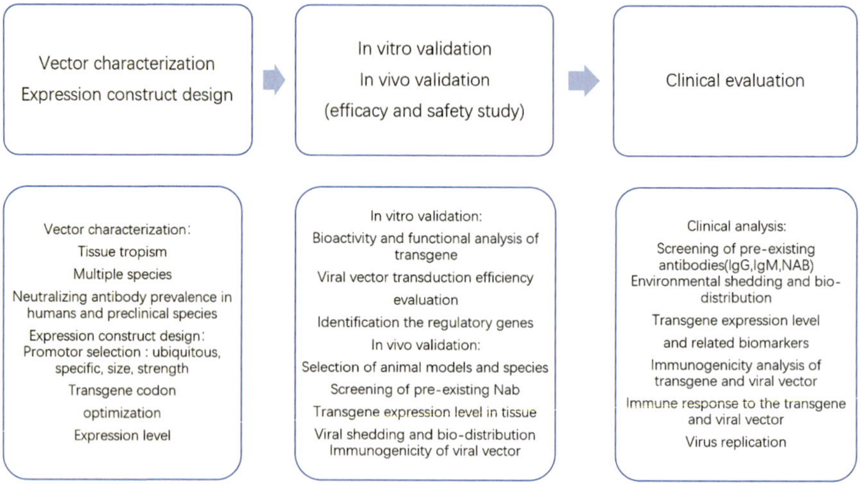

Fig. 8.2 Development process of gene therapy drugs

BAC can accommodate large DNA and RNA viral genomes of up to 300 kb in length. The BAC vector also includes an antibiotic resistance gene, which allows for easy screening of recombinant viruses in *E. coli*. Additionally, many BAC vectors contain fluorescent genes that enable visualization of gene expression in transfected cells [22]. This feature is helpful for identifying recombinant viruses containing BACs in mammalian cells.

The CRISPR/Cas9 system technology has been used to knock out the eGFP gene in herpes simplex virus, and the resulting recombinant virus has been verified by sequencing. The CRISPR system is a simpler method compared to the BAC system; however, it is limited in the manipulation of genes necessary for viral replication. Thus, the choice of system needs to be tailored based on specific requirements for each application [23].

In gene therapy, the presence of preexisting antibodies can hinder the efficiency of viral vectors. To surmount this challenge, further optimization of viral vectors is required, such as capsid modification. Capsid modification plays a key role in the application of AAV in gene therapy [24]. Capsid modification can be achieved through directed evolution and rational design. Compared with directed evolution, a complex and time-consuming method, rational design is more efficient and is thus widely used. Specifically, AAV binds to cell surfaces by attaching to primary receptors or coreceptors [25]. The receptor-binding domains of some AAV serotypes have been identified, and studies of AAV capsid sequences and structures provide detailed information about AAV transduction mechanisms. This knowledge enables the rational design of AAV vectors with enhanced transduction efficiency by inserting amino acids or specific peptides that bind to receptors or by modifying exposed amino acids on the capsid surface. Given that the transduction efficiencies depend on AAV serotypes and cell types, it is evident that optimizing capsid design holds the potential to align with specific disease types and objectives [6, 26].

8.3.2 Proof of Concept for Viral Vectors Through In Vitro and In Vivo Experiments

Once an optimized viral vector design has been obtained, several characteristics of the vector can be evaluated through in vitro experiments. These evaluations include assessing the infectivity and replication characteristics of the vector itself. For instance, the TCID50 assay can be employed to gauge the infectious potential and transduction efficacy of AAV. Similarly, for oncolytic virus products, the replication ability of the virus can be evaluated by analyzing the growth curve of the modified virus. These in vitro experiments can provide valuable insights into the overall performance of the viral vector, allowing researchers to further refine and optimize the vector design to achieve better outcomes in gene therapy [27].

After evaluating the characteristics of the viral vector, the target gene can be evaluated at both the mRNA and protein levels. Complex modifications, such as codon optimization or nonessential gene deletion, may impact the expression of the target gene at these levels [28]. Once the characteristics of the viral vector and the target gene have been evaluated, functional validation is necessary. This validation includes assessing the functionality of the viral vector and the functional activity and mechanism of the target gene [21]. Furthermore, in vitro experiments can be conducted to explore the effects of tumor-killing cytokines, which can guide the selection of appropriate biomarkers for subsequent in vivo pharmacodynamic studies. The evaluation of viral vector functionality and target gene mechanisms can provide essential guidance for animal experimentation and subsequent studies [29].

8.3.3 Drug Clinical Evaluation

When evaluating a viral vector in a clinical study, its efficacy, pharmacokinetics, immunogenicity, and immunotoxicity are the main areas of focus. However, analyzing clinical samples requires a more complex and comprehensive approach to methodological development and validation [30]. This involves considering various factors such as the matrix effect, precision, accuracy, sensitivity, selectivity, robustness, and stability. These parameters are crucial to ensure that the results obtained from clinical samples are reliable and accurate. Therefore, a rigorous and well-designed methodology is essential to evaluate the safety and efficacy of viral vectors in clinical settings [31].

8.3.4 Current Status of Gene Therapy Drugs in China

Gene therapy has a history that dates back to the 1960s, but it wasn't until the 1990s that it entered the clinical stage. Over the years, with advancements in genome sequencing and vector technology, gene therapy has made significant progress in terms of safety and efficacy. The advent of breakthrough technologies such as CRISPR has further enriched the gene therapy technology system and opened up new avenues for its development [32]. In recent years, gene therapy has experienced rapid advancement and has emerged as a promising novel field within biomedicine, alongside small molecules and large molecules. Its potential to cure genetic disorders and other diseases has generated a great deal of interest and excitement in the scientific community [33].

As of September 2020, the US Food and Drug Administration (FDA) has approved 15 gene therapy products, each falling into one of four categories: CAR-T therapy, antisense oligonucleotides (ASOs), plasmid-based DNA, and siRNA. ASOs are the most well-established product type, with the most approved products and the earliest approvals dating back to 1998. CAR-T therapy and RNAi drugs began later but have made rapid progress [34].

Gene therapy products have mainly been developed for two types of diseases: hereditary rare diseases and cancer. CAR-T therapy products have primarily been used in cancer treatment, while other gene therapy products have mainly been used to address rare genetic disorders [35]. As of the end of 2018, gene therapy clinical trials have shown that the most common indications for gene therapy are tumors and monogenic diseases, accounting for 80% of all clinical trials. Many of these drugs have achieved significant breakthroughs in drug therapy for these indications, thus addressing the critical medical needs of patients with rare diseases [36] (Fig. 8.3).

China has been actively pursuing research in gene therapy for almost two decades, with a significant milestone achieved in 1991 when the world's second gene therapy clinical trial for hemophilia B patients was conducted by Professor Xue Jinglun's research group at the Institute of Genetics of Fudan University in China. Using retroviruses to transfect fibroblasts in vitro, they successfully treated two patients and became the second group in the world to carry out human gene

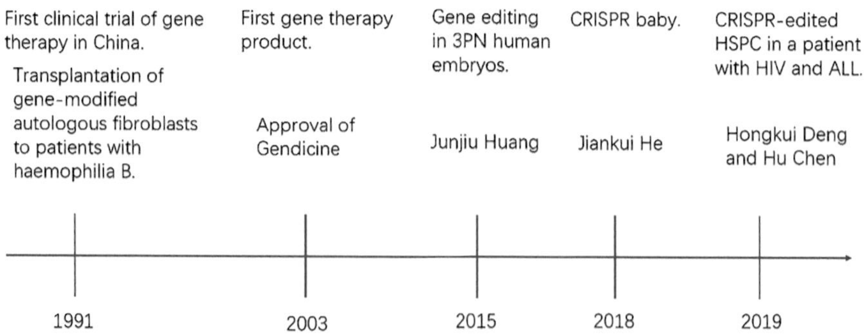

Fig. 8.3 Gene therapy trials for cancer treatment

therapy trials, just a year after the ADA-SCID trial in the United States. In 2003, Professor Wu Xiaobing's team collaborated with Professor Xue Jinglun's group and received approval for a Phase I clinical trial of gene therapy drugs for rAAV2-hFIX injection in the treatment of hemophilia B. This trial was conducted at Tianjin Hematology Hospital, where the low-dose group of two patients completed multipoint intramuscular injection therapy. Today, two gene therapy drugs, independently developed in China, have gained significant attention from the global medical community [37].

In 2003, China also made history by approving Gendicine, the world's first gene therapy product. Since then, China has been continuously exploring the field of gene therapy, with more than 20 clinical trials currently underway [38, 39]. Two CAR-T drugs, FKC876 and Relma-cel, have received priority review and breakthrough therapy designation, respectively. Additionally, Cilta-cel, which is currently being examined in a Phase II clinical trial, has also received breakthrough therapy designation and is expected to undergo an accelerated review process. While gene therapy in China is primarily aimed at rare diseases, such as hemophilia and thalassemia, and tumor diseases, like melanoma, the approved gene therapies are expected to be rapidly introduced into the market as "new drugs urgently needed in clinical practice." [40] For instance, Spinraza received marketing approval without the necessity for domestic clinical trials. Furthermore, approximately 20 ongoing domestic gene therapy clinical trials showcase a robust dedication to advancing gene therapy research within China. In fact, China accounts for almost half (46.7%) of all registered gene therapy clinical trial protocols in Asia, with around 70 protocols currently registered on the Clinical Trial website [41].

Although China still lags behind the international market in terms of the number of approved gene therapies, it is anticipated that gene therapy will become more prevalent in the domestic market shortly, bringing significant benefits to cancer patients and those suffering from rare diseases.

8.4 Representative Gene Therapy Drugs Developed in China

8.4.1 Gendicine

Gendicine, a recombinant human p53 adenovirus, was developed by Shenzhen Sibiono Gene Technology Co., Ltd. and received approval from the China Food and Drug Administration (CFDA) in October 2003 for treating head and neck squamous cell carcinoma (HNSCC). This groundbreaking approval of the first gene therapy drug and its subsequent commercialization caused mixed reactions [42]. While the international gene therapy community was once again excited about the potential of such novel therapies after being overshadowed by unexpected clinical events in late 1999, concerns were raised about the clinical trial data for Gendicine. Some questioned whether the data collection methods were comparable to the good clinical practice standards of the US FDA. One of the issues surrounding Gendicine is that while adenovirus-p53 can express the P53 gene in vivo at the first injection, it is difficult to express the P53 gene after subsequent continuous intratumoral injections over a long period [43]. Due to these concerns, the approval and marketing of the drug have been controversial, and there has been little clinical promotion since 2008 [44]. Nonetheless, the safety and efficacy of Gendicine have reignited interest in investigational new drugs and clinical trials of other gene therapies [45].

8.4.2 *Oncorine*

In recent years, oncolytic viral drugs have become a hot topic in cancer therapy. An example of such a drug is Recombinant Human Adenovirus Type 5 Injection, also known as Oncorine, which is currently the only oncolytic virus product available on the market in China. Previous studies have shown that Oncorine has significant potential in treating various malignant tumors such as nasopharyngeal carcinoma, esophageal cancer, and gastric cancer [46].

Oncorine can selectively infect cancer cells due to its ability to knock down the adenovirus type 5 E1B gene. This gene is essential for adenovirus replication and also inhibits the function of p53, a protein that plays a critical role in triggering apoptosis, or programmed cell death. However, in tumor cells, the p53 protein is absent, making it easier for Oncorine to replicate within the cancer cells. Conversely, in normal cells, viruses that lack the E1B gene are unable to inhibit the p53 pathway, leading to apoptosis of the host cell and failure to replicate [47]. Oncorine's unique mechanism of selective infection allows it to effectively target and replicate within cancer cells, making it a promising treatment option for certain types of cancer.

8.5 Gene Therapy Drugs Under Clinical Trials

Multiple gene therapy drugs are currently in the progress of clinical trials. The Academy of Military Medical Sciences has developed a gene therapy product called Ad-HGF Injection for the treatment of myocardial infarction, which is now in Phase II clinical trials [48]. In collaboration with Humanwell, they are also developing a naked plasmid drug called recombinant plasmid-hepatocyte growth factor injection (pUDK-HGF) for the treatment of limb rest pain caused by severe lower limb ischemic diseases [49]. This drug is currently undergoing Phase III clinical trials (CTR20181274). Meanwhile, Helixmith has developed a recombinant human hepatocyte growth factor naked plasmid injection (NL-003), which is being tested in clinical trials worldwide. In China, the development of this drug is being conducted by Beijing Northland Biotechnology Co., Ltd., and it is currently undergoing Phase III clinical trials (CTR20190746 and CTR20190750) for the treatment of lower limb ischemic diseases.

Multiple teams in China are conducting clinical trials for tumor treatment. For example, Huazhong University of Science and Technology has developed a cancer gene therapy product called ADV-TK, which has shown significant effectiveness in treating liver cancer and refractory and recurrent head and neck cancer. ADV-TK is currently undergoing a multicenter Phase III clinical trial [50]. Another team, including Sun Yat-sen University, has developed a product called recombinant human endostatin adenovirus injection (E-10A), which has shown efficacy in treating advanced head and neck squamous cell carcinoma. E-10A has already undergone Phase III clinical trials in both China and North America and has promising development prospects. Chengdu Kanghong Biology has developed KH901, an engineered oncolytic adenovirus gene therapy preparation that has completed a Phase II clinical trial for the treatment of head and neck cancer [51]. The team at Sichuan University has developed EDS01, a gene therapy product that targets tumor angiogenesis and is currently undergoing a Phase II clinical trial.

In particular, China has emerged as a leader in the field of gene editing therapy, with significant breakthroughs being reported by Chinese scientists in recent years. In 2015, Huang Jun of Sun Yat-sen University conducted the first-ever gene editing operation using CRISPR technology on human embryonic cells. Subsequently, in September 2017, another milestone achievement was attained when Huang's team employed a single-base editing system to accurately rectify specific types of single-base mutations within the human embryonic genome, particularly addressing thalassemia HBB-28 [52]. More recently, in August 2022, Shanghai Bangyao Biotechnology Co., Ltd. and Central South University collaborated to use CRISPR technology to edit the expression of γ-globin activated by BCL11A erythroid-specific enhancer [53]. The results were promising, as the reinfused autologous hematopoietic stem cells effectively relieved the symptoms of β0/β0 severe thalassemia in two pediatric patients who were able to escape transfusion dependence for up to 2 years. Based on this success, Bangyao Biotechnology has developed BRL-101, a gene editing therapeutic that was approved by the CDE to enter the clinical phase on August 22, and a Phase 1/2 trial was initiated in October of the same year. Overall, these breakthroughs demonstrate China's commitment to advancing the field of gene editing therapy and improving the lives of patients suffering from genetic disorders such as thalassemia. These achievements also have the potential to pave the way for further advancements in gene editing technology and its applications in treating a wide range of diseases [54].

China has also made great progress in the treatment of ophthalmic diseases. On June 29, 2021, Wuhan Neurophth made a significant announcement that its newly developed ophthalmic in vivo gene therapy drug, NR082 (R&D code NFS-01), had been successfully administered to the first patient in China as part of a Phase 1/2/3 clinical trial for Leber hereditary optic neuropathy (LHON) caused by the ND4 mitochondrial gene mutation. The operation was performed by Wei Wenbin, vice president of Beijing Tongren Hospital, Capital Medical University, and director of ophthalmology. This marks a groundbreaking moment in the field of ophthalmic in vivo gene therapy in China, as it represents the first administration of a registered clinical study of such therapy in the country. This development is particularly noteworthy as it brings renewed hope to LHON patients who currently have limited treatment options. In 2022, there were additional exciting developments in the field of gene therapy for eye diseases in China. Both VGR-R01 by Vitalgen and ZVS101e by Beijing Zhongyin Technology were approved to enter clinical trials for crystal-like retinal degeneration caused by the CYP4V2 gene mutation. Gene therapy also presents a promising new approach for treating age-related macular degeneration (AMD). In this regard, KH631 by Chengdu Hongji Biotechnology Co., Ltd. (Kanghong Pharmaceutical Group Co., Ltd.) has received clinical approval both in China and the United States for treating wet AMD (wet-AMD). Overall, these developments are significant and offer new hope for patients suffering from various forms of eye diseases.

8.6 Gene Therapy Adverse Events

The safety of gene therapy is often questioned, particularly when using lentiviral vectors. These vectors are used to deliver a "normal gene" into the target cells, but there is a risk that it may bind to the wrong location on the chromosome, potentially causing genetic damage or even cancer [55]. Additionally, incomplete removal of the viral components in the vector may result in the virus being infectious and potentially transmitted to other individuals or future generations. Scientists are actively engaged in developing more precise vector viruses that can be utilized safely and efficiently in gene therapy [56]. Nevertheless, these vectors may still trigger an immune response in patients, potentially resulting in unfavorable side effects or even treatment ineffectiveness. To address this issue, researchers are modifying the vectors themselves and incorporating "inhibitors" to prevent adverse immune responses during in vivo treatments. These measures aim to minimize the risks associated with gene therapy and increase its effectiveness as a treatment option.

References

1. Tang R, Xu Z. Gene therapy: a double-edged sword with great powers. Mol Cell Biochem. 2020;474:73–81.
2. Brody H. Gene therapy. Nature. 2018;564:S5.
3. Wirth T, Parker N, Yla-Herttuala S. History of gene therapy. Gene. 2013;525:162–9.
4. Dunbar CE, High KA, Joung JK, et al. Gene therapy comes of age. Science. 2018;359:eaan4672.
5. Sha S, Maloney AJ, Katsikis G, et al. Cellular pathways of recombinant adeno-associated virus production for gene therapy. Biotechnol Adv. 2021;49:107764.
6. Wang D, Tai PWL, Gao G. Adeno-associated virus vector as a platform for gene therapy delivery. Nat Rev Drug Discov. 2019;18:358–78.
7. Sharma G, Sharma AR, Bhattacharya M, et al. CRISPR-Cas9: a preclinical and clinical perspective for the treatment of human diseases. Mol Ther. 2021;29:571–86.
8. Song X, Liu C, Wang N, et al. Delivery of CRISPR/Cas systems for cancer gene therapy and immunotherapy. Adv Drug Deliv Rev. 2021;168:158–80.

9. Wang D, Zhang F, Gao G. CRISPR-based therapeutic genome editing: strategies and in vivo delivery by AAV vectors. Cell. 2020;181:136–50.
10. Carmignotto GP, Azzoni AR. On the expression of recombinant Cas9 protein in E. coli BL21(DE3) and BL21(DE3) Rosetta strains. J Biotechnol. 2019;306:62–70.
11. Wang SW, Gao C, Zheng YM, et al. Current applications and future perspective of CRISPR/Cas9 gene editing in cancer. Mol Cancer. 2022;21:57.
12. Gaj T, Gersbach CA, Barbas CF 3rd. ZFN, TALEN, and CRISPR/Cas-based methods for genome engineering. Trends Biotechnol. 2013;31:397–405.
13. Waterman DP, Haber JE, Smolka MB. Checkpoint responses to DNA double-strand breaks. Annu Rev Biochem. 2020;89:103–33.
14. Li J, Sun H, Huang Y, et al. Pathways and assays for DNA double-strand break repair by homologous recombination. Acta Biochim Biophys Sin Shanghai. 2019;51:879–89.
15. Mondal M, Guo J, He P, et al. Recent advances of oncolytic virus in cancer therapy. Hum Vaccin Immunother. 2020;16:2389–402.
16. Wang G, Kang X, Chen KS, et al. An engineered oncolytic virus expressing PD-L1 inhibitors activates tumor neoantigen-specific T cell responses. Nat Commun. 2020;11:1395.
17. Kaufman HL, Kohlhapp FJ, Zloza A. Oncolytic viruses: a new class of immunotherapy drugs. Nat Rev Drug Discov. 2015;14:642–62.
18. Petrov G, Dymova M, Richter V. Bacteriophage-mediated cancer gene therapy. Int J Mol Sci. 2022;23:14245.
19. Shirley JL, de Jong YP, Terhorst C, et al. Immune responses to viral gene therapy vectors. Mol Ther. 2020;28:709–22.
20. Ginn SL, Amaya AK, Alexander IE, et al. Gene therapy clinical trials worldwide to 2017: an update. J Gene Med. 2018;20:e3015.
21. Zu H, Gao D. Non-viral vectors in gene therapy: recent development, challenges, and prospects. AAPS J. 2021;23:78.
22. Kakirde KS, Wild J, Godiska R, et al. Gram negative shuttle BAC vector for heterologous expression of metagenomic libraries. Gene. 2011;475:57–62.
23. Memi F, Ntokou A, Papangeli I. CRISPR/Cas9 gene-editing: research technologies, clinical applications and ethical considerations. Semin Perinatol. 2018;42:487–500.
24. Naso MF, Tomkowicz B, Perry WL 3rd, et al. Adeno-Associated Virus (AAV) as a vector for gene therapy. BioDrugs. 2017;31:317–34.
25. Zolotukhin S, Vandenberghe LH. AAV capsid design: a goldilocks challenge. Trends Mol Med. 2022;28:183–93.
26. Li C, Samulski RJ. Engineering adeno-associated virus vectors for gene therapy. Nat Rev Genet. 2020;21:255–72.
27. Evgin L, Kottke T, Tonne J, et al. Oncolytic virus-mediated expansion of dual-specific CAR T cells improves efficacy against solid tumors in mice. Sci Transl Med. 2022;14:eabn2231.
28. Bae H, Coller J. Codon optimality-mediated mRNA degradation: linking translational elongation to mRNA stability. Mol Cell. 2022;82:1467–76.
29. Bulcha JT, Wang Y, Ma H, et al. Viral vector platforms within the gene therapy landscape. Signal Transduct Target Ther. 2021;6:53.
30. Marchini A, Bonifati S, Scott EM, et al. Oncolytic parvoviruses: from basic virology to clinical applications. Virol J. 2015;12:6.
31. Hajba L, Guttman A. Recent advances in the analysis full/empty capsid ratio and genome integrity of adeno-associated virus (AAV) gene delivery vectors. Curr Mol Med. 2020;20:806–13.
32. Zhang B. CRISPR/cas gene therapy. J Cell Physiol. 2021;236:2459–81.
33. Dugger SA, Platt A, Goldstein DB. Drug development in the era of precision medicine. Nat Rev Drug Discov. 2018;17:183–96.
34. Wang D, Wang K, Cai Y. An overview of development in gene therapeutics in China. Gene Ther. 2020;27:338–48.
35. Lin H, Cheng J, Mu W, et al. Advances in universal CAR-T cell therapy. Front Immunol. 2021;12:744823.

36. Kaufmann KB, Buning H, Galy A, et al. Gene therapy on the move. EMBO Mol Med. 2013;5:1642–61.
37. Peng JQ, Dong XY, Peng M, et al. Preparation of rAAV2/hFIX and experimentally application to gene therapy for hemophilia B. Zhonghua Xue Ye Xue Za Zhi. 2004;25:513–8.
38. Blaese RM. The ADA human gene therapy clinical protocol. Hum Gene Ther. 1990;1:327–62.
39. Lu DR, Zhou JM, Zheng B, et al. Stage I clinical trial of gene therapy for hemophilia B. Sci China B. 1993;36:1342–51.
40. Liu D. CAR-T "the living drugs", immune checkpoint inhibitors, and precision medicine: a new era of cancer therapy. J Hematol Oncol. 2019;12:113.
41. Cao Y, Liao L, Liu X, et al. Trend of drug clinical trials in mainland China from 2009 to 2020. Curr Med Res Opin. 2022;38:1499–507.
42. Wilson JM. Gendicine: the first commercial gene therapy product. Hum Gene Ther. 2005;16:1014–5.
43. Li Y, Li B, Li CJ, et al. Key points of basic theories and clinical practice in rAd-p53 (Gendicine) gene therapy for solid malignant tumors. Expert Opin Biol Ther. 2015;15:437–54.
44. Peng Z. Current status of gendicine in China: recombinant human Ad-p53 agent for treatment of cancers. Hum Gene Ther. 2005;16:1016–27.
45. Lundstrom K. Viral vectors in gene therapy: where do we stand in 2023? Viruses. 2023;15:698.
46. Liang M. Oncorine, the world first oncolytic virus medicine and its update in China. Curr Cancer Drug Targets. 2018;18:171–6.
47. Buonaguro FM, Tornesello ML, Izzo F, et al. Oncolytic virus therapies. Pharm Pat Anal. 2012;1:621–7.
48. Liu J, Wu P, Wang H, et al. Necroptosis induced by Ad-HGF activates endogenous C-Kit+ cardiac stem cells and promotes cardiomyocyte proliferation and angiogenesis in the infarcted aged heart. Cell Physiol Biochem. 2016;40:847–60.
49. Gu Y, Cui S, Liu C, et al. pUDK-HGF gene therapy to relieve CLI rest pain and ulcer: a phase II, double-blind, randomized placebo-controlled trial. Hum Gene Ther. 2021;32:839–49.
50. Wang N, Li X, Liu X, et al. Clinical efficacy and safety of AdV-tk gene therapy for patients with cervical squamous intraepithelial lesion: a prospective study. Hum Gene Ther. 2023;34:1033–40.
51. Peng W, Li J, Yin XG, et al. Adenovirus KH901 promotes 5-FU antitumor efficacy and S phase in LoVo cells. Front Biosci (Elite Ed). 2012;4:2389–95.
52. Liang P, Ding C, Sun H, et al. Correction of beta-thalassemia mutant by base editor in human embryos. Protein Cell. 2017;8:811–22.
53. Frangoul H, Altshuler D, Cappellini MD, et al. CRISPR-Cas9 gene editing for sickle cell disease and beta-thalassemia. N Engl J Med. 2021;384:252–60.
54. Gupta D, Bhattacharjee O, Mandal D, et al. CRISPR-Cas9 system: a new-fangled dawn in gene editing. Life Sci. 2019;232:116636.
55. Ertl HCJ. Immunogenicity and toxicity of AAV gene therapy. Front Immunol. 2022;13:975803.
56. Day JW, Finkel RS, Chiriboga CA, et al. Onasemnogene abeparvovec gene therapy for symptomatic infantile-onset spinal muscular atrophy in patients with two copies of SMN2 (STR1VE): an open-label, single-arm, multicentre, phase 3 trial. Lancet Neurol. 2021;20:284–93.

Chapter 9
Biosimilar

Ya Wang, Qinqin Xu, and Xiangyu Zhang

Abstract Biosimilars in cancer treatment represent a significant development, offering cost-effective alternatives to existing biologic therapies without compromising efficacy or safety. Biologics, including monoclonal antibodies and other complex molecules, have been instrumental in cancer treatment, but their high cost limits accessibility. Biosimilars are highly similar to their reference biologic drugs but are produced at a lower cost, making cancer treatment more accessible to a broader patient population. The introduction of biosimilars in oncology not only reduces treatment costs but also widens patient access to advanced therapies. As regulatory pathways for biosimilars become more streamlined and their acceptance within the medical community grows, they are poised to play an increasingly vital role in global cancer care strategies, offering a sustainable and equitable approach to treatment.

Keywords Biosimilar · Cost-effective alternatives · Accessibility

The use of biologicals has revolutionized cancer treatment strategies, offering targeted approaches that were previously unattainable with conventional chemotherapeutics. Specifically, biologicals include a diverse range of products such as monoclonal antibodies, growth factors, cytokines, cell therapies, and monoclonal

---

Y. Wang
Department of Medical Oncology, Lung Cancer and Gastrointestinal Unit, Hunan Cancer Hospital/The Affiliated Cancer Hospital of Xiangya School of Medicine, Central South University, Changsha, China
e-mail: wangya@hnca.org.can

Q. Xu
Qinghai Provincial People's Hospital, Xining, China

X. Zhang (✉)
Department of Respiratory and Critical Care Medicine, The Third Xiangya Hospital, Changsha, China
e-mail: 218302029@csu.edu.cn

© The Author(s), under exclusive license to Springer Nature Singapore Pte Ltd. 2024
Y. Zhang, N. Yang (eds.), *New Anti-cancer Drug Development and Evaluation*,
https://doi.org/10.1007/978-981-97-7274-2_9

antibody-drug toxin combinations. Biologicals have become increasingly popular in oncology for their remarkable efficacy and specificity, accounting for approximately 40% of the current cancer therapies. However, due to their complex manufacturing process and the extensive research and development (R&D) required, biologicals are often expensive, limiting their accessibility and burdening healthcare systems.

The introduction of biosimilars into the market aims to provide more affordable alternatives to expensive biologicals, thereby increasing accessibility to these life-saving treatments [1, 2]. Biosimilars are akin to generic versions of biologicals. According to the Food and Drug Administration (FDA) definition, biosimilar refers to a product as highly similar but not identical to a reference product, i.e., the original biological, in terms of efficacy, safety, and quality [3]. In China, the definition of biosimilar was first specified by the National Medical Products Administration (NMPA) in 2015, along with the announcement of Technical Guidelines for the Development and Evaluation of Biosimilars [4] (Fig. 9.1). It is worth mentioning that biosimilars are not the same as small-molecule generic drugs, which have exactly the same chemical structures as their reference products. In contrast, biosimilars are produced by living systems and may be subtly different from the reference biologicals. The regulatory pathways for biosimilars can ensure their

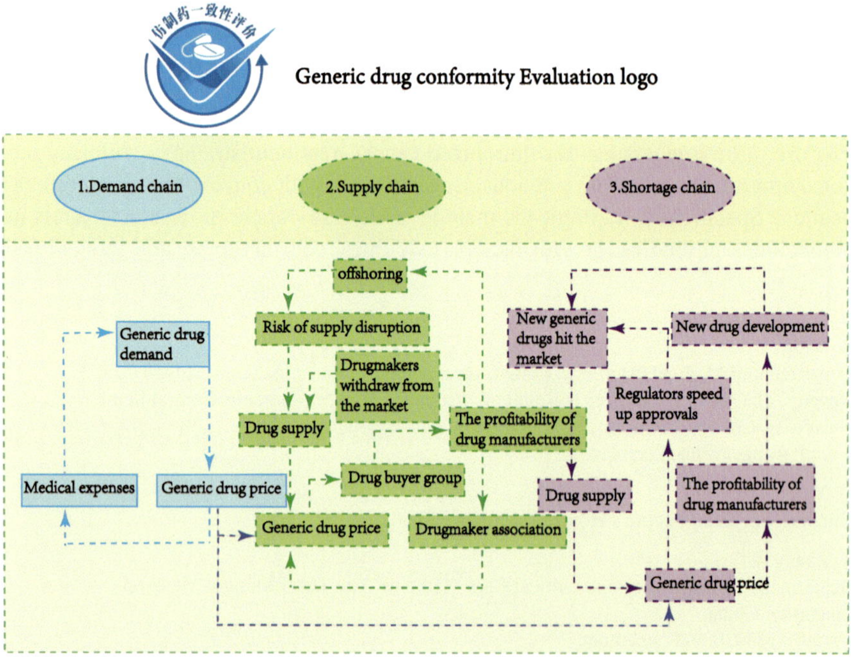

Fig. 9.1 Technical guidelines for the development and evaluation of biosimilars

comparability to the original biologicals, thus maintaining treatment standards while addressing the issue of cost.

The biosimilar market in China has witnessed a remarkable surge, primarily due to the expiration of patents for numerous biological products. By the end of 2019, the Chinese biosimilar industry boasted a robust pipeline with 391 biosimilars under R&D. This momentum continued into 2020, culminating in the NMPA approving 11 biosimilars for marketing within China, 6 of which are dedicated to cancer treatment [5]. These approvals mark a significant step in making advanced cancer therapies more accessible and affordable in China. In this chapter, the R&D of major biosimilars for oncology therapeutics in China is introduced, with special emphasis on the main clinical research design, efficacy, and adverse reactions.

9.1 Trastuzumab Biosimilar

Trastuzumab (Herceptin®, Genentech, Inc./Roche Diagnostics, GmbH) is a humanized monoclonal antibody that targets the human epidermal growth factor receptor 2 (HER2) [6, 7]. Trastuzumab is specifically indicated for treating HER2-positive breast cancer and HER2-positive metastatic gastric or gastroesophageal junction adenocarcinoma. Since receiving approval over two decades ago, trastuzumab has established itself as the cornerstone of treatment for metastatic HER2-positive breast cancer. Its clinical benefits are well documented, including significant tumor regression and improved survival rates, whether used as a monotherapy or in combination with other therapeutic agents [6].

Trastuzumab biosimilars have undergone rigorous evaluations to establish their equivalence to the original trastuzumab, particularly for treating metastatic HER2-positive breast cancer. Recent systematic reviews underscore the suitability of trastuzumab biosimilars for both early stage and metastatic breast cancer, highlighting their crucial role in expanding patient access to essential cancer treatments. Key studies on biosimilars such as MYL-1401O (Biocon/Mylan), BCD-022 (BIOCAD), and PF-05280014 (Pfizer) have reinforced their therapeutic equivalence. Notably, the HLX02 biosimilar, the first trastuzumab biosimilar developed in China, underwent extensive efficacy and safety evaluations, confirming its similarity to trastuzumab in clinical settings.

The phase I clinical trial for HLX02 (NCT02581748) was a randomized, double-blind, parallel-group study. In this study, HLX02's bioequivalence was evaluated against two reference drugs: CN-trastuzumab (manufactured in China) and EU-trastuzumab (manufactured in the EU). The study involved healthy Chinese male participants who received a 6 mg/kg dose IV infusion of these drugs. Bioequivalence between HLX02 and each reference drug was assessed based on the 90% confidence intervals (CIs) of the estimated geometric least squares mean ratios (GLSMRs) for the primary pharmacokinetic (PK) endpoints, AUC_{inf} (area under the concentration-time curve from zero to infinity), and secondary PK endpoints, AUC_{last} (area under the concentration-time curve to the last observable concentration), and C_{max} (peak serum concentration). These endpoints were compared against the standard bioequivalence range of 0.8–1.25. The study found no significant differences in the median time to reach maximum concentration (T_{max}) and its variability across the test and reference drugs. The 90% CIs for GLSMRs of all primary and secondary endpoints fell within the accepted bioequivalence margin, leading to the conclusion that HLX02 is bioequivalent to both CN-trastuzumab and EU-trastuzumab. Furthermore, this trial's PK parameter selection and bioequivalence margins aligned with those used in previous studies of marketed trastuzumab biosimilars, including PF-05280014 (Pfizer Ltd.), MYL-1401O (Mylan and Biocon Ltd.), ABP980 (Amgen Ltd.), (Teva Pharmaceutical Industries Ltd.), and SB3 (Samsung Biopsies Ltd.).

HLX02, along with the two reference drugs, demonstrated a favorable safety profile among the participants. In the first part of the study, no serious adverse events (AEs) were reported, while two participants reported at least one treatment-emergent adverse event (TEAE). The three AEs reported (ventricular dilatation, decreased ejection fraction, and left atrial dilatation) were consistent with previous studies of trastuzumab. In the second part of the study, while most TEAEs were mild, three participants in the CN-trastuzumab group experienced at least one severe TEAE. However, no severe TEAEs led to discontinuation in any group, and no severe TEAEs were reported for the HLX02 and EU-trastuzumab groups. This safety profile also mirrors previous findings from trastuzumab studies.

In a comprehensive multicenter, double-blind phase III trial, HLX02 was examined for its therapeutic equivalence to reference trastuzumab in patients with recurrent or metastatic breast cancer. The primary measure for equivalence was based on the 95% CIs of the intergroup difference in objective response rate at 24 weeks (ORR24) relative to the prespecified equivalence margin of ±13.5%. There was no statistically significant difference between HLX02 and reference trastuzumab across all evaluated parameters, including efficacy endpoints, PKs, safety, and immunogenicity, confirming that HLX02 has a comparable therapeutic effectiveness and safety profile in treating these patients.

9.2 Bevacizumab Biosimilar

Bevacizumab (Avastin), a recombinant humanized immunoglobulin G1 monoclonal antibody, is a notable antitumor and antiangiogenic drug. It works by inhibiting the activity of vascular endothelial growth factor (VEGF) to suppress tumor angiogenesis, modulate the tumor microenvironment, and enhance chemosensitivity. Originally developed by Roche and marketed as Avastin®, bevacizumab was first approved in the United States in 2004 for treating advanced colorectal cancer, marking the inception of widespread antiangiogenic therapy in advanced cancer management. Later, the indications for bevacizumab have expanded to include eight types of cancer: ① metastatic colorectal cancer (mCRC), in combination with fluoropyrimidine-based chemotherapy; ② metastatic breast cancer, combined with paclitaxel or capecitabine; ③ first-line non-squamous non-small cell lung cancer (NSCLC), administered alongside carboplatin and paclitaxel; ④ recurrent glioblastoma, as monotherapy; ⑤ metastatic renal cell carcinoma (RCC), combined with interferon α; ⑥ persistent, recurrent, or metastatic cervical cancer, in combination with either paclitaxel and cisplatin or paclitaxel and topotecan; ⑦ epithelial ovarian cancer, fallopian tube cancer, or primary peritoneal cancer, combined with paclitaxel; and ⑧ first-line liver cancer, combined with atezolizumab.

Several biosimilars of bevacizumab have been developed and demonstrated to be as safe and effective as the original drug in clinical trials. Some of these biosimilars have also been approved by regulatory bodies such as the US FDA and the European Medicines Agency (EMA) for use in treating various types of cancer.

QL1101 is the first biosimilar of bevacizumab in China, developed by Qilu Pharmaceutical. Prior to its clinical trials, QL1101 underwent extensive production process research, quality analysis, and preclinical pharmacological and toxicological studies. It is produced using Chinese hamster ovary (CHO) cell lines, with the manufacturing process encompassing cell culture, harvest, and purification steps. Preclinical evaluations have shown that QL1101 exhibits safety, efficacy, and PK profiles similar to those of the reference bevacizumab product.

The biosimilarity of QL1101 to bevacizumab was further assessed in a randomized, double-blind, single-dose study involving healthy male subjects, comparing the PKs of QL1101 with the reference bevacizumab product [8]. The study successfully demonstrated that QL1101 has PK equivalence to Avastin®. At a dosage of 3 mg/kg administered intravenously, QL1101 was found to be safe and well-tolerated in healthy Chinese subjects, providing a strong foundation for its continued clinical evaluation as a viable bevacizumab biosimilar.

The efficacy and safety of QL1101, a bevacizumab biosimilar, were rigorously tested in a phase III randomized, double-blind clinical trial involving Chinese patients with untreated locally advanced non-squamous NSCLC [9]. The study enrolled 675 patients, of whom 535 were eligible and randomized into two groups: 269 patients received QL1101, and 266 received bevacizumab. The objective response rates (ORRs) were closely matched, with 52.8% in the QL1101 group and 56.8% in the bevacizumab group. Additionally, key parameters such as progression-free survival (PFS), overall survival (OS), disease control rate (DCR), and adverse events (AEs) were comparable between the two groups. This similarity persisted even after stratifying the data based on epidermal growth factor receptor (EGFR) mutation status or smoking history. These results affirm that QL1101 exhibits a safety and efficacy profile similar to that of bevacizumab in the treatment of NSCLC.

Innovent's IBI305 is another promising biosimilar to bevacizumab. Its PK equivalence to bevacizumab was assessed in a phase I, randomized, double-blind, single-dose study involving healthy male subjects. The study's results indicated that key PK parameters, including the area under the curve from time zero to the last measurable concentration ($AUC_{0\text{-}t}$), AUC_{inf}, peak serum concentration (C_{max}), half-life ($T_{1/2}$), drug clearance, and volume of distribution, were similar for subjects treated with IBI305 and bevacizumab. Specifically, the 90% confidence intervals for the ratios of geometric means for $AUC_{0\text{-}t}$, AUC_{inf}, and C_{max} were all within the bioequivalence range of 0.80–1.25, affirming IBI305's bioequivalence to bevacizumab. Furthermore, the study reported no significant differences in adverse reactions between the two treatment groups. These adverse reactions included gastrointestinal symptoms such as nausea, vomiting, diarrhea, and inflammation; respiratory reactions such as cough, shortness of breath, and pneumonia; neurological effects including headache, dizziness, and inattention; and other general symptoms such as fever, fatigue, and muscle pain. It is important to highlight that while IBI305 has shown promising similarity in PKs, immunogenicity, and safety profiles to bevacizumab, its safety and efficacy continue to be evaluated. As with any medication, patients considering IBI305 should consult their healthcare providers to discuss any potential concerns and to stay informed about the ongoing research and any newly identified side effects.

BAT1706, another proposed biosimilar of bevacizumab (Avastin®), has undergone a global phase I clinical study (NCT03030430) to evaluate its safety and PK profile. Conducted on healthy male subjects, this study demonstrated that BAT1706 exhibits PK equivalence, safety, and immunogenicity comparable to both EU- and US-manufactured bevacizumab after a single intravenous (IV) infusion [10]. The findings of this study are paving the way for further investigation, with a phase III clinical trial currently in progress.

In addition to BAT1706, the bevacizumab biosimilars include other candidates, such as TRS003 and SCT510, which are also progressing through various stages of clinical trials. These ongoing studies are part of a broader effort to expand the availability of effective and affordable biosimilar options for cancer treatment.

9.3 Denosumab Biosimilar

Denosumab, a fully human monoclonal antibody that targets the receptor activator of nuclear factor kappa-B ligand (RANKL), has been a significant advancement in the treatment of bone metastases from solid tumors, multiple myeloma, and bone giant-cell tumors [11]. Amgen, based in Thousand Oaks, USA, developed and patented denosumab, commercializing it under the brand name Xgeva® [12].

In China, the market has seen the introduction of its first denosumab biosimilar, Boyoubei®, produced by Boan Biotech. This biosimilar has been approved specifically for the treatment of postmenopausal osteoporosis. Additionally, Boan Biotech has developed another denosumab biosimilar, BA1102, targeting the treatment of bone metastases from solid tumors and multiple myeloma. BA1102 is currently in the premarketing phase, with a phase III clinical trial actively underway. The application for its listing has already been submitted to the China NMPA, indicating significant progress toward its potential market availability.

Three additional denosumab biosimilars are currently in the premarket phase, including QL1206 (QiLu Pharmaceutical), MW032 (Jiangsu T-mab BioPharma), and HS-20090 (Hansoh Pharma). Phase I clinical trials have demonstrated that

QL1206 possesses PK and pharmacodynamic (PD) properties comparable to the original drug in healthy Chinese subjects (CTR20181448) [13]. Following this, a phase III clinical trial (NCT04550949, CTR20191911) was conducted to assess the efficacy and safety of QL1206 compared to denosumab. Between September 2019 and January 2021, the study enrolled 717 patients, randomly allocating 357 to receive QL1206 and 360 to receive denosumab. The results indicated no significant differences in primary and secondary endpoints, adverse events, immunogenicity, and PKs between the two groups [14]. In addition, another phase III clinical trial (CTR20190726) evaluated QL1206's efficacy and safety in postmenopausal Chinese women with osteoporosis and a high risk of fractures, reporting favorable outcomes. These comprehensive clinical studies support the anticipation that QL1206 will soon be approved for marketing, thereby expanding treatment options for patients with conditions treated by denosumab [15].

The phase I clinical trial for MW032 has successfully established its similarity to denosumab in terms of PKs, PDs, safety, and immunogenicity in healthy Chinese subjects (CTR20190835) [16]. Building on these promising results, a phase III clinical trial is currently underway to evaluate the efficacy and safety of MW032 compared with Xgeva® in patients suffering from bone metastases due to solid tumors (CTR20200407).

Similar to MW032, the phase I clinical trial for HS-20090 has confirmed its similarity to Xgeva® in PKs, PDs, safety, and immunogenicity in healthy Chinese subjects (NCT04494373) [17].

9.4 Rituximab Biosimilar

Rituximab, a human/murine chimeric and glycosylated immunoglobulin (Ig) G1-κ monoclonal antibody (mAb), targets CD20, a transmembrane protein found on B-lymphocytes. Developed and patented by F. Hoffmann-La Roche Ltd. under the brand name MabThera®, rituximab has been approved for treating patients with CD20 positive stage I–IV follicular non-Hodgkin's lymphoma and chronic lymphocytic leukemia [18].

Hanlikang®, the first rituximab biosimilar in the Chinese market, was developed by Henlius. Its bioequivalence to the reference rituximab was established in a phase III study (CTR20150583), particularly for treating diffuse large B-cell lymphoma [19]. This study confirmed similar efficacy and safety profiles between HLX01 (Hanlikang®) and reference rituximab, both in combination with the standard CHOP therapy (cyclophosphamide, adriamycin, Oncovin, and prednisolone). The study revealed that Rituximab and Hanlikang had comparable overall response rates (ORRs) (H-CHOP 94.1%; R-CHOP 92.8%), incidences of treatment-emergent adverse events (H-CHOP 99.5%, R-CHOP 99.0%), and serious adverse events (H-CHOP 34.0%, R-CHOP 32.5%). Common adverse events included hematological issues like decreased white blood cell and neutrophil counts, as well as anemia.

Real-world data analysis further supported HLX01 as a cost-effective alternative to reference rituximab and is thus more suitable for Chinese patients [20]. The NMPA has approved Hanlikang® for various indications, including: ① untreated stage I–IV follicular non-Hodgkin's lymphoma, ② single-drug maintenance therapy for follicular lymphoma, ③ recurrent or chemotherapy-resistant follicular lymphoma, ④ CD20-positive diffuse large B-cell non-Hodgkin's lymphoma (DLBCL) in combination with standard CHOP chemotherapy, and ⑤ untreated or relapsed/refractory chronic lymphocytic leukemia (CLL) in combination with fludarabine and cyclophosphamide. Post-marketing surveillance has noted adverse reactions such as leukopenia, chills, fever, and in rare cases, severe cutaneous reactions and cardiac events.

HALPRYZA® (IBI301), co-developed by Innovent and Eli Lilly, has emerged as a promising rituximab biosimilar. Its phase I trial (CTR20140762) suggested good tolerability [21], and a subsequent multicenter phase II trial (NCT02945215) compared IBI301 with rituximab in patients with CD20+ B-cell lymphoma [22]. The results showed similar treatment-related adverse events in both groups: the treatment-related adverse events were reported in 50 (56.2%) and 56 (61.5%) patients in the IBI301 group and rituximab group, respectively. The most common adverse events were decreased WBC count (27.0% vs. 23.1%), decreased neutrophil count (22.5% vs. 19.8%), and decreased lymphocyte count (9.0% vs. 4.4%) (IBI301 vs. rituximab). The PDs, PKs, and immunogenicity of IBI301 were found to be similar to those of reference rituximab. Furthermore, a phase III trial (NCT02867566) comparing IBI301 with rituximab in untreated DLBCL patients demonstrated comparable efficacy and safety, with ORRs of 89.9% for IBI301 vs. 93.8% for rituximab, and similar rates of treatment-emergent adverse events (IBI301 vs. rituximab: 100% vs. 99.0%) [23].

A number of other rituximab biosimilars are currently in various stages of clinical development, including:

- H02, advancing through phase III clinical trials (CTR20200889, CTR20170502)
- HL03, also in phase III clinical trials (CTR20190424, CTR20171351)
- TQB2303, progressing in phase III clinical trials (CTR20182377, CTR20171394)
- GB241, at the phase III clinical trial stage (CTR20181465)
- HS006, undergoing extensive phase III clinical trials (CTR20180855, CTR20140901, CTR20160466, CTR20160456)
- WBP263, currently in phase I clinical trials (CTR20171351)
- LZM002C, at the phase I clinical trial stage (CTR20171007)
- IBI301, progressing through phase III clinical trials (CTR20160770, CTR20140762, CTR20160493)
- SCT400, also in phase III clinical trials (CTR20160368, CTR20150086, CTR20132164)

These biosimilars represent ongoing efforts to expand the range of rituximab options available, with each at different stages of R&D, primarily in clinical trials.

9.5 Cetuximab Biosimilar

Cetuximab, a human/mouse chimeric monoclonal antibody targeting the epidermal growth factor receptor (EGFR), was developed by ImClone Systems Inc. under the brand name Erbitux®. It has been approved for treating metastatic colorectal cancer with a wild-type RAS gene and squamous cell carcinoma of the head and neck. Despite its clinical significance, cetuximab biosimilars have yet to receive marketing approval in China [24]. Currently, KL-140, developed by KeLun-Biotech, is progressing through a phase III clinical trial (CTR20202451). Additionally, other cetuximab biosimilar candidates, such as CDP1 (CTR20212382) and CPGJ-602 (CTR20170331), are undergoing phase I clinical trials. Given these developments, it is anticipated that cetuximab biosimilars will soon become more widely available in China, offering additional therapeutic options for patients.

9.6 Pertuzumab Biosimilar

Pertuzumab, marketed under the brand name Perjeta, is a monoclonal antibody designed to target the human epidermal growth factor receptor 2 (HER2). Developed by Genentech, it has been approved for both the treatment and neoadjuvant treatment of HER2-positive metastatic breast cancer [25]. Currently, the development of pertuzumab biosimilars in China is progressing, with two biosimilars in phase I clinical trials and five others in the preclinical stage.

The regulatory framework for biosimilars in China has been evolving, particularly since the country's entry into the International Council for Harmonization of Technical Requirements for Pharmaceuticals for Human Use (ICH). The "Technical Guidelines for the Development and Evaluation of Biosimilars (Trial)" issued by the NMPA in 2015 marked a significant step by defining "biosimilar" for the first time in the Chinese context. In China, the approval process for biosimilars mirrors that of innovative bioproducts, aligning with international standards. Despite this progress, the R&D of biosimilars still faces numerous regulatory challenges, indicating that there is considerable work ahead to streamline their path to market.

References

1. Bennett CL, Chen B, Hermanson T, et al. Regulatory and clinical considerations for biosimilar oncology drugs. Lancet Oncol. 2014;15:e594–605.
2. Hirsch BR, Lyman GH. Will biosimilars gain momentum? J Natl Compr Cancer Netw. 2013;11:1291–7.
3. Nahleh Z, Lyman GH, Schilsky RL, et al. Use of biosimilar medications in oncology. JCO Oncol Pract. 2022;18:177–86.

4. Liu JW, Yang YH, Wu N, et al. Biosimilar monoclonal antibodies in China: a patent review. Bioengineered. 2022;13:14503–18.
5. Yang J, Zhao X, Li J, et al. Creating China's biosimilar drugs regulatory system: a calculated approach. Front Pharmacol. 2022;13:815074.
6. Harries M, Smith I. The development and clinical use of trastuzumab (Herceptin). Endocr Relat Cancer. 2002;9:75–85.
7. Petricevic B, Laengle J, Singer J, et al. Trastuzumab mediates antibody-dependent cell-mediated cytotoxicity and phagocytosis to the same extent in both adjuvant and metastatic HER2/neu breast cancer patients. J Transl Med. 2013;11:307.
8. Liu YN, Huang J, Guo C, et al. A randomized, double-blind, single-dose study to evaluate the biosimilarity of QL1101 with bevacizumab in healthy male subjects. Cancer Chemother Pharmacol. 2020;85:555–62.
9. Chu T, Lu J, Bi M, et al. Equivalent efficacy study of QL1101 and bevacizumab on untreated advanced non-squamous non-small cell lung cancer patients: a phase 3 randomized, double-blind clinical trial. Cancer Biol Med. 2021;18:816–24.
10. Wu X, Wynne C, Xu C, et al. A global phase I clinical study comparing the safety and pharmacokinetics of proposed biosimilar BAT1706 and bevacizumab (Avastin((R))) in healthy male subjects. BioDrugs. 2019;33:335–42.
11. Kostenuik PJ. Osteoprotegerin and RANKL regulate bone resorption, density, geometry and strength. Curr Opin Pharmacol. 2005;5:618–25.
12. Kendler DL, Cosman F, Stad RK, et al. Denosumab in the treatment of osteoporosis: 10 years later: a narrative review. Adv Ther. 2022;39:58–74.
13. Zhang H, Wu M, Zhu X, et al. A phase I, randomized, single-dose study to evaluate the biosimilarity of QL1206 to denosumab among Chinese healthy subjects. Front Pharmacol. 2020;11:01329.
14. Li H, Huang Y, Chen Z, et al. Efficacy and safety of denosumab biosimilar QL1206 versus denosumab in patients with bone metastases from solid tumors: a randomized phase III trial. BioDrugs. 2023;37:259–69.
15. Zhang H, Gu JM, Chao AJ, et al. A phase III randomized, double-blind, placebo-controlled trial of the denosumab biosimilar QL1206 in postmenopausal Chinese women with osteoporosis and high fracture risk. Acta Pharmacol Sin. 2023;44:446–53.
16. Hou J, Hu Z, Xu W, et al. The similarity of pharmacokinetics, pharmacodynamics, safety, and immunogenicity between recombinant fully human anti-RANKL monoclonal antibody injection (MW032) and denosumab (Xgeva®) in healthy Chinese subjects: a single-center, randomized, double-blind, single-dose, parallel-controlled clinical study. Int Immunopharmacol. 2022;107:108666.
17. Lin Y, Yang H, Yang X, et al. Biosimilarity of HS-20090 to denosumab in healthy Chinese subjects: a randomized, double-blinded, pharmacokinetics/pharmacodynamics study. Expert Opin Investig Drugs. 2022;31:1125–32.
18. Salles G, Barrett M, Foà R, et al. Rituximab in B-cell hematologic malignancies: a review of 20 years of clinical experience. Adv Ther. 2017;34:2232–73.
19. Shi Y, Song Y, Qin Y, et al. A phase 3 study of rituximab biosimilar HLX01 in patients with diffuse large B-cell lymphoma. J Hematol Oncol. 2020;13:38.
20. Deng W, Yang S, Yang C, et al. Rituximab biosimilar HLX01 versus reference rituximab in the treatment of diffuse large B-cell lymphoma: real-world clinical experience. J Oncol Pharm Pract. 2022;3:10781552221110470.
21. Jiang B, Qi JY, Sun MY, et al. [Tolerance and pharmacodynamics phase I clinical trial study of chimeric anti-CD20 monoclonal antibody IBI301 in Chinese patients with CD20-positive non-Hodgkin's lymphoma]. Zhonghua Xue Ye Xue Za Zhi. 2018;39:320–4.
22. Jiang B, Ke X, Zhang Q, et al. Pharmacokinetics and safety of IBI301 versus rituximab in patients with CD20(+) B-cell lymphoma: a multicenter, randomized, double-blind, parallel-controlled study. Sci Rep. 2020;10:11676.

23. Song Y, Zhou H, Zhang H, et al. Efficacy and safety of the biosimilar IBI301 plus standard CHOP (I-CHOP) in comparison with rituximab plus CHOP (R-CHOP) in patients with previously untreated diffuse large B-Cell lymphoma (DLBCL): a randomized, double-blind, parallel-group, phase 3 trial. Adv Ther. 2021;38:1889–903.
24. Vincenzi B, Zoccoli A, Pantano F, et al. Cetuximab: from bench to bedside. Curr Cancer Drug Targets. 2010;10:80–95.
25. Dean L, Kane M. Pertuzumab therapy and ERBB2 genotype. In: Pratt VM, Scott SA, Pirmohamed M, et al., editors. Medical genetics summaries. Bethesda: National Center for Biotechnology Information (US); 2012.

Chapter 10
New Insights on Success and Failed Drugs

Ziyi Sun and Yuling Zhou

Abstract The emergence of molecular targeted therapy and immunotherapy has revolutionized the treatment approach for numerous cancers. Compared with traditional chemotherapy and radiotherapy, targeted therapy and immunotherapy provide enhanced treatment efficacy and lower toxicity. Nonetheless, designing and developing these innovative drugs is fraught with challenges. While some drugs have demonstrated promising efficacy, others have failed to meet their anticipated outcomes. This chapter reviews the clinical trials of several successful and failed targeted therapies and immunotherapies, aiming to distill critical insights and learnings that can inform and guide the development of future drugs in this rapidly evolving field. Specifically, the critical factors involved in the design of clinical trials are emphasized.

Keywords Successful drugs · Failed drugs · Insight

10.1 Successful Drugs

10.1.1 Targeted Therapy

Targeted therapy employs small-molecule drugs or antibodies to directly inhibit cancer cell proliferation or induce cancer cell death. In contrast to chemotherapy and radiotherapy, which often cause significant collateral damage to normal somatic cells, targeted therapy agents are designed to be more selectively toxic to cancer

Z. Sun (✉)
Department of Oncology, Beijing Electric Power Hospital, Beijing, China
e-mail: sunziyi@hnca.org.cn

Y. Zhou
Department of Medical Oncology, Lung Cancer and Gastrointestinal Unit, Hunan Cancer Hospital/The Affiliated Cancer Hospital of Xiangya School of Medicine, Central South University, Changsha, China

© The Author(s), under exclusive license to Springer Nature Singapore Pte Ltd. 2024

Y. Zhang, N. Yang (eds.), *New Anti-cancer Drug Development and Evaluation*,
https://doi.org/10.1007/978-981-97-7274-2_10

cells. This specificity minimizes harm to healthy cells, making targeted therapy a more precise and potentially less harmful option in the treatment of cancer [1].

10.1.1.1 Selecting the "Most-Benefiting" Patient Cohorts

Epidermal growth factor receptor (EGFR), a member of the ErbB family of receptor tyrosine kinases, plays a pivotal role in the pathogenesis of non-small cell lung cancer (NSCLC). EGFR mutation is one of the leading mutations that induce NSCLC development. Gefitinib, an EGFR tyrosine kinase inhibitor (TKI), selectively targets and binds to the ATP-binding site of EGFR, inhibiting its antiapoptotic activity and, hence, inhibiting the proliferation of NSCLC cells [2, 3]. Due to its targeted mechanism of action and efficacy, gefitinib has been approved for first-line treatment in patients with NSCLC who exhibit specific EGFR mutations (Fig. 10.1).

The IPASS study is a classic clinical study that underscored the significance of EGFR-TKIs in NSCLC treatment. This pivotal study contrasted the effectiveness of gefitinib with standard first-line chemotherapy (carboplatin plus paclitaxel) in a specific cohort of over 1200 East Asian patients. These participants were predominantly nonsmokers or light smokers diagnosed with advanced-stage lung adenocarcinoma. Researchers also employed amplification refractory mutation system-polymerase chain reaction (ARMS-PCR) to identify EGFR mutations in the selected patients [4].

A key finding of the IPASS study was that patients harboring positive EGFR mutations experienced markedly improved progression-free survival (PFS) when treated with gefitinib compared to chemotherapy. It should be noted that the EGFR mutation rate is relatively high among the selected patient cohort. This result highlights the potential impact of patient selection on clinical findings, suggesting that a different patient cohort might have yielded different results. Gefitinib's success, therefore, can be attributed not only to the identification of EGFR as a key oncogenic driver in NSCLC but also to the careful selection of patients most likely to respond to the treatment.

The success of osimertinib in treating NSCLC can also be attributed to the strategic selection of target patients. Osimertinib is particularly effective in NSCLC patients who have both sensitizing EGFR mutations and the T790M resistance mutation, which is the most prevalent mutation associated with acquired resistance to first-generation EGFR-TKIs. In the AURA3 study, researchers specifically enrolled patients with T790M-positive advanced NSCLC who had developed resistance to first-line EGFR-TKIs. This precise patient selection led to significant findings: the median progression-free survival (PFS) for patients in the osimertinib group was considerably longer than for those receiving platinum therapy plus pemetrexed (10.1 months vs. 4.4 months). Moreover, while first-generation EGFR-TKIs had demonstrated poor efficacy in patients with brain metastases in previous trials, osimertinib demonstrated encouraging results even in this subgroup. The subgroup analysis revealed that osimertinib was effective for patients with central nervous

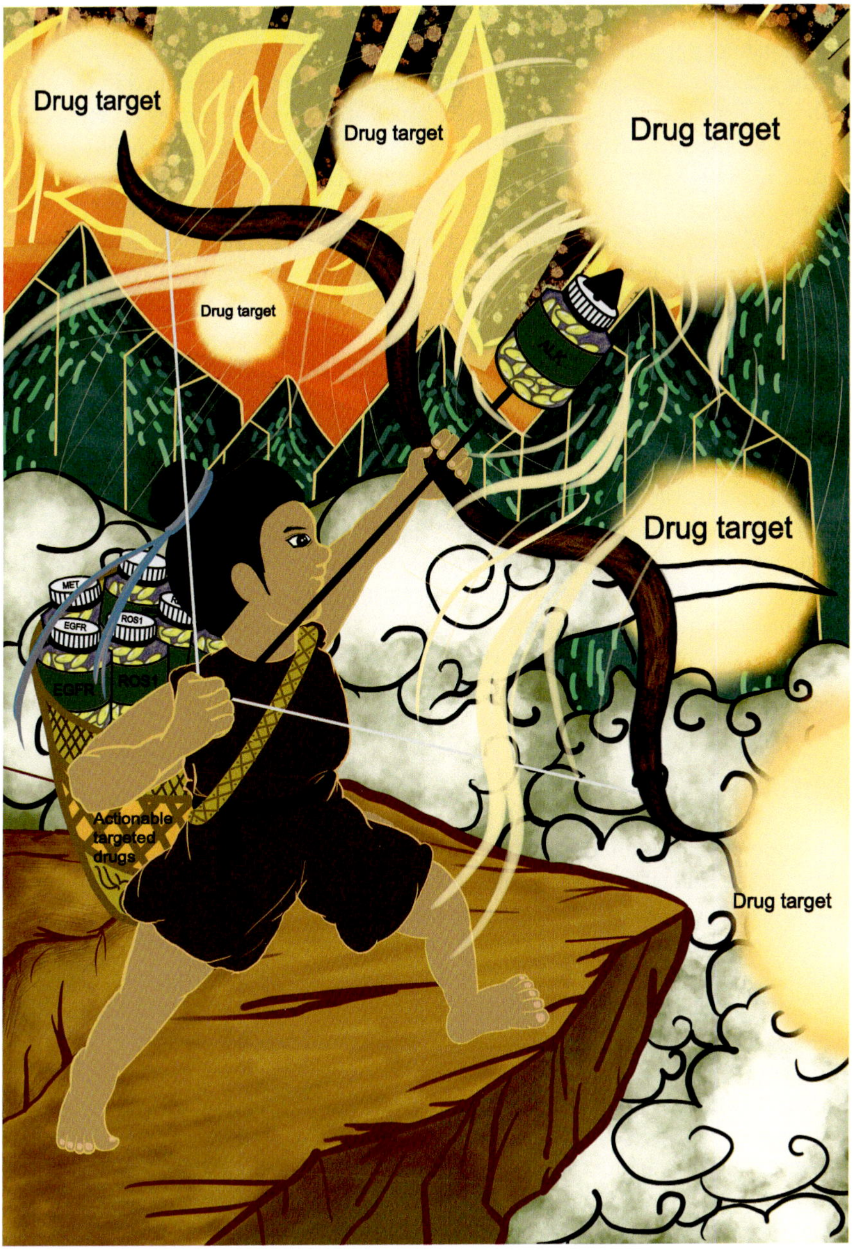

Fig. 10.1 Successful drug

system (CNS) metastases, further emphasizing the drug's efficacy in a carefully chosen patient population [5].

The critical role of patient population selection has been reaffirmed in the clinical trials of bevacizumab and cetuximab, which are targeted therapies for metastatic colorectal cancer (mCRC). In the FIRE-3 trial, enrollment was strategically limited to patients with KRAS exon 2 wild-type status, a criterion chosen to align with the specific molecular characteristics the study aimed to investigate. This trial revealed that combining FOLFIRI, a standard chemotherapy regimen for colorectal cancer, with bevacizumab led to an extended median overall survival (OS) compared to a combination of FOLFIRI and cetuximab in patients with KRAS wild-type mCRC [6]. Moreover, the CALGB/SWOG 80405 study shed light on how the tumor's anatomical location significantly influences the effectiveness of targeted treatments. It was discovered that cetuximab is more efficacious for patients with left-sided colon cancer, whereas bevacizumab shows greater suitability for right-sided colon cancer. These findings underscore the importance of patient selection based on molecular and anatomical criteria to optimize the efficacy of targeted therapies in mCRC [7].

To summarize, the precise selection of patients can catalyze the clinical success of molecularly targeted agents. Meanwhile, the emergence of novel drugs may be inspired by careful subgroup analysis. As our understanding of cancer biology and molecular characteristics deepens, we are increasingly equipped to utilize targeted therapies effectively, enhancing patient outcomes through more personalized and effective treatment strategies.

10.1.1.2 Timing of Treatment

Determining the optimal timing for administering first-, second-, and third-line treatments is crucial for enhancing patient outcomes in cancer therapy. Typically, new drugs are developed to overcome drug resistance encountered with first- or second-line treatments. For example, a new drug is often introduced when its predecessor has become ineffective due to drug resistance in cancer therapy. However, this conventional approach has been increasingly challenged by findings from recent clinical trials, suggesting a need to rethink and potentially revise this strategy in drug development and patient care. In contrast, some drugs may exhibit better efficacy or provide more overall benefit at later stages of cancer. Hence, careful investigation is needed to determine the most appropriate time to introduce a specific drug into a patient's treatment regimen. Understanding the unique dynamics and interactions of different therapies at various stages of cancer progression is key to optimizing treatment plans and improving patient outcomes.

In the FLAURA study, osimertinib was directly compared with first-generation EGFR-TKIs in patients with advanced NSCLC harboring EGFR mutations. The results showed that osimertinib significantly improved progression-free survival (PFS) across all patient subgroups compared to the first-generation EGFR-TKIs. Notably, even though about one-third of patients in the control group received crossover therapy to osimertinib, the group initially treated with osimertinib still demonstrated a marked benefit in overall survival (OS), extending it by nearly 7 months. These findings suggest that introducing osimertinib earlier in the treatment regimen could be more advantageous than reserving it for use after first-line therapies have failed. As a result, osimertinib is now recommended as a first-line therapy for advanced NSCLC patients with EGFR-sensitive mutations [8].

Maintenance treatment in first-line therapy for ovarian cancer involves subsequent treatment for patients who have achieved either complete or partial clinical remission following their initial therapy. The primary objective of this approach is to postpone disease relapse and enhance overall survival rates. The SOLO1 study explored the effectiveness of olaparib, a PARP inhibitor, as a first-line maintenance therapy in ovarian cancer. Complementarily, the SOLO2 study assessed olaparib's efficacy as a maintenance therapy in cases of platinum-resistant ovarian cancer. Both studies conclusively demonstrated that olaparib significantly benefited patients with BRCA-mutated ovarian malignancies, whether platinum-sensitive or platinum-resistant. Both studies showed that olaparib provided significant benefits to patients with BRCA-mutated platinum-sensitive and platinum-resistant ovarian malignancies. These results raise a critical question: what is the best time to introduce olaparib in maintenance therapy? A comparative analysis of the two studies revealed a significant difference in PFS benefits: in the SOLO1 study, patients experienced an extension of PFS by over 3 years, while in SOLO2, the PFS extension was only 13.6 months [9, 10].

Bevacizumab, as previously discussed, is employed in the first-line treatment for metastatic colorectal cancer (mCRC) but encounters the inevitable challenge of drug resistance. Recently, the TML study (ML18147) has gained attention for exploring the potential of using bevacizumab in cross-line treatment. Specifically, patients who had failed first-line treatment with bevacizumab were randomly assigned to receive or not receive bevacizumab in second-line treatment. Notably, the results showed that continuing treatment with bevacizumab led to improved PFS and overall survival (OS) [11]. In a parallel development, a large retrospective study in China demonstrated that for mCRC patients with wild-type KRAS, cross-line treatment with cetuximab provided greater benefits in both PFS and OS compared to chemotherapy alone. These studies challenge the conventional belief that drugs lose their effectiveness once a patient develops resistance to them; instead, they suggest the potential benefits of reusing the same drug at different treatment stages, even after resistance has occurred [12].

Apatinib, a pioneering small-molecule antiangiogenic tyrosine kinase inhibitor, stands out as the first angiogenesis inhibitor completely and independently developed in China. Apatinib has demonstrated remarkable efficacy across a wide spectrum of cancer types, including digestive tract tumors, breast cancer, and melanoma. The AHELP study is the first phase III study to recommend apatinib as a second-line or later treatment for patients with advanced hepatocellular carcinoma. In particular, the AHELP study focused on patients in more advanced stages of cancer, typically characterized by complex disease conditions such as prevalent vascular invasion, extrahepatic metastasis, and a high rate of HBV positivity (over 80%). The results showed that apatinib significantly extended the OS and PFS while maintaining good tolerability and safety compared with the placebo. It should be noted that the success of apatinib lies not only in its high selectivity for inhibiting VEGFR-2 tyrosine kinase activity but also in the unique study design, which was tailored for patients with late-stage tumors and HBV infection [13].

In summary, the clinical study design of targeted drugs should overcome traditional and rigid thought patterns. The development and application of various treatment modalities, including first-line, cross-line, and late-stage treatments, require a profound understanding of different cancer types and drugs. This approach ensures that treatment strategies evolve in line with the complexities and specificities of cancer care.

10.1.1.3 Think Out of the Box: Innovation and Optimization in Drug Design

Antibody-drug conjugates (ADCs) represent a class of innovative targeted therapies that combine a cytotoxic drug with a monoclonal antibody (mAb). This mAb specifically targets cell surface antigens present on cancer cells. Once the ADC binds to these antigens, the drug is internalized into the cancer cell through endocytosis, followed by lysosomal degradation. This process eventually leads to the release of the toxic payload within the cancer cells, effectively inhibiting their proliferation or inducing apoptosis [14, 15].

The first approval of an ADC in cancer therapy can be traced back to 2013, when the US Food and Drug Administration (FDA) approved T-DM1 for treating HER2-positive advanced breast cancer. T-DM1 is a stable ADC comprising trastuzumab, a mAb that targets the HER2 receptor, linked to DM1, a small-molecule drug that inhibits microtubule assembly [16]. This combination leverages the precise targeting ability of trastuzumab with the powerful cytotoxic activity of DM1, thereby enhancing the overall effectiveness of the treatment while simultaneously reducing side effects.

T-DXd, also known as trastuzumab deruxtecan, is an upgraded version of T-DM1. While both T-DXd and T-DM1 incorporate trastuzumab as their monoclonal antibody (mAb) component, there are two major differences between T-DXd and T-DM1. Firstly, the cytotoxic payload in T-DM1 is replaced in T-DXd with camptothecin, a topoisomerase-I inhibitor. Secondly, T-DXd employs a cleavable tetrapeptide-based linker, in contrast to the non-cleavable thioether linker used in T-DM1. In the DESTINY-Breast03 study, T-DXd was compared head-to-head with T-DM1 as a second-line treatment for HER2-positive advanced breast cancer. The results showed that patients treated with T-DXd experienced notable improvements in survival rates for HER2-positive advanced breast cancer [17]. In addition, T-DXd demonstrated promising efficacy in treating patients with low HER2 expression in advanced breast cancer. The effectiveness of T-DXd in treating advanced breast cancer was further validated by results from the DESTINY-Breast04 study, which revealed that T-DXd significantly improved both the PFS and OS of patients compared to the chemotherapy group [18].

The remarkable efficacy of T-DXd can be attributed to its well-balanced combination and sophisticated design. DXd, serving as the cytotoxic payload in T-DXd, demonstrates high inhibitory activity against topoisomerase I, while exhibiting lower myelotoxicity compared to DM1, the payload used in T-DM1. In addition, the drug-to-antibody ratio (DAR) of T-DXd is measured to be approximately 8, which is the maximum drug loading number for ADCs that are currently available on the market. DAR is a crucial and distinctive feature of ADC drugs, indicating the average number of cytotoxic molecules conjugated to an antibody. A lower DAR in ADCs typically results in reduced efficacy due to fewer drug molecules entering the cell, while a higher DAR often correlates with increased instability and toxicity of the ADC. Despite its high DAR, T-DXd maintains a stable pharmacokinetic profile due to its innovative drug-linker system. Specifically, the linker-payload system in T-DXd contains an aminomethylene (AM) moiety, which increases the DAR while reducing the hydrophobicity of the ADC, thus improving its overall stability in the systemic circulation. These factors collectively explain why T-DXd has demonstrated superior efficacy and safety in both fundamental research and clinical studies [19]. The success of T-DXd has catalyzed a surge in research on HER2-ADCs. Inspired by the designs of T-DM1 and T-DXd, many Chinese pharmaceutical companies have embarked on similar developmental paths. For instance, BAT8010 has already received clinical approval for use in locally advanced solid tumors. Similarly, SHR-A811 has rapidly progressed to phase III trials.

The success of HER2-ADCs exemplifies the broader trend of innovation in drug design. Driven by the ongoing technological advancements and increasingly sophisticated approaches to drug design, a wave of novel pharmaceuticals is expected to enter the market in the coming decades. To achieve this, researchers must thoroughly investigate the pathogenesis of cancer and the mechanisms underlying drug resistance by continuously refining research methodologies, leveraging pharmacokinetics to inform preclinical experiments, and striving to balance drug efficacy with the minimization of adverse reactions.

10.1.2 Immunotherapy

Different from targeted therapy, which employs small-molecule drugs or antibodies to directly inhibit cancer cells, immunotherapy aims to activate the immune system to eradicate these cells. Among the leading strategies in immunotherapy are immune checkpoint inhibition and adoptive cell therapy (ACT). Immune checkpoint therapy works by releasing the immune system's inherent potential to fight cancer, which involves countering the immunoinhibitory effects that cancer cells often exert on the immune system [20]. In contrast, adoptive cell therapy, also known as T cell transfer therapy, involves extracting T cells from the patient, modifying and amplifying these cells ex vivo, and then reintroducing them into the patient's body to target and destroy cancer cells [21]. As a relatively novel approach compared to targeted therapy, immunotherapy has shown immense potential and holds great promise for future advancements in cancer treatment.

10.1.2.1 Novel Targets and Careful Design

In 1996, James P. Allison demonstrated for the first time that cytotoxic T-lymphocyte-associated protein 4 (CTLA-4) antibodies could cure malignant tumors in laboratory mice [22]. CTLA-4 acts as an immune checkpoint that suppresses the immune system and prevents overreaction; hence, antibodies that target CTLA-4 can "release the brake" on the immune system, promoting the proliferation and activity of T cells. It was not until 1999 that researchers developed fully humanized CTLA-4 antibodies; later, in 2011, the US FDA approved ipilimumab (Yervoy), a mAb of CTLA-4, for the treatment of melanoma, marking the first approved immune checkpoint inhibitor (ICI) in the world [23].

Following the discovery of CTLA-4, another critical pair of molecules in the cancer-immune system interaction, namely programmed cell death protein 1(PD-1) and its ligand PD-L1, has gained significant attention. PD-1 is a transmembrane protein found on T cells, while PD-L1 is present on certain healthy cells as well as cancer cells. During a T cell's encounter with a cancer cell, the T cell receptor (TCR) on the T cell recognizes the major histocompatibility complex (MHC) on the cancer cell, leading to T cell activation. An activated T cell can induce apoptosis in the cancer cell. However, this apoptotic process can be inhibited by the PD-1/PD-L1 interaction. When PD-1 binds to PD-L1, it triggers an immunosuppressive response in the T cell, preventing it from inducing apoptosis in the cancer cell. Thus, by inhibiting the PD-1/PD-L1 interaction, PD-1 or PD-L1 antibodies can reinvigorate T cell activity against tumor cells, normalizing the suppressed immune response and facilitating an antitumor effect [24].

Targeting PD-1/PD-L1 is considered more advantageous than targeting CTLA-4. While PD-1/PD-L1 primarily influences the immune response at the effector stage in peripheral tissues, CTLA-4 is mainly involved in the early phase of T cell activation and central tolerance. Therefore, CTLA-4 inhibitors may excessively activate T cells, leading to autoimmune reactions and a range of uncontrollable adverse events; whereas inhibiting the PD-1/PD-L1 interaction may specifically activate the immune response against cancer cells. Consequently, recent developments in immune checkpoint therapy have increasingly favored PD-1/PD-L1 as a target, aiming for a more precise and safer modulation of the immune response in the fight against cancer [25–27].

In 2014, a significant advancement in immunotherapy was marked by the US FDA's approval of two anti-PD-1 antibodies, pembrolizumab (keytruda) and nivolumab (opdivo), for clinical use [23, 28]. On June 15, 2018, nivolumab was officially approved by the National Medical Products Administration (NMPA) of China based on the excellent outcomes of the CheckMate-078 study, marking China's entry into the era of immuno-oncology (I-O) [29]. Following this, the research and development of PD-1 inhibitors rapidly accelerated within the country.

In 2018, China's pharmaceutical industry also witnessed a landmark with the marketing of toripalimab, the first independently developed anti-PD-1 monoclonal antibody in China. This achievement catalyzed the launch of other ICIs, including sintilimab, camrelizumab, and tislelizumab.

Tislelizumab is an antihuman PD-1 monoclonal IgG4 antibody, which is also the PD-1 drug with the most approved indications to date in China. It has received NMPA approval for the treatment of ten different malignant tumors, including lymphoma, urothelial carcinoma, lung cancer, and hepatocellular carcinoma. Based on the traditional PD-1 antibody, tislelizumab has undergone molecular optimization to enhance its efficacy. Specifically, while other PD-1 antibodies, such as nivolumab and pembrolizumab, bind to the N-terminal region of PD-1, tislelizumab binds to the CC′ loop on the front β-sheet face of PD-1, significantly blocking the binding of PD-1 and PD-L1. Meanwhile, tislelizumab has a slow dissociation rate from PD-1, which enhances its affinity and ensures sustained antitumor activity [30]. Moreover, tislelizumab's F_c fragment has been genetically engineered to avoid binding to FcγR on macrophages, thereby eliminating antibody-dependent cellular phagocytosis (ADCP), and avoiding the potential reduction in therapeutic efficacy due to T cell exhaustion. The success of tislelizumab is not a matter of chance but the result of strategic planning, which considers the selection of the ICI target, the molecular structure optimization of the drug, and the methodical expansion of its indications.

It is crucial for Chinese pharmaceutical companies to avoid the pitfalls of blindly following prevailing trends in new drug research and development. As China's biopharmaceutical industry experiences rapid growth, it is essential for researchers to stay focused on the significance of strategic planning in the development of anticancer drugs. This involves independently crafting research programs that are not only innovative but also specifically tailored to align with the unique requirements of China's clinical practice.

10.1.2.2 Optimal Targeting Strategy

Adoptive cell therapy (ACT) is another pivotal element of immunotherapy that involves expanding immune cells ex vivo and reintroducing them into the patient to kill cancer cells directly or indirectly. ACT involves three primary categories of T cells, including tumor-infiltrating lymphocytes (TILs), chimeric antigen receptor T (CAR-T) cells, and T cell receptor (TCR) engineered T cells [31]. Among these, CAR-T cell immunotherapy has emerged as a focal point in the realm of adoptive T cell therapy due to its groundbreaking potential and effectiveness. The key to CAR-T cell therapy is to genetically modify the patient-extracted T cells so that they express chimeric antigen receptors (CARs) on their surface. These CARs are specially designed to recognize specific antigens found on the surface of cancer cells. Once these CAR-T cells are reintroduced into the patient's body, they seek out and bind to these antigens on the cancer cells, thereby eradicating them [32].

CAR-T therapy has become a promising treatment option for cancer patients, particularly those with B-cell malignancies. Among the various CAR-T therapies, those targeting the CD19 antigen have been widely utilized and have shown exceptional efficacy in treating B-cell lymphomas and acute lymphoblastic leukemia [33, 34]. Another significant area of research in CAR-T therapy pertains to multiple myeloma (MM), the second most prevalent hematologic malignancy [35]. A key focus here is the B-cell maturation antigen (BCMA), a molecule vital for the proliferation of MM cells, thus serving as an important biomarker for this disease. In 2015, Chinese researchers launched a clinical trial using cilta-cel, a CAR-T therapy that targets BCMA. The cilta-cel CAR-T cells are designed to express two single-domain antibodies against BCMA, enhancing T cell activation and proliferation. Based on the critical phase Ib/II CARTITUDE-1 study results, cilta-cel received US FDA approval in 2022. This approval, granted for the treatment of patients with relapsed/refractory multiple myeloma (R/R MM) who have undergone at least four prior lines of therapy, marks a significant success in the field. The success of cilta-cel in MM treatment underscores the vital role of targeting optimal antigens with CAR-T cells [36]. Also, this achievement represents a major milestone in China's journey in cancer immunotherapy research.

In addition to targeting B-cell maturation antigen (BCMA), researchers are investigating other potential targets for CAR-T therapy. These include G Protein-Coupled Receptor, Class C Group 5 Member D (GPRC5D) and CD138, both of which show promise in expanding the scope and efficacy of CAR-T cell treatments [37, 38]. Furthermore, there is a growing focus on clinical studies exploring dual-targeted CAR-T cell therapies. Such studies aim to enhance the precision and effectiveness of CAR-T cells in targeting cancer cells, potentially offering more robust treatment options. China is at the forefront of these developments in CAR-T therapy. As of November 15, 2021, an impressive number of clinical studies, totaling 714, related to CAR-T cells have been registered in the country.

It should be emphasized that CAR-T therapy is not without drawbacks. CAR-T therapy is inherently a highly personalized approach to treating cancer because the T cells are individually derived from each patient. This customization makes the production of CAR-T cells both costly and time-consuming, posing significant challenges to its broader application. To address this limitation and make it accessible to more patients, efforts are being directed toward developing a universal CAR-T cell therapy. The fundamental concept behind universal CAR-T cell therapy is to engineer tumor antigen-specific T cells from healthy allogeneic (unrelated) donors, hence bypassing the need to produce patient-specific T cells. This approach involves gene editing techniques to disrupt the T cell receptor (TCR) and HLA class I genes, thus mitigating graft vs. host disease, a common complication in donor-derived cell therapies. Relevant research and clinical trials for universal CAR-T cell therapy are currently in their early stages. It may take a considerable amount of time before these therapies are clinically available, as they undergo rigorous testing and development processes to ensure safety and efficacy [39].

Another challenge faced by CAR-T therapy is its efficacy in treating solid tumors. The heterogeneity of tumor antigens and the suppression of the host immune system within the tumor microenvironment are major impediments to the effectiveness of CAR-T cell therapy in solid tumors. Additionally, the physical barrier of the tumor often hampers CAR-T cells' ability to infiltrate solid tumor tissues via the bloodstream. In early 2023, the US FDA granted orphan drug designation (ODD) to China's self-developed universal CAR-T cell therapy product, MT027, which targets B7-H3, for the treatment of recurrent high-grade gliomas, a type of solid tumor. This breakthrough marks a critical step forward in extending the efficacy of CAR-T therapy beyond hematological malignancies to solid tumors. It underscores the ongoing efforts and progress in enhancing the scope and accessibility of CAR-T therapy for a broader range of cancer patients [40].

Reflecting on the trajectory of CAR-T therapy, it becomes evident that immunotherapy heavily relies on identifying highly specific biomarkers. The ideal scenario is to target antigens that are predominantly, if not exclusively, expressed on the surface of tumor cells and not on healthy cells, or only minimally so. This targeted approach is crucial for maximizing antitumor efficacy while minimizing potential adverse effects. However, the effectiveness of immunotherapy extends beyond the specificity of the target. It also depends on the functional status of the patient's endogenous T cells and the unique attributes of the tumor microenvironment. Consequently, immunotherapy is not typically effective as a standalone treatment in the battle against tumors; instead, it is increasingly viewed as a pivotal component of future cancer treatment strategies, expected to play a synergistic role alongside other therapeutic modalities.

10.2 Failed Drugs

Drug discovery and development is a lengthy, expensive, and high-risk endeavor, typically spanning 10–15 years and costing an average of $1–2 billion for each new drug to receive clinical approval [41]. However, the overall success rate of clinical drug development remains low: more than 90% of the drug candidates would fail during the preclinical stage, phase I, II, III clinical trials, or during the final drug approval process [42]. An analysis of clinical data from 2000 to 2017 shows that leading factors for failure in drug clinical development include lack of clinical efficacy, unmanageable toxicity, poor drug properties, lack of commercial demand, and poor strategic planning [43, 44]. These challenges highlight the complexities and uncertainties inherent in the drug development process, emphasizing the importance of careful planning and strategic foresight in drug development.

10.2.1 Targeted Therapy

10.2.2 Inadequate Number of Patients

Anaplastic lymphoma kinase (ALK) is a transmembrane receptor tyrosine kinase implicated in 3–7% of NSCLC cases due to its rearrangement. Specifically, the dysfunction of ALK is known to mediate dysregulation in several critical signaling pathways, including JAK-STAT, MAPK/ERK, PLCγ, and PI3K-AKT pathways, which play vital roles in cell cycle progression, cellular proliferation, and apoptosis/cell survival processes. Consequently, ALK-TKIs have been approved by the US FDA as first-line treatments for NSCLC patients with ALK rearrangements, increasing the PFS by over 20 months and OS by over 30 months [45, 46].

RF-A089, an ALK-TKI developed by Renfu Pharmaceutical in China, entered phase I clinical trials in 2018, targeting patients with locally advanced or metastatic NSCLC featuring ALK rearrangements. Unfortunately, the trial was prematurely terminated in 2021 due to an insufficient number of participants. Another major factor contributing to the discontinuation of this trial was the market presence of seven other approved drugs targeting the same protein, which positioned RF-A089 in a less competitive landscape.

10.2.2.1 Inappropriate Target

The Kirsten rat sarcoma viral oncogene (KRAS) protein, a small membrane-bound GTPase, acts as a key switch regulating multiple cellular signaling pathways. Mutations in KRAS can constantly activate the MAPK and PI3K pathways, resulting in uncontrolled cellular proliferation and survival [47, 48]. Notably, KRAS mutations are present in 25–35% of newly diagnosed cases of NSCLC, with the G12C mutation being the most common. Here, three drugs for treating patients harboring the $KRAS^{G12C}$ mutation are compared: sotorasib, adagrasib, and abemaciclib. Specifically, both sotorasib and adagrasib are irreversible, direct inhibitors of the $KRAS^{G12C}$ protein, whereas abemaciclib is a cell cycle inhibitor targeting cyclin-dependent kinases CDK4 and CDK6, which are downstream effectors of $KRAS^{G12C}$.

The efficacy and safety of sotorasib were evaluated against standard-of-care treatment in a randomized, open-label phase III trial (NCT04303780). Sotorasib showed a significant increase in the PFS for NSCLC patients with the $KRAS^{G12C}$ mutation, achieving a median PFS of 5.6 months compared to 4.5 months in the control group. However, there was no significant difference in OS in the sotorasib-treated group [49]. Adagrasib showed promising results in the phase II clinical trial (NCT03785249), achieving a median PFS of 6.5 months and a median OS of

12.6 months [50]. Consequently, both sotorasib and adagrasib have received US FDA approval for treating NSCLC with the $KRAS^{G12C}$ mutation.

The efficacy of abemaciclib was investigated in the JUNIPER study, a phase III, multicenter, randomized, open-label trial. The study found that abemaciclib showed no improvement in the primary endpoint, with a median OS of 7.4 months compared to 7.8 months for erlotinib, a US FDA-approved EGFR inhibitor [51]. Although abemaciclib showed a prolonged PFS (median PFS for abemaciclib vs. erlotinib: 3.6 months vs. 1.9 months), it failed to gain approval for treating NSCLC patients with the $KRAS^{G12C}$ mutation. Abemaciclib's failure in this study may be attributed to the selection of an inappropriate target, i.e., the downstream effectors of $KRAS^{G12C}$ instead of the KRAS protein itself. These results suggest that precision-targeted drugs may be a more effective choice for cancer patients harboring specific driver-gene mutations.

10.2.3 Immunotherapy

10.2.3.1 Inappropriate Clinical Trial Design

Sintilimab, a domestically produced fully human IgG4 monoclonal antibody against PD-1, attracted much attention for being the first approved mAb by the NMPA for the treatment of classical Hodgkin's lymphoma (HL) in patients who have relapsed or are refractory after receiving two or more lines of systemic chemotherapy [52]. Subsequently, based on the results of the ORIENT-11 and ORIENT-12 trials, sintilimab received NMPA approval for use in NSCLC in combination with chemotherapy as a first-line therapy [53, 54].

However, sintilimab's journey in the international market, particularly in the US, encountered a setback. The US FDA, with a vote of 14 to 1, declined its approval for NSCLC treatment, citing issues with the clinical trial design. The key concerns raised about the ORIENT-11 and ORIENT-12 trials included:

1. Population representativeness: Both trials predominantly involved Asian patients, a demographic significantly different from the diverse racial composition in the US. This lack of representativeness in the patient population raised questions about the generalizability of the trial results to the US population.
2. Trial endpoints: The trials used PFS as the primary endpoint rather than OS. The US FDA and US medical standards typically prefer OS as a more definitive endpoint, questioning the trials' alignment with US regulatory standards and medical practices.
3. Patient demographics: The age and gender distribution of patients in the clinical trials differed from the typical characteristics of NSCLC patients in the US, highlighting the issue of the applicability of the trial results to the US patient population.

The US FDA's decision not to approve sintilimab for the US market underscores the importance of designing clinical trials with a global perspective. For a drug aiming for international marketing, clinical trials should be designed with a broader scope that accommodates diverse demographic characteristics. Including patients from multiple research centers across different regions is also advantageous, as it ensures a more representative and inclusive study population.

10.3 Conclusion

In summary, both small-molecule drugs and immunotherapies have shown varying levels of success and failure in clinical trials. Successes can be attributed to key factors such as careful patient selection, precise timing of treatment, innovative drug design, identification of novel targets, and effective targeting strategies. On the other hand, failures have often been linked to challenges such as insufficient patient numbers, inappropriate targeting, and flawed clinical trial designs.

The success of clinical trials in oncology depends on a wide range of critical factors. For future oncology trials in China, it is imperative for both academia and industry to thoughtfully consider the selection of appropriate patient populations and drugs. Learning from past experiences, including both successes and failures, and staying open to emerging technologies and products are critical steps to reduce the risk of failure. This approach will ensure a more strategic and informed pathway in the development of new oncological treatments, potentially leading to more effective and targeted therapies for cancer patients.

References

1. Baudino TA. Targeted cancer therapy: the next generation of cancer treatment. Curr Drug Discov Technol. 2015;12(1):3–20. PMID: 26033233.
2. Lynch TJ, Bell DW, Sordella R, et al. Activating mutations in the epidermal growth factor receptor underlying responsiveness of non-small-cell lung cancer to gefitinib. N Engl J Med. 2004;350(21):2129–39. PMID: 15118073.
3. Mok TS, Wu Y-L, Thongprasert S, et al. Gefitinib or carboplatin-paclitaxel in pulmonary adenocarcinoma. N Engl J Med. 2009;361(10):947–57. PMID: 19692680.
4. Fukuoka M, Wu Y-L, Thongprasert S, et al. Biomarker analyses and final overall survival results from a phase III, randomized, open-label, first-line study of gefitinib versus carboplatin/paclitaxel in clinically selected patients with advanced non-small-cell lung cancer in Asia (IPASS). J Clin Oncol. 2011;29(21):2866–74. PMID: 21670455.
5. Papadimitrakopoulou VA, Mok TS, Han J-Y, et al. Osimertinib versus platinum-pemetrexed for patients with EGFR T790M advanced NSCLC and progression on a prior EGFR-tyrosine kinase inhibitor: AURA3 overall survival analysis. Ann Oncol. 2020;31(11):1536–44. PMID: 32861806.
6. Heinemann V, von Weikersthal LF, Decker T, et al. FOLFIRI plus cetuximab versus FOLFIRI plus bevacizumab as first-line treatment for patients with metastatic colorectal cancer

(FIRE-3): a randomised, open-label, phase 3 trial. Lancet Oncol. 2014;15(10):1065–75. PMID: 25088940.
7. Lenz H-J, Ou F-S, Venook AP, et al. Impact of consensus molecular subtype on survival in patients with metastatic colorectal cancer: results from CALGB/SWOG 80405 (Alliance). J Clin Oncol. 2019;37(22):1876–85. PMID: 31042420.
8. Soria J-C, Ohe Y, Vansteenkiste J, et al. Osimertinib in untreated EGFR-mutated advanced non-small-cell lung cancer. N Engl J Med. 2018;378(2):113–25. PMID: 29151359.
9. Moore K, Colombo N, Scambia G, et al. Maintenance olaparib in patients with newly diagnosed advanced ovarian cancer. N Engl J Med. 2018;379(26):2495–505. PMID: 30345884.
10. Pujade-Lauraine E, Ledermann JA, Selle F, et al. Olaparib tablets as maintenance therapy in patients with platinum-sensitive, relapsed ovarian cancer and a BRCA1/2 mutation (SOLO2/ENGOT-Ov21): a double-blind, randomised, placebo-controlled, phase 3 trial. Lancet Oncol. 2017;18(9):1274–84. PMID: 28754483.
11. Bennouna J, Sastre J, Arnold D, et al. Continuation of bevacizumab after first progression in metastatic colorectal cancer (ML18147): a randomised phase 3 trial. Lancet Oncol. 2013;14(1):29–37. PMID: 23168366.
12. Feng Q, Wei Y, Ren L, et al. Efficacy of continued cetuximab for unresectable metastatic colorectal cancer after disease progression during first-line cetuximab-based chemotherapy: a retrospective cohort study. Oncotarget. 2016;7(10):11380–96. PMID: 26863631.
13. Qin S, Li Q, Gu S, et al. Apatinib as second-line or later therapy in patients with advanced hepatocellular carcinoma (AHELP): a multicentre, double-blind, randomised, placebo-controlled, phase 3 trial. Lancet Gastroenterol Hepatol. 2021;6(7):559–68. PMID: 33971141.
14. Hafeez U, Parakh S, Gan HK, et al. Antibody-drug conjugates for cancer therapy. Molecules. 2020;25(20):4764. PMID: 33081383.
15. Gogia P, Ashraf H, Bhasin S, et al. Antibody-drug conjugates: a review of approved drugs and their clinical level of evidence. Cancers (Basel). 2023;15(15):3886. PMID: 37568702.
16. Verma S, Miles D, Gianni L, et al. Trastuzumab emtansine for HER2-positive advanced breast cancer. N Engl J Med. 2012;367:1783–91.
17. Cortes J, Kim SB, Chung WP, et al. Trastuzumab deruxtecan versus trastuzumab emtansine for breast cancer. N Engl J Med. 2022;386:1143–54.
18. Modi S, Jacot W, Yamashita T, et al. Trastuzumab deruxtecan in previously treated HER2-low advanced breast cancer. N Engl J Med. 2022;387:9–20.
19. Ogitani Y, Aida T, Hagihara K, et al. DS-8201a, a novel HER2-targeting ADC with a novel DNA topoisomerase I inhibitor, demonstrates a promising antitumor efficacy with differentiation from T-DM1. Clin Cancer Res. 2016;22:5097–108.
20. Pardoll DM. The blockade of immune checkpoints in cancer immunotherapy. Nat Rev Cancer. 2012;12(4):252–64. PMID: 22437870.
21. Rosenberg SA, Restifo NP. Adoptive cell transfer as personalized immunotherapy for human cancer. Science. 2015;348(6230):62–8. PMID: 25838374.
22. Krummel MF, Allison JP. CD28 and CTLA-4 have opposing effects on the response of T cells to stimulation. J Exp Med. 1995;182(2):459–65. PMID: 7543139.
23. Hodi FS, O'Day SJ, McDermott DF, et al. Improved survival with ipilimumab in patients with metastatic melanoma. N Engl J Med. 2010;363(8):711–23. PMID: 20525992.
24. Zou W, Wolchok JD, Chen L. PD-L1 (B7-H1) and PD-1 pathway blockade for cancer therapy: Mechanisms, response biomarkers, and combinations. Sci Transl Med. 2016;8(328):328rv4. PMID: 26936508.
25. Topalian SL, Taube JM, Anders RA, et al. Mechanism-driven biomarkers to guide immune checkpoint blockade in cancer therapy. Nat Rev Cancer. 2016;16(5):275–87. PMID: 27079802.
26. Buchbinder EI, Desai A. CTLA-4 and PD-1 pathways: similarities, differences, and implications of their inhibition. Am J Clin Oncol. 2016;39(1):98–106. PMID: 26558876.
27. Topalian SL, Drake CG, Pardoll DM. Immune checkpoint blockade: a common denominator approach to cancer therapy. Cancer Cell. 2015;27(4):450–61. PMID: 25858804.

28. Kwok G, Yau TCC, Chiu JW, et al. Pembrolizumab (Keytruda). Hum Vaccin Immunother. 2016;12(11):2777–89. PMID: 27398650.
29. Wu Y-L, Lu S, Cheng Y, et al. Nivolumab versus docetaxel in a predominantly Chinese patient population with previously treated advanced NSCLC: CheckMate 078 randomized phase III clinical trial. J Thorac Oncol. 2019;14(5):867–75. PMID: 30659987.
30. Zhang T, Song X, Xu L, et al. The binding of an anti-PD-1 antibody to FcgammaRIota has a profound impact on its biological functions. Cancer Immunol Immunother. 2018;67:1079–90.
31. Katiyar V, Chesney J, Kloecker G. Cellular therapy for lung cancer: focusing on chimeric antigen receptor T (CAR T) cells and tumor-infiltrating lymphocyte (TIL) therapy. Cancers (Basel). 2023;15(14):3733. PMID: 37509394.
32. Singh AK, McGuirk JP. CAR T cells: continuation in a revolution of immunotherapy. Lancet Oncol. 2020;21(3):e168–78. PMID: 32135120.
33. Maude SL, Teachey DT, Porter DL, et al. CD19-targeted chimeric antigen receptor T-cell therapy for acute lymphoblastic leukemia. Blood. 2015;125(26):4017–23. PMID: 25999455.
34. Chong EA, Alanio C, Svoboda J, et al. Pembrolizumab for B-cell lymphomas relapsing after or refractory to CD19-directed CAR T-cell therapy. Blood. 2022;139(7):1026–38. PMID: 34496014.
35. Cappell KM, Kochenderfer JN. Long-term outcomes following CAR T cell therapy: what we know so far. Nat Rev Clin Oncol. 2023;20(6):359–71. PMID: 37055515.
36. Berdeja JG, Madduri D, Usmani SZ, et al. Ciltacabtagene autoleucel, a B-cell maturation antigen-directed chimeric antigen receptor T-cell therapy in patients with relapsed or refractory multiple myeloma (CARTITUDE-1): a phase 1b/2 open-label study. Lancet. 2021;398(10297):314–24. PMID: 34175021.
37. Smith EL, Harrington K, Staehr M, et al. GPRC5D is a target for the immunotherapy of multiple myeloma with rationally designed CAR T cells. Sci Transl Med. 2019;11(485):eaau7746. PMID: 30918115.
38. van der Schans JJ, Wang Z, van Arkel J, et al. Specific targeting of multiple myeloma by dual split-signaling chimeric antigen receptor T cells directed against CD38 and CD138. Clin Cancer Res. 2023;29(20):4219–29. PMID: 37527004.
39. Depil S, Duchateau P, Grupp SA, et al. 'Off-the-shelf' allogeneic CAR T cells: development and challenges. Nat Rev Drug Discov. 2020;19(3):185–99. PMID: 31900462.
40. Shang X, et al. An exploratory investigator-initiated trial via intrathecal or intracerebroventricular delivery of B7H3-specific allogeneic universal CAR-T cells in patients with recurrent high-grade gliomas. JCO. 2024;42:23. https://doi.org/10.1200/JCO.2024.42.23_suppl.23.
41. Hinkson IV, Madej B, Stahlberg EA. Accelerating therapeutics for opportunities in medicine: a paradigm shift in drug discovery. Front Pharmacol. 2020;11:770.
42. Dowden H, Munro J. Trends in clinical success rates and therapeutic focus. Nat Rev Drug Discov. 2019;18:495–6.
43. Harrison RK. Phase II and phase III failures: 2013–2015. Nat Rev Drug Discov. 2016;15:817–8.
44. Waring MJ, Arrowsmith J, Leach AR, et al. An analysis of the attrition of drug candidates from four major pharmaceutical companies. Nat Rev Drug Discov. 2015;14:475–86.
45. Golding B, Luu A, Jones R, et al. The function and therapeutic targeting of anaplastic lymphoma kinase (ALK) in non-small cell lung cancer (NSCLC). Mol Cancer. 2018;17:52.
46. Mok T, Camidge DR, Gadgeel SM, et al. Updated overall survival and final progression-free survival data for patients with treatment-naive advanced ALK-positive non-small-cell lung cancer in the ALEX study. Ann Oncol. 2020;31:1056–64.
47. Hofmann MH, Gerlach D, Misale S, et al. Expanding the reach of precision oncology by drugging all KRAS mutants. Cancer Discov. 2022;12:924–37.
48. Drosten M, Barbacid M. Targeting the MAPK pathway in KRAS-driven tumors. Cancer Cell. 2020;37:543–50.
49. de Langen AJ, Johnson ML, Mazieres J, et al. Sotorasib versus docetaxel for previously treated non-small-cell lung cancer with KRAS(G12C) mutation: a randomised, open-label, phase 3 trial. Lancet. 2023;401:733–46.

50. Janne PA, Riely GJ, Gadgeel SM, et al. Adagrasib in non-small-cell lung cancer harboring a KRAS(G12C) mutation. N Engl J Med. 2022;387:120–31.
51. Goldman JW, Mazieres J, Barlesi F, et al. A randomized phase III study of abemaciclib versus erlotinib in patients with stage IV non-small cell lung cancer with a detectable KRAS mutation who failed prior platinum-based therapy: JUNIPER. Front Oncol. 2020;10:578756.
52. Hoy SM. Sintilimab: first global approval. Drugs. 2019;79:341–6.
53. Yang Y, Sun J, Wang Z, et al. Updated overall survival data and predictive biomarkers of sintilimab plus pemetrexed and platinum as first-line treatment for locally advanced or metastatic nonsquamous NSCLC in the phase 3 ORIENT-11 study. J Thorac Oncol. 2021;16:2109–20.
54. Zhou C, Wu L, Fan Y, et al. Sintilimab plus platinum and gemcitabine as first-line treatment for advanced or metastatic squamous NSCLC: results from a randomized, double-blind, phase 3 trial (ORIENT-12). J Thorac Oncol. 2021;16:1501–11.

Chapter 11
The Road from Laboratory to Patient

Yongchang Zhang and Yangqian Chen

Abstract Drug development is a multifaceted process aimed at enhancing patient health outcomes, involving collaborative efforts from researchers, regulatory bodies, and industry stakeholders. It begins with identifying disease-related biomolecules and validating potential drug candidates, followed by optimizing these leads for efficacy, safety, and pharmacokinetics. Subsequent preclinical tests evaluate safety and efficacy in animal and human models, leading to clinical trials that assess the drug's safety, therapeutic efficacy, and patient impact across three phases. Despite rigorous testing and collaboration, the success rate in clinical drug development hovers around 10–15%. Major challenges contributing to the high failure rate include lack of efficacy, excessive toxicity, and suboptimal drug characteristics. Consequently, refining drug development approaches is essential to improve success probabilities, underscoring the intricate and demanding nature of bringing new therapeutic solutions from the lab to the market.

Keywords Drug discovery · Lead compound · Clinical evaluation · Lab · Market

---

Y. Zhang
Department of Medical Oncology, Lung Cancer and Gastrointestinal Unit, Hunan Cancer Hospital/The Affiliated Cancer Hospital of Xiangya School of Medicine, Central South University, Changsha, China
e-mail: zhangyongchang@csu.edu.cn

Y. Chen (✉)
Department of Medical Oncology, Lung Cancer and Gastrointestinal Unit, Hunan Cancer Hospital/The Affiliated Cancer Hospital of Xiangya School of Medicine, Central South University, Changsha, China

Department of Medical Oncology, Graduate Collaborative Training Base of Hunan Cancer Hospital, Hengyang Medical School, University of South China, Hengyang, China
e-mail: chenyangqian@hnca.org.cn

© The Author(s), under exclusive license to Springer Nature Singapore Pte Ltd. 2024

Y. Zhang, N. Yang (eds.), *New Anti-cancer Drug Development and Evaluation*,
https://doi.org/10.1007/978-981-97-7274-2_11

11.1 Overview

Developing a drug is a multifaceted endeavor that spans from identifying a potential drug molecule to its final approval and market release. The core objective of this process is to transition promising therapeutic discoveries into clinical applications, thereby enhancing patient health outcomes. Specifically, this process requires the collaborative efforts of diverse teams, encompassing basic and clinical researchers, regulatory bodies, and industry stakeholders.

The first stage in drug development involves target identification and lead validation. This entails identifying crucial biomolecules or cellular pathways associated with the disease in question and identifying a potential drug candidate, known as a lead compound, that precisely targets them. Once the lead compound's viability is affirmed, it undergoes optimization to enhance its efficacy, safety, and pharmacokinetic profile. These preliminary stages of drug development are largely fundamental exploratory and can span several years.

The second stage involves rigorous preclinical tests to assess the safety and efficacy of the candidate drug in both animals and humans. Initially, the pharmacokinetic and toxicological profiles of the candidate drug are assessed in animal models. If these results prove promising, the candidate progresses to clinical trials. Typically, clinical trials involve three phases: in the phase I clinical trial, the drug is administered to a small cohort of healthy volunteers to ascertain its safety and gather pharmacokinetic data. In phase II trials, the drug is evaluated among a group of patients to evaluate its therapeutic efficacy and safety. In phase III trials, the candidate undergoes comprehensive testing on a broader patient base to confirm its efficacy, tolerability, potential side effects, and any interactions with other medications. The results of these studies are then evaluated by regulatory agencies, such as the National Medical Products Administration (NMPA), which determines the drug's suitability for human use.

The final stage of drug development is commercialization. In this phase, the approved drug undergoes manufacturing, marketing, and distribution to deliver its therapeutic advantages to patients. Specifically, this stage involves securing regulatory endorsements, strategizing pricing, and setting up efficient distribution networks to guarantee the drug's availability to its intended recipients.

To summarize, drug development is an intricate journey demanding meticulous planning, stringent testing, and synergistic collaboration to seamlessly transition novel therapies into clinical application. The progression in this field has introduced groundbreaking treatments for various diseases, such as cancer. However, despite substantial efforts and resources invested in drug discovery, the overall success rate for clinical drug development hovers around a mere 10–15% [1]. A review of clinical trial data spanning 2010–2017 revealed four primary contributors to the staggering 90% clinical failure rate in drug development: lack of clinical efficacy (40–50%), excessive toxicity (30%), suboptimal drug characteristics (10–15%), and a combination of insufficient commercial demand and strategic missteps (10%) [2].

Consequently, the refinement and judicious selection of drug development approaches are crucial to augment the overall success probability.

11.2 Drug Discovery

11.2.1 Target Discovery and Validation

Drugs achieve their therapeutic effects by interacting with specific biomolecules in the human body, such as proteins, polysaccharides, lipids, or nucleic acids [3]. Predominantly, both small-molecule drugs and biotherapeutics act by perturbing the function of proteins, as they often lack specificity against other biomolecules. Out of the >20,000 protein-coding genes in humans, not all yield proteins amenable to drug interactions, and an even smaller subset qualify as viable drug targets [4]. The proteins that allow the binding of ligand molecules are defined as the "druggable proteome."[5]. Yet, only those that have a direct connection to disease mechanisms and don't significantly interfere with vital biological processes are considered promising drug targets. In drug discovery, the first step is to identify the target protein. In practice, several approaches have been employed to identify potential drug targets [4], including genome-wide association studies (GWAS), CRISPR-based studies, in silico prediction, and chemical proteomics, as detailed below.

Given that a large number of diseases are linked to certain mutations, identifying disease-relevant mutations is a major task in drug discovery. GWAS involve scanning large sets of genetic information to statistically associate specific genetic variants, referred to as single nucleotide polymorphisms, with the risk of a disease or its progression.

CRISPR-based studies identify the target genes of a drug by systematically silencing or activating large numbers of candidate genes. Perturbations that enhance or attenuate the efficacy of the drug may indicate potential drug targets. For example, through CRISPR-Cas9 genetic screening, researchers were able to determine that nicotinamide phosphoribosyltransferase (NAMPT) was the molecular target of the clinical-stage anticancer compound KPT-9274 [6].

In silico prediction leverages computational models to mine extensive databases for potential targets of chemical compounds or, alternatively, to predict the structures of compounds capable of inhibiting disease-associated proteins. For example, DTINet is a computational pipeline that can predict novel drug-target interactions using a heterogeneous neural network that integrates existing drug-disease-associated information [7]. Using this approach, researchers discovered and validated novel interactions between the drugs and COX proteins.

Chemical proteomics is a method for both target identification and validation, usually applied when the drug structure is known. Specifically, chemical proteomics identifies the protein targets of an existing drug through affinity chromatography coupled with high-resolution mass spectrometry [8]. In this process, a protein mixture, such as cell lysates, is passed through a drug-embedded column. The proteins that bind to the drug are "pulled down," subsequently eluted, and identified via mass spectrometry. The utility of chemical proteomics has been exemplified by the discovery of rapamycin's target. Originally recognized as a macrolide with immunosuppressive properties, rapamycin's precise mechanism was decoded with chemical proteomics, revealing its binding to FKBP12 [1]. Further exploration of the rapamycin-FKBP12 complex exposed its role in interacting with the mammalian target of rapamycin (mTOR), and by extension, the mTOR signaling pathway [9]. The identification of this novel target led to the development of small-molecule derivatives of rapamycin, such as everolimus and temsirolimus, which offer improved pharmacokinetic profiles and reduced immunosuppressive effects and have been approved for the treatment of cancer [9].

Target validation is a crucial step following target discovery in drug development, as it helps mitigate off-target effects that could lead to safety concerns and, ultimately, the failure of the drug, particularly in the context of poorly characterized diseases. The target validation step involves two critical parts: verifying the role of the target protein in the disease process and confirming the specific interaction between the drug and the target protein [10–16]. The first part may be achieved using a wide range of genetic or genomic methods; however, discrepancies can arise between cellular, animal, and human studies due to complex protein interaction networks [17]. In reality, a molecular target is not fully validated until a successful drug is developed, which poses challenges for first-in-class drug discovery and development.

The second part of target validation is usually achieved through structure–activity relationship (SAR) studies and affinity/selectivity characterization, such as chemical proteomics [12–16]. The pharmacological effects of the drug can also be confirmed by comparing with the effects of genetic alteration of the target protein using small interfering RNA (siRNA) knockdown or CRISPR gene editing in cells or animal models [17, 18]. Note that some drugs may exert their activities by targeting unknown molecules instead of their intended targets [18], which may affect the subsequent drug optimization process. Interestingly, some drugs have been successfully developed even though their targets differ from their intended targets, as reported previously [18]. Despite the complexities, these methods of target validation are essential, albeit they contribute to the high attrition rates in clinical drug development [10, 11].

11.2.2 Lead Compound Identification and Optimization

Lead compounds are chemical compounds that show desired pharmacologic activity against specific targets in preliminary experiments. These compounds often serve as the foundational structures for subsequent drug optimization efforts aimed at enhancing therapeutic efficacy, improving pharmacokinetics, and minimizing toxicity [1].

The predominant source of lead compounds is natural products, i.e., active molecules extracted from plants, fungus, or animals that show medicinal properties. Many modern drugs are derivatives or analogs of natural lead compounds [19]. For instance, the opioid analgesic morphine, initially derived from the opium poppy in the nineteenth century, has led to the development of related analgesics such as codeine, hydromorphone, oxycodone, and hydrocodone [19]. Similarly, teprotide is a nanopeptide isolated from the venom of *Bothrops jararaca*, a Brazilian pit viper. Teprotide was the lead compound for the development of the first angiotensin converting-enzyme inhibitor, captopril [20]. In addition, the *Pleurotus ostreatus* (oyster mushroom) metabolite, lovastatin, provided the base structure for an entire class of lipid-lowering medications, including atorvastatin, fluvastatin, rosuvastatin, and simvastatin [21]. From one natural lead compound, modern combinatorial chemistry methods have enabled the synthesis of hundreds to thousands of different compounds that share a similar motif, functional group, or reaction sequence [22], among which drug candidates with more favorable properties can be selected.

In addition to natural products, synthetic compound libraries have emerged as a crucial source of lead compounds. Specifically, compound libraries targeting certain oncoproteins and their variants, such as KRAS and the $KRAS^{G12C}$ mutant, have been developed for large-scale screening [23]. In addition to these exclusively designed libraries, major pharmaceutical companies have established broad proprietary libraries after decades of drug development. These comprehensive archives are invaluable for the identification of novel lead compounds, propelling the development of new therapeutic agents [24].

Advancements in computational modeling, particularly due to machine learning innovations, have significantly augmented traditional experiment-based methods in drug development. For target proteins whose 3D structures have been resolved through X-ray crystallography, molecules with potential affinity to these targets can be generated through molecular simulation. For example, by analyzing the crystal structure of renin-inhibitor complexes, lead compounds that are predicted to specifically bind to the renin S1/S3 pocket are designed and synthesized [25]. Among these in silico lead compounds, the most effective molecule was further developed into aliskiren, marking it as the first direct renin inhibitor to be used therapeutically.

High-throughput screening (HTS) is a pivotal technique where libraries composed of diverse structures, whether sourced from nature, synthesized in the lab, or designed using computational methods, are rapidly evaluated for their effectiveness against specific biological targets. HTS is an automation-powered process designed to expedite the identification of initial "hit series" from which more potent and drug-like candidates can be developed [26]. The process relies heavily on simplistic, high-automation assay techniques, advanced robotics for sample manipulation, and sophisticated data analysis systems to handle the voluminous data generated. Key assays employed in HTS include biochemical assays to assess enzymatic reactions and receptor-ligand interactions, cell-based assays utilizing functional or reporter genes for response measurement, and organism-based screens (e.g., the two-hybrid yeast assay), each integral for quickly parsing through potentially hundreds of thousands of compounds daily.

Following HTS, the subsequent phase is the meticulous optimization process, which aims at improving the lead compound's biological activity, physicochemical and metabolic properties, and minimizing toxicity [1]. This process often involves structural modification of the original compound. The pharmacophore responsible for binding to the molecular target is rarely altered; however, adhesion groups improve the affinity and biological activity, and lipophilic groups enhance the absorption, distribution, metabolism, and excretion (ADME) profile.

One major aspect of biological activity is affinity and specificity. A critical parameter in assessing biological activity is the drug's affinity and specificity for its target, as measured by the inhibitor constant (Ki) or the half maximal inhibitory concentration (IC_{50}). Optimizing these values into the low nanomolar (nM) or even picomolar (pM) range is paramount, ensuring that the administered dose is both effective in inhibiting the target and has a diminished likelihood of eliciting off-target effects, thereby reducing potential toxicity.

Moreover, the physicochemical and metabolic properties of a drug are crucial for reaching and being retained in target organs or tissues at effective concentrations over the required duration.

Part of the optimization process is to enhance the compound's "drug-likeness," which encompasses attributes such as solubility, membrane permeability, and bioavailability. These features are important in the context of the "free drug hypothesis," which claims that only free, unbound drug in plasma can distribute to disease-targeted tissues to interact with its molecular targets. Thus, sustaining adequate plasma concentrations and ensuring optimal permeability are critical for the drug's therapeutic effectiveness. The traditional method to evaluate "drug-likeness" is Lipinski's rule of five (RO5), which states that an orally active drug is more likely to be successful if it exhibits no more than one violation of the following criteria: ① no more than five hydrogen bond donors, ② no more than 10 hydrogen bond acceptors, ③ a molecular mass less than 500 Da, and ④ an octanol-water partition coefficient (Clog P) equal to or smaller than 5 [26]. In addition, compounds with a polar surface area of less than 140 A^2 are also sought after. While there are notable exceptions to this guiding principle, candidate drugs that conform to RO5 have lower attrition rates during clinical trials [27]. On the other hand, the metabolic properties of the drug are characterized by in vivo pharmacokinetics data, including bioavailability (F), drug exposure, peak serum concentration (C_{max}), half-life ($t_{1/2}$), clearance (CL), and volume of distribution (V_d). Typically, drugs with in vitro microsomal stability $t_{1/2}$ of over 45–60 min, in vivo half-life $t_{1/2}$ of over 4–6 h, bioavailability F of over 30%, and CL of below 25% of hepatic blood flow (Q) are preferred [28].

Besides activity and pharmacokinetic properties, the toxicity of the drug is another critical aspect of drug optimization, since unmanageable clinical toxicity is one of the leading causes of drug development failure. Drug toxicity could result from either off-target or on-target inhibition of the molecular targets. To prevent off-target toxicity, the selectivity of the drug needs to be screened among a series of proteins other than its designated target, particularly those within the same family as the intended target [29, 30]. This is especially critical for kinase inhibitors, which should be screened against hundreds of kinases to ascertain a selectivity profile, ideally demonstrating a tenfold or greater preference for the disease-related kinase over others, as indicated by IC_{50} ratios. On the other hand, on-target toxicity may occur because the inhibited protein plays roles not only in the disease but also in other essential physiological processes. Unfortunately, the solution is limited for on-target toxicity: titration of the dose regimen must be performed to minimize the disruption of normal physiological processes.

Additionally, some drugs may exhibit toxicity against vital organs or biomolecules. For example, in vitro and in vivo hERG assays are usually performed as predictive markers of cardiotoxicity, specifically lethal torsade de pointes arrhythmia, of the lead compounds [31]. Some drugs may also exhibit toxicity by forming nonspecific drug-protein or drug-DNA adducts, which may potentially translate into genotoxicity and carcinogenicity. These risks are often quantified using a series of in vitro or in vivo assays. Finally, the accumulation of drugs or their metabolic products can lead to temporary or permanent organ damage; however, strategies to counteract such accumulation are still underdeveloped. To mitigate these potential toxicities, drug candidates during the optimization phase undergo comprehensive testing in multiple animal species to assess chronic and acute toxicity and to establish appropriate dosing regimens. These rigorous evaluations are critical to ensure that drug candidates advancing to clinical trials have a maximized safety profile [32].

11.3 Preclinical Development

Upon the successful identification and refinement of a lead compound, it enters an intensive phase of preclinical development, followed by a sequence of clinical trials. The preclinical development aims to collect safety data for a novel drug and to determine a starting safe dose for the first-in-human study. During this stage, the compound's efficacy, pharmacodynamics, and toxicological attributes are scrutinized through rigorous testing in diverse animal models, typically including both rodent and non-rodent species. These studies are critical for determining the appropriate dosage, administration route, and dosing frequency for future clinical trials. Meanwhile, the synthetic route of the lead compound is optimized to pave the way for mass production. This stage culminates in the submission of an Investigational New Drug (IND) application to regulatory bodies such as the US FDA [33].

11.3.1 Clinical Trials

Clinical trials are multistage, rigorous evaluations of novel drugs for a given indication [34] and are critical steps that decide whether a drug can finally be pushed to the market. Clinical trials typically involve three phases with distinct aims and scales.

11.3.1.1 Phase I

Phase I clinical trials serve as the initial step in evaluating the safety, dosage range, and potential adverse effects of a new drug in humans. These trials generally enroll a small group of participants (<100), often healthy individuals, although oncology trials may recruit patients with cancer. Typically, no control group or placebo group is set for phase I trials.

China has witnessed a surge in phase I trials, but the landscape reveals significant challenges. A total of 180 phase I trials were performed, but they were concentrated in only 18 facilities. Of these studies, 107 (59%) were completed by five study sites only. In addition, 132 (73%) of these studies were conducted in either Beijing, Shanghai, or Guangzhou, the three biggest cities in China, while the rest of the studies were also performed in other major cities in China. This concentration not only introduces potential regional biases in study outcomes but also points to an underlying inefficiency that could hinder China's ambition to become a leader in drug innovation [35]. The repetitive study designs in phase I trials may also impede China's advancement in the pharmaceutical area.

The Chinese phase I Oncology Trial Consortium, established in June 2017, serves as a collaborative nexus, uniting premier cancer centers, prominent contract research organizations, and both international and domestic biopharmaceutical enterprises. This initiative streamlines the exchange of insights and best practices. For studies targeting less common carcinogenic mutations, the consortium assists in patient recruitment by referring patients with specific mutations to corresponding clinical sites. Every 6 months, the consortium summit is held to address challenges in current phase I trials and to review recent advances in anticancer drug R&D with experts from the National Center for Drug Evaluation. Under this concerted framework, there is a noticeable pivot within Chinese biopharmaceutical entities toward original drug research and development, as evidenced by a threefold increase in investigational new drug applications submitted to the center [35].

11.3.1.2 Phase II

Phase II clinical trials focus on assessing the drug's initial efficacy by contrasting the therapeutic effects observed in a treatment cohort with those in a placebo-controlled group, comprised of patient participants rather than healthy individuals. Enrolling between 100 and 500 patients, phase II trials are exclusively designed to offer a preliminary but robust evaluation of the new drug's efficacy and safety through randomized, blinded, and controlled methodologies, or customized settings depending on the specific purpose. Overall, the outcomes from phase II trials are critical for shaping the structure of phase III trials and for fine-tuning the dosage strategies for further investigation.

11.3.1.3 Phase III

Phase III clinical trials represent the critical final stage of testing prior to a drug's application for market approval, often referred to as the confirmatory phase for validating therapeutic efficacy. These trials typically involve 1000–5000 outpatient and inpatient participants recruited from multiple centers, aiming to evaluate the drug's safety, efficacy, and tolerability, as well as identify side effects and interactions with other drugs during an extended treatment duration of 6 months to over a year. These studies are typically double-blinded to eliminate biases to the greatest extent.

Furthermore, phase III clinical trials can also include comparative studies, which compare the new drug or therapeutic approach against existing, approved treatment standards. For submission to the US FDA, at least two well-constructed, randomized phase III clinical trials are generally required to establish a solid basis for the new drug application. The US FDA will then meticulously review these data and assess the suitability of the drug for the treatment of the disease. Drugs that demonstrate non-inferiority, or ideally, superiority, in terms of efficacy, safety, or cost-effectiveness are poised for approval, paving the way for their commercial distribution and clinical use.

Concurrent with phase III clinical trials, the active pharmaceutical ingredient (API) and formulation process studies also advance to the appropriate stage. During this phase, establishing a commercially viable manufacturing process for the API is critical. Typically, a commercially produced API manufacturing process should account for the following factors: ensuring consistent quality of the product, maintaining safety in the manufacturing environment, optimizing production costs, minimizing environmental impact, achieving stable manufacturing operations, and ensuring long-term sustainability.

It should be noted that under certain circumstances, phase II and phase III clinical trials may be merged into one trial. This approach is typically considered in scenarios such as ① addressing an urgent global health crisis, such as a pandemic; ② developing treatments for rare diseases; and ③ expanding the indications of already approved drugs to cover additional diseases. These combined trials are conducted in several phases: an initial phase focusing on ascertaining the drug's preliminary promise for further investigation, followed by a later phase where the investigational drug is compared against a control group. The combined phase II/III design offers several benefits. It can lead to a reduction in the sample size required, conserve time and resources, and decrease the overall duration of the study.

11.4 Approval to Launch

The journey of a drug from phase I–III clinical trials to market approval is meticulous and highly regulated. Pharmaceutical companies are obliged to adhere strictly to regulatory guidelines for submitting their application materials and must engage proactively with the regulatory agency's review process. After thorough review and evaluation of the clinical trial data, the drug regulatory authority decides whether to approve the drug for marketing. This decision hinges on critical data pertaining to the drug's efficacy and safety. If the drug meets the necessary standards, the regulatory body issues a drug approval number, thereby granting the pharmaceutical company the right to commercialize the drug.

Once a drug receives clearance from the regulatory authority, it is authorized for official distribution to healthcare professionals and patients, an important milestone for any drug. However, this approval is not the end of the road. The pharmaceutical company must continuously provide the regulator with up-to-date information regarding the drug's side effects and quality management records. Additionally, for certain medications, the regulator may mandate a phase IV clinical trial to monitor long-term side effects.

Phase IV clinical trials, also known as post-marketing surveillance, are crucial for evaluating a drug's long-term risks and benefits in a large population. Based on the findings from this phase, drug regulatory authorities may mandate updates or revisions to the drug's usage instructions. This phase often includes research on drug interactions, exploring the effects of combining the drug with other medications, and identifying any new contraindications. An important aspect of phase IV is the detection of severe adverse reactions that may not have been evident in earlier trial phases. If significant risks are identified, such as an unexpected increase in the incidence of a serious condition like cardiovascular disease among users, regulatory authorities can require the addition of warning labels to the drug, or in extreme cases, demand its withdrawal from the market. A notable example of this was the withdrawal of Merck's anti-arthritis drug Vioxx in 2004, which was taken off the market due to concerns over an increased risk of cardiovascular disease. The phase IV clinical trials serve as a critical safeguard, ensuring that any new risks associated with a drug are identified and managed promptly to protect public health.

Prior to the release of the "Opinions on the Reform of the Drug and Medical Device Evaluation and Approval System" by the State Council of the People's Republic of China, the Chinese drug evaluation and approval system faced significant challenges, including lengthy approval times and low efficiency in the process of introducing new drugs to the market. Therefore, a comprehensive revision of the "Drug Registration Management Regulations" (DRR) was deemed necessary [36]. This initiative, spearheaded by the National Medical Products Administration, came into effect on July 1, 2020. Specifically, four drug acceleration programs were launched: breakthrough therapy drugs, conditional approval, priority review, and special approval processes. Under these programs, drugs that qualify for accelerated market access are supported by regulatory authorities and professional technical institutions through policy and technical assistance, with minimized evaluation timeframes. As of October 1, 2022, China had conditionally approved 77 drugs (counted by indication), with 60 of these pertaining to oncology treatments. Thus, oncological drugs have emerged as frontrunners in utilizing and benefiting from the conditional approval pathway, showcasing the effectiveness of these accelerated approval processes in facilitating timely access to critical treatments [36].

11.5 Conclusion

11.5.1 The Importance of New Antitumor Drugs

In 2016, China had 4.064 million new cases of cancer, with a standardized incidence rate of 186.46/100,000. By 2020, the number of new cancer cases had risen to 4.57 million, with deaths attributable to cancer reaching 3 million [37]. These figures underscore the significant challenge that cancer poses to China, particularly as the issue of an aging population becomes more pressing.

Pharmacotherapy plays a critical role in helping cancer patients gain extended survival time. Common treatment options for tumors include surgery, chemotherapy, radiation therapy, targeted therapy, and immunotherapy. Surgery is typically the first-line therapy for early stage cancers, whereas other treatments are selected based on postoperative pathological types and immunohistochemical results. Anticancer drugs have always been the mainstream treatment strategy for locally advanced or metastatic solid tumors that cannot be removed. However, due to the high costs of research and development, only a limited number of high-cost drugs have been approved, creating a significant financial burden for many patients who cannot afford them [38, 39]. Therefore, the timely approval of new antitumor drugs is not just a regulatory issue but a critical step in saving lives, as it provides more accessible treatment options for patients battling cancer.

Regulatory agencies in China have strived to approve new antitumor drugs in a timely manner. The New Drug Application (NDA) processing times for oncology drugs tend to be shorter compared to those for non-oncology drugs. This is consistent across various categories, whether the drug is marked for priority review, classified as clinically urgent overseas drugs, or subjected to standard review procedures. A primary factor influencing the acceleration of reviews, particularly for priority review status, is the significant clinical benefit that new drugs potentially offer. In November 2021, the Center for Drug Evaluation (CDE) issued the "Guiding Principles for Clinical Research and Development of Antitumor Drugs Guided by Clinical Value," the first regulatory guide in China for patient-centered drug development, demonstrating the powerful motivation to accelerate review and improve access to new antitumor drugs for cancer patients.

11.5.2 Eliminate the Lag in Drug Approval: Concerns and Efforts

Despite the high unmet medical need of patients with cancer in China, the pace of oncology drug approvals has historically been slower than in Western countries, notably the United States and Europe. While a range of oncology drugs, including tyrosine kinase inhibitors (TKIs) and monoclonal antibodies, are available in China, their approval timelines have typically trailed those in other nations. For example, the approval of TKI and monoclonal antibody cancer treatments in China has, on average, occurred approximately 3 years after their approval in the United States. This delay is also evident with newer agents, such as those targeting the PD-1/PD-L1 pathways. By 2016, only 4 of the 42 (about 10%) novel and innovative oncology products globally approved between 2011 and 2015 were available in China, highlighting a significant healthcare disparity.

The lag in drug approval primarily results from inherent complexities. China has a high prevalence of cancers with poor prognosis that differ in etiology and/or follow a more aggressive course than in other populations. The heterogeneity in disease epidemiology, etiology, pathobiology, and clinical manifestations can pose challenges in the evaluation of drugs across ethnic groups, complicating the development of medicines in China. Hence, ethnic sensitivities to drug exposure, efficacy, and safety must be carefully considered in China's drug approval process. Moreover, the standards of care for various tumor types can differ from those in other regions, impacting the clinical context in which drugs are utilized. Taken together, these complexities may contribute to the challenges in China's drug approval, underscoring the need for specific consideration in study design and data interpretation (Fig. 11.1).

The China Food and Drug Administration (CFDA) has introduced significant reforms aimed at expediting the drug development and approval processes. These

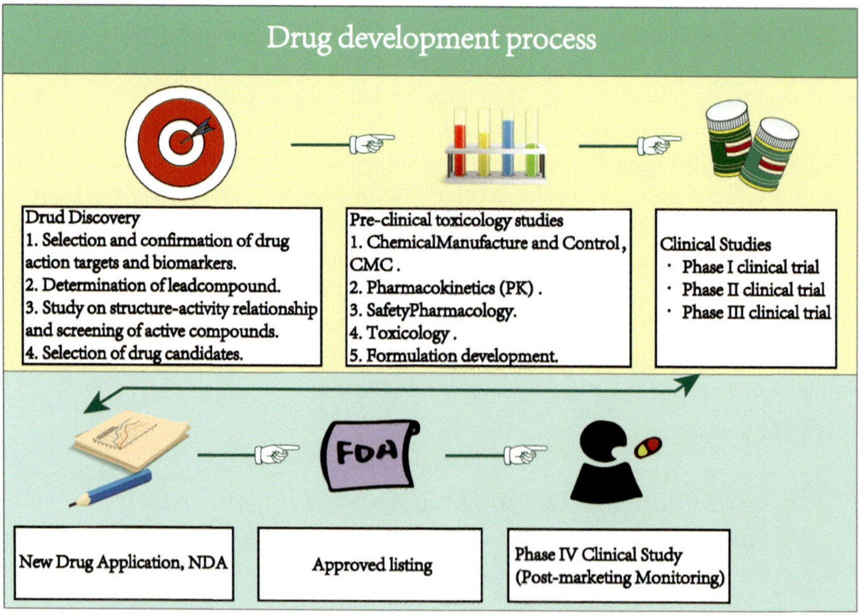

Fig. 11.1 Drug development process

reforms take into account the evolving understanding of ethnic factors, disease etiology, and variations in standards of care, creating substantial opportunities to enhance the oncology drug development process in China. For example, while ethnic factors remain a concern for some oncology drug classes, such as small molecules or TKIs, most monoclonal antibodies are ethnically insensitive. Hence, the CFDA has relaxed the requirements for phase I/II pharmacokinetics data and safety studies for these therapies. Additionally, China has shifted from a China-centric approach to an East Asian development strategy, thereby addressing the existing disparities in drug development compared to Western countries. These scientific, clinical, and regulatory advancements collectively pave the way for both international and Chinese pharmaceutical companies to narrow the development gap between China and the West. The ultimate goal is to facilitate the co-development of new oncology drugs through globally integrated programs. This approach not only accelerates the introduction of novel treatments in China but also offers hope for delivering advanced oncology care to Chinese patients more swiftly [40].

11.5.3 Trends in Oncology Drug Innovation in China

China is currently witnessing an unprecedented era in pharmaceutical development, marked by a significant shift from generic to innovative drug research and development, with oncology leading this transformative journey. Between 2018 and August 2020, of the 44 new cancer drugs approved in China, an impressive count of 12 originated domestically. It should be mentioned that the development of these drugs is driven by the high burden of cancer, as indicated by disease-specific disability-adjusted life years (DALYs). For instance, lung cancer, having the highest DALY burden in China, had the most candidate drugs, predominantly me-too drugs. In contrast, cancers like esophageal, gastric, and hepatic cancers, despite having a high DALY burden, had fewer candidate drugs but a higher proportion of first-in-class drugs, reflecting the lack of validated targets for these cancers. While a majority of these approvals were for me-too drugs, which follow established drug classes, the emergence of first-in-class drug candidates signifies a notable trend. This overview of the domestic oncology drug pipeline in China sheds light on the evolving landscape of the pharmaceutical ecosystem and highlights current trends in research and development, underscoring China's growing impact in the field of innovative oncology therapies [41].

As of January 2020, China's oncology drug development landscape showcased a significant focus on addressing unmet medical needs, with 821 investigational anticancer drug candidates in the pipeline. This includes 404 me-too drugs and 359 first-in-class agents. Among the me-too drugs, there were 56 CD19-directed CAR T-cell therapies, 83 targeting EGFR or HER2, and 32 monoclonal antibodies targeting PD-1/PD-L1.

While me-too drugs offer moderate market competition and potential affordability for patients, they also pose challenges such as resource inefficiency and risks to